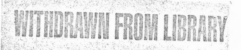

AMERICAN CHILDREN
THROUGH THEIR BOOKS

MY CHILDHOOD.
by Mr. UPTON.
Perfect Inocence.

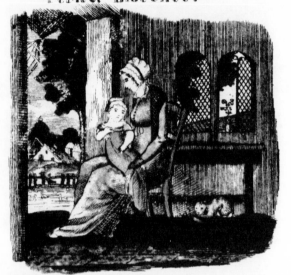

When first my eyes discovered day,
And quite a senseless lump I lay,
What did my wond'ring looks display?
　　　My Childhood

AMERICAN CHILDREN

through their

BOOKS

1700 — 1835

By MONICA KIEFER

FOREWORD

By DOROTHY CANFIELD FISHER

PHILADELPHIA

SBN:8122-7007-X

Printed in the United States of America

For
DR. RICHARD HARRISON SHRYOCK
Scholar, Mentor, and Friend

FOREWORD

THIS admirably conceived and skillfully executed book comes to break a historical impasse between the new modern, serious interest in children, and the pretty complete absence of authentic material about the boys and girls who grew up to be our great-great-grandfathers and grandmothers. Here for the first time we see the book-diet of those long-ago children, and get a glimpse of the psychological pressures put upon them.

The reader's first impression on looking into this unique volume is surprise that it was not written earlier. His second thought is great satisfaction that nobody did it before, because it might not have been done as well. Children were not, by our ancestors, even by our relatively speaking modern fathers, let alone grandfathers, considered important enough phenomena for able intellectuals to pay much attention to them; or to write down and have printed what little they had observed of them. But modern psychology tells us that children are the future of the race, that what children are *now* decides what human society will be twenty years from now; that the experiences of boys and girls influence and mold them far more intimately, more unescapably than what happens to them in later life. This fact was well known centuries ago to those skilled educators, the Jesuits. Longer ago than mere centuries, every mother intuitively felt it. But only of late years have real scientists, real educators, lent the weight of their prestige to such a feeling.

It is now an axiom that the way the children of any generation are treated deeply colors the life of the next generation. But now it is too late for historians to find reliable information about how little boys and girls were treated long ago; because mostly children were left to the care of women, and mostly in those days women were either illiterate or silenced by the prevalent idea that what women thought was of no consequence save to their own families.

Here, in this volume, we find fresh and authentic material on this point. For the first time we can look over the shoulders of those children of the past and see what they saw. More people than ever before now know something about interpreting data connected with child life. We shall never have more interesting material to try to interpret and understand than is offered us in this book.

DOROTHY CANFIELD FISHER

PREFACE

My chief pleasure in writing this book lies in the opportunity it affords
to acknowledge indebtedness to the numerous persons who have helped
in the research. It is my first desire to express sincere gratitude to Dr.
Richard Harrison Shryock, of the University of Pennsylvania, under
whose inspiration and guidance this work was begun, and whose criticism
and encouragement have been invaluable in its completion. Had it not
been for the generosity of Dr. A. S. W. Rosenbach, who permitted me
to use his valuable collection of early American children's books, this
study could hardly have been written. I wish, therefore, to thank him
sincerely for the privilege of handling these treasures. For providing
ready access to the Rosenbach collection, as well as a convenient study
in which to examine the books, I am deeply indebted to the courtesy
of Mr. F. H. Price of the Free Library of Philadelphia and to the efficient
services of the staff of Pepper Hall. I wish also to express my gratitude
to the staff of the Children's Department of the New York Public Library,
of the Boston Public Library, and of the Library of Congress, as well
as to the librarians of the rare book department of the Yale University
Library, the Ohio Archeological and Historical Library, and the University of Pennsylvania Library, for their coöperation and assistance in
locating materials.

M. K.

Albertus Magnus College
New Haven, Connecticut
November, 1947

CONTENTS

ILLUSTRATIONS

AMERICAN CHILDREN
THROUGH THEIR BOOKS

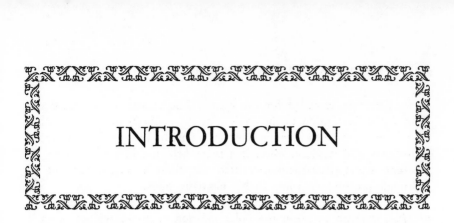

INTRODUCTION

THIS study is an attempt to trace the changing status of the American child in the Colonial and early national periods as it is revealed in juvenile literature. The general movement of the child's escape from a submerged position in an adult setting at the beginning of the eighteenth century advances slowly towards the recognition of his rights as a distinct personality by 1835. This evolution is traced through the record of the various aspects of child life, including religion, manners and morals, education, health, and recreation, in the hope of determining the place of the child in the church, in the home, in the school, and in the community at large. In analyzing these trends, the author has consciously invoked the European heritage and the American setting as the two major forces at work. An attempt has been made to distinguish the influences of the several European traditions and to take into account the sectional differences of the American colonies and states. Recent scholarship has given increased attention to the history of the family as a vital part of social history. For this reason a study of the status of the child within the family is an essential part of that record. If one were to judge by the scant attention paid in historical works to the child in the past, his emergence from oblivion would seem to have been delayed by the traditional indifference under which childhood languished in the early eighteenth century.

It is necessary to set boundaries to an almost limitless field, hence this study is confined to the period from 1700 to 1835. The analysis of the emancipation of the child from his early status of "total depravity" to his position as a cherished factor in the social life of the nation falls naturally into two parts. The first, from the beginning of the eighteenth century to the opening of the Revolution, marks the theological age— an era of stern pietism—during which the child was constantly impressed with the fact that he "was born not to live but to dy," and that his time and talents were to be focused on the proper fulfillment of this eternal end. The note of fear and repression, which dominated every phase of Colonial childhood, is clearly apparent to the most casual reader of the literature provided for the young. The second period, from the close of the Revolution to the middle of the eighteen thirties, describes the influence of a utilitarian philosophy. This trend, stressing the value of industry and wisdom. fostered a more benign and worldly view of life—one which humanely permitted the child a certain amount of legitimate pleasure en route to his heavenly home.

Status, sociologically defined by Ralph Linton in his work, *The Study of Man,* is taken to mean the polar position of an individual or of a group in reciprocal behavior patterns. According to Linton, status in this study may mean the position of a child in a particular social group, or the sum of all his participations in various groups. Simply stated, the status of the child will be treated as the aggregate of those rights and duties which commonly found expression in some special set of circumstances and thus shaped his mode of existence. Thus the status of a juvenile member of early American society will be derived from his relative position as a member of a family and of a church, as a pupil in a school, as a playmate among his equals, and as a potential citizen of the nation.[1]

Students of society have recently emphasized the significance of status systems in the development of American culture, in the study of personality, and in the socialization of the child. In regard to the changing status of the child in the last half century, Professor James H. S. Bossard of the Department of Sociology at the University of Pennsylvania asserts that the outstanding change in the recent history of children has occurred in the minds of their elders, but that this change is "so significant as to take its place among the great revolutions of history."[2]

Although child study was an unknown science in Colonial days, and the American society of 1700 was probably unconscious of such characteristics, recent scholarship has defined two types of statuses in the early social system. The achieved statuses of individuals or those requiring special qualities were not assigned at birth, but left open to be attained later in life through competition and personal effort. Ascribed statuses, on the other hand, were those assigned to individuals without reference to native abilities. Both Linton and Davis emphasize the ascribed statuses and take them to be the socially defined goals of childhood as ordered to systems of age, sex, and family relationships.[3]

Since the ascription of statuses with relation to sex was basic in Colonial and early American society, this study will examine the different attitudes and activities prescribed for boys and for girls. It will be noted that in the family, church, and school, as well as in community life, the male was trained for the superordinate roles, while the female was generally assigned to subordinate positions. This training was accomplished by universal insistence upon sex-appropriate language, clothes, work, and recreation.

Closely allied to sex as a point of reference in establishing status was age. Like most social groups, the early Americans recognized three age levels: child, adult, and old. In most considerations of age, cultural factors predominated in determining the content of status. This fact was best illustrated by the accepted status of the child in the home, where it will be found he was expected to be seen but not heard, where he slept in a trundle bed or on a straw tick in a loft, and where he ate his single dish, seated on a stool at a side table, while his elders and betters enjoyed the limited luxuries of the times as well as the obsequious deference of the young.

Birth placed the child immediately within the range of a variety of social patterns which related him to his parents, to his brothers and sisters, and to his parents' families. Since the life of the early American child, for the most part, was restricted by lack of communication and travel to intercourse with this narrow circle of blood relatives, his status in the family was of prime importance and will accordingly be treated in its various phases.

Class relationships were but the extensions of intimate family and clique connections, and thus narrowed the environment of the child's training to those groups with whom he could freely associate. Even in this limited scope, the number of class controls which the child had to maintain in order to satisfy the demands of his family's status as a unit will probably seem formidable enough to the modern reader. Class training ranged from the various types of educational opportunities presented by the home, the church, and the school to the proper style of dress and address or to the accepted types of recreation permitted the child.

No attempt has been made to define the term "child" in the sense of exact age-limits. As a matter of common sense, these limits have been so set as to begin at the time when a small child could talk and understand a simple conversation, and are then carried through to include early adolescence. But the phraseology in this respect seems to have changed, for such references as "young people" or "youth" were once applied to boys and girls in their childhood. It is to be understood that the use of these phrases here implies this older connotation. The limitations of space permit only the position of white children to be considered in the discussions of this study, with no reference to the status of the Indian or Negro child.

An attempt has been made to analyze and interpret the mass of contemporary juvenile literature by an examination of hundreds of tiny volumes written especially for children and for their training, but the author is under no illusions that this is a complete estimate of child life. A definite study would have to employ further types of sources, such as technical, legal, and medical works, as well as material relevant to child labor and to institutional care; but the limitations of time and space again did not admit of these in the present work. For the same reason, travel books and general biographical material have not been used; but this loss may not be so great as at first supposed, since most foreign travelers failed fully to record juvenile life in America; and the section devoted to youth in most biographies relating to these periods is brief and unsatisfactory. Other types of literature, pertinent to the history of the child in the period following 1835, had no considerable development until after that date. This is notably true of juvenile magazines; for even the *Youth's Companion,* which was first issued in 1827, was concerned in its early years mainly with morbid accounts of dead or dying children, and it was not until after 1835 that it provided domestic stories about a family of real boys and girls. *Our Young Folks* and *Saint Nicholas* also offer the historian of this later period a wealth of material on child life. At the earlier date, the delightful autobiographical works, such as the New England reminiscences of Thomas Bailey Aldrich or such stirring adventures of frontier youth as sketched by Mark Twain, were also lacking.

In terms of the sources actually used—children's books and guides for parents—other limitations of research may be readily conceived. The scarcity of juvenile books at this period, the customary habit of passing the most popular ones in turn to each new member of the family, and the traditional vandalism of most children as far as books are concerned, combine to explain the absence of some valuable materials from this study.

Certain definite impressions of bygone days are lost in a study of this type, because it is impossible to reproduce adequately, even to a sympathetic reader, the soul of these little books and the message imparted by their very physical make-up. Titles, quotations, and prefaces, while quaint and informative, do not suffice to carry the scent of old ink, the feel of faded leaves, the lack of perspective in the grotesque illustrations, and the curious flowered or gilt bindings of these tiny treasures; nor can they reproduce the touching inscriptions and crude sketches made long ago by childish hands on flyleaves or margins. Even with this loss the books are used as valued sources, for they reflect more accurately than any other class of literature the spirit of the times and the lives and customs of their young owners.

[1]Ralph Linton, *The Study of Man,* p. 113.

[2]Kingsley Davis, "The Child and the Social Structure," *The Journal of Educational Sociology* (December 1940) pp. 217, 230; Allison Davis, "American Status Systems and the Socialization of the Child," *American Sociological Review* (June 1941), pp. 345-54.

[3]Linton, *loc. cit.;* Allison Davis, "American Status Systems and the Socialization of the Child," pp. 347-50.

Mental Pabulum

OF

GODLY CHILDREN

THE changing status of the early American child may be given tangible expression by the books provided the "little men and women" for the period 1700 to 1835. The very appearance of the small volumes indicates not only an evolution in American tastes and customs but also a transition in adult response to the needs of childhood. The content of juvenile publications depicts even more clearly the formal, tortured existence of these "godly children."

The earliest coverless works with their crooked, faded lettering and crude woodcuts bear such religious titles as *Remember Thy Creator in the Days of Thy Youth* and *Spiritual Milk for Boston Babes.* These fragile relics are followed by others more securely bound in curious wooden covers with backs of coarse leather and burdened by such long, quaint titles as *War with the Devil; or The Young Man's Conflict with the Powers of Darkness.* Fascinating miniatures or thumb books in silver, gilt, or variegated bindings eclipse their less imposing neighbors and hold the stories children cherished from Revolutionary days to the end of the century. *The History of Goody Twoshoes, with the Means by Which She Acquired Learning and Wisdom* is among the most attractive works of this class.

A brilliant array of yellow, blue, pink, and marbled covers for fairy stories and "histories" such as *Mother Goose's Melody* or *Sonnets for the Cradle* stand next in line. These charming works are succeeded by the drab cloth bindings of such anemic moral tales as *The History of Betsey Brown, the Robber's Daughter: Shewing the Utility of Sunday Schools.* This drabness was relieved only at rare intervals by such works as *Peter Piper* in its bright orange wrapper, or by the Peter Parley tales bound in cream boards and red leather backs. A pall of dejection encompassed nearly all juvenile books until the days of *Alice in Wonderland,* whose sheer nonsense and fantastic illustrations broke the spell of gloom.

The only literary diversion recommended for children before the American Revolution was the reading of stories of a purely religious nature or tales of a didactic and moral character.[1] Such tales as *Jack the Giant Killer, Tom Thumb,* and *Guy of Warwick* were, at least orally, a common tradition of the first colonists. They were probably used as bedtime stories by many mothers in the South, even though they were frowned upon in the other colonies.[2] Among the Puritans and Quakers and other pietist sects of the Middle Colonies any books that provided entertainment, or that stimulated the child's imagination by opening the door even a little to the "Land of Make-Believe," were looked upon as vain and wordly.[3] John Croker, a Quaker, warned his children in 1721: "Read not in foolish books, with which the nation abounds, but read in the Holy Scriptures in which there is a great deal of comfort."[4] In a Puritan publication of the same period, a father gave his six-year-old child this solemn advice: "Child, the Bible is your rule of life . . . which being the Word of God, you are to read it with reverence, regard it with faith as the word of God and obey it as your rule."[5]

No period in the history of American juvenile literature is therefore so bleak and uninspiring as the first seventy-five years of the eighteenth century. During this time no real effort was made either in the colonies or in England to provide suitable reading material for the young. Children everywhere were treated not as undeveloped beings but as ignorant men and women, and nothing was written especially for the needs of the immature mind. Instead, little ones were expected to digest as best they could the heavy literary diet of adults. Even those few writers who did devote some of their time to the writing of primers and "pabulum" were apologetic for thus wasting their talents. John Bunyan, for instance, in 1688, began his *Book for Boys and Girls* with the words:

> To those who are in years but Babes I bow
> My Pen to teach them what the letters be,
> And how they may improve their A B C.[6]

Almost eighty years later Isaac Watts wrote in reference to his *Divine Songs for the Use of Children:* "Some of my friends imagine that my time is employed in too mean a service while I write for babes."[7]

None but the most arbitrary distinctions can be made between English and American literature for children at this time, because a majority of the publications used in the Colonies were prepared in England, and the few American productions current followed British models so closely as to have no distinct individuality. This barrenness in the field of American juvenile literature is readily understood, for not only did the colonists lack the tradition of providing reading material at the child's level, but the intense physical activity necessary for the successful planting of the Colonies destroyed any literary aspirations they may have had.[8] Native authors, in those rare moments given to writing, produced books of an instructive type. Catechisms, primers, spellers, Latin grammars, and books of good manners were among our first American publications.[9]

Attempts were made by some publishers to adapt English works to the American scene, as shown in the preface of the *American Instructor, or the Young Man's Best Companion,* in which the printers, "B. Franklin and D. Hall," have written: "In the British Edition of this Book, there were many Things of little or no Use in these Parts of the World: In this Edition those Things are omitted, and in their Room many other Matters inserted, more useful to us Americans."[10]

No change was made in the general character of these works, for even the arithmetics and spellers were permeated with a morbid pietism which confined the childish imagination to those channels connected with the awful duty of an early conversion as the prelude to an untimely death. An excellent example of this type is found in Cotton Mather's *A Family Well-Ordered; or, An Essay to Render Parents and Children Happy in One Another:* "You must know Parents that your Children are by your Means born under the dreadful Wrath of God: and if they are not New-Born before they dy it has been good for them, that they had never been born at all."[11]

Mather also gave expression to the educational aims of his time and indicated the types of books needed for Colonial children:

Tis very pleasing to our Lord Jesus Christ, that our Children should be well formed with, and well informed in the Rules of Civility, and not be left a Clownish, and Sottish and Ill-bred sort of Creatures. An unmannerly Brood is a Dishonour to Religion. And there are many points of a good education that we should bestow on our Children; They should Read, and Write, and Cyphar, and be put into some agreeable Calling: not only our Sons but our Daughters should also be taught such things as will afterwards make them useful in their Places. Acquaint them with God and Christ and the Mysteries of Religion, and the Doctrines and Methods of the Great Salvation.[12]

Books to carry out this program were a costly luxury, since colonists had to import most of them from England. After 1775 they printed their own and some pirated works on the presses of Boston, Philadelphia, and New York. Following the counsel of men like Mather, and in keeping with the advice of John Locke, who knew no study aids "out of the ordinary road of the Psalter, the New Testament, and the Bible," the colonists used hornbooks and primers of a rudimentary sort, reprints of sermons, miniature Bibles, and catechisms "expounding the precepts of the Christian religion" to prod the child up the weary road to learning. These guides, Locke said, "engage the liking of children and tempt them to read."[13] If youthful climbers faltered in the ascent, they had but to cast their eyes on such popular selections as the following to spur their lagging steps:

> Let all backsliders of me warning take,
> Before they fall into the Stygian Lake;
> Yea, and return and make with God their peace
> Before the Days of Grace and Mercy cease;
> For mine are past forever, Oh! condole
> My sad Estate and miserable Soul.
> My Days will quickly end, and I must lie
> Broyling in Flames to all Eternity.[14]

The Bible was in every home not only the chief source of religious instruction, but also the text used for teaching reading and spelling. The Scriptures were indeed the "key of instruction" by which the children were taught to worship God, to order their conversation aright, and to perform their duty to their neighbor.[15] In the course of this training, little thought was given to the devastating effect which some passages of the Bible might have on the nervous system of a sensitive child. Indeed, there were a few who studied versions of the *Children's Bible,* but the usual method of reading the Scriptures for children as well as adults was to begin with the first book of the Old Testament and to proceed by stated assignments to the end, with no expurgations.

Next to the Bible, the *New England Primer* was another fruitful source of theological knowledge. This tiny text, just big enough to fit snugly in a child's pocket, was immensely popular in all the Colonies and went through numerous editions even in the nineteenth century. Although this primer, too, was deeply religious in tone, the crude woodcuts and the cruder rhymes illustrating the alphabet must have been a welcome diversion to children forced otherwise to study reprints of drowsy sermons of interminable length. Added charm lay in the primer's few extremely pious stories of such martyrs as John Rogers, or in some of Watts's hymns, even though the search for such treasures led through exhortations not to lie, not to cheat at play, not to be a dunce, and to love school.[16]

Michael Wiggleworth's *Day of Doom,* as a supplement to the *New*

England Primer, reflected the same somber aspects of religion and education for children. This book, printed on sheets like a common ballad and hawked about the country, apparently held out but one small hope to unregenerate "infants":

> You sinners are, and such a share as sinners may expect,
> Such you shall have; For I do save none but mine own elect . . .
> Therefore in bliss you may not hope to dwell,
> But unto you I shall allow the easiest room in Hell.[17]

The *Book of Martyrs* by Fox was deemed a most desirable work for children in Colonial days, and was repeatedly recommended for use in schools. Other works especially intended for the young introduced martyrologies with a wealth of revolting detail.[18]

The almanac, which held place with the Bible and the *New England Primer* as an integral factor of the Colonial library, was published by local printers in great variety. The abundance of almanacs and the great diversity of important and useful data packed between their covers, probably tempted children to read them with the same avidity as did their parents and elders. Benjamin Franklin's "Poor Richard" deeply engraved pithy maxims on the minds and hearts of young Americans, and helped in no small measure to establish those habits of prudence and thrift characteristic of the new nation.[19]

English-speaking children since 1700 have taken for their exclusive use four world-famous books not intended originally by the authors as juvenile literature. The first of these, Bunyan's *Pilgrim's Progress,* published in 1688 for adults, was eagerly seized upon by children. Its illustrations and forthright style particularly pleased them, while Pilgrim's difficulties in the Slough of Despond or with the Giant Despair were agreeable contrasts to the martyrs' deaths and the horrors of fire and sword in their usual reading.[20] *Robinson Crusoe,* appearing in 1714, was immediately appropriated by the little folk in the same way.[21] *Gulliver's Travels* was composed by Swift in 1726 for satirical purposes, but children reveled in the controversy of the foolish Big Endian and Little Endian which agitated the kingdom of Lilliput, "wherein eleven thousand persons suffered death rather than break an egg at the smaller end."[22] Finally, *Munchausen* in 1785 derided the extravagances of travelers' tales; but again, children responded to its extraordinary adventures and made it their own.[23]

English chapbooks or reprints of the little volumes sold by wandering British peddlers began to deluge America about the middle of the eighteenth century. The wide range of subjects covered may have been

responsible for the popularity of these works. In the chapman's pack
could be found A B C books, nursery rhymes, fairy stories, fables, primers,
riddle books, song and hymn books, lives of heroes, historical abridgments, travels, religious histories, and abstracts of popular novels. This
motley array reflected the moral tone of the times, for many of the
earlier chapbooks were crude in thought as well as inartistic in physical
design. The incongruity of giving abridgments of such novels as Field-
ing's *Tom Jones* to children who were denied *Mother Goose* is difficult
to comprehend. Peerless among the shorter stories unfit for children's
reading was the *Prodigal Daughter; or a strange and wonderful relation,
shewing how a gentleman of vast estate in Bristol, had a proud and
disobedient Daughter, who because her Parents would not support her
in all her extravagance, bargained with the Devil to poison them. How
an Angel of the Lord informed her parents of her Design. How she lay
in a trance for four days; and when she was put into the grave, she came
to life again, etc.*[24] Other books treating of witchcraft and fortune-telling
may have left their mark on certain inhuman proceedings in the history
of those times.

The majority of books were in small octavo, about five-and-one-half
by four-and-one-half inches, but those particularly designed for children
were even smaller or about two-and-one-half by three-and-one-half inches.
One of the first of these miniatures, published in Boston, was printed
by William Secker, and had the amazing title: *A Wedding Ring Fit for
the Finger; or the Salve of Divinity on the Sore of Humanity.* These
little books contained four or a multiple of four pages, up to twenty-four
or thirty-two, were printed in a rude manner on very coarse paper,
bound in wall-paper wrappers, and "adorned" with woodcuts which
had at best only a remote reference to the text. Engravers were scarce
in the colonies, and the art of woodcutting little practised; so the same
cut was used over and over again, sometimes with grotesque results.
The History of the Holy Jesus, published in Boston in 1749, showed the
cut of the "Wise Men Come from the East," consisting of a group of
Puritan men gazing through telescopes at a comet but not noticing the
moon or stars that filled the rest of the sky. Another extraordinary cut
in the same work, representing Christ teaching the multitude, depicted
Him in the gown and bands of a Puritan preacher in a pulpit before
which stood three Puritan men on one side and three Puritan women
on the other.

The waning of Puritan fervor and the ferment of skepticism about
the middle of the eighteenth century caused the emphasis in juvenile
literature to shift from works of a purely theological character to more

practical books of moral instruction in which stern dogma was supplanted by humorous examples of right living. To supply children with this new type of reading material John Newbery, the famous printer of St. Paul's Churchyard, London, in 1744 began the publication of dozens of quaint rhymes and stories filled with playful humor. Many of these books that would amuse as well as instruct have maintained their popularity with boys and girls to the present. It is believed that Dr. Johnson and Oliver Goldsmith assisted Newbery in his venture into the land of youthful mirth and nonsense. Newbery frequently referred in his little gilt volumes to his friend Goldsmith as "the very great writer of very little books."[25] Goldsmith, on the other hand, has described Newbery's infectious enthusiasm for the mass production of "interesting and amusing little books for children": "He was no sooner alighted but he was in haste to be gone; for he was ever on business of the utmost importance, and was at that time actually compiling materials for the history of one Mr. Thomas Trip."[26]

Dr. Johnson, during his interest in Newbery's publications, records an incident in which he "withdrew his attention" from a noted contemporary who bored him and "thought about Tom Thumb." Johnson's escape was not only from dull facts into a dream-world, but from formalism of words into simple realism; for to him, as to children, the experiences of the tiny creature, Tom Thumb, were logical. The great and the childish mind alike could grasp the magic of the dwarf who not only slept in a walnut shell, or feasted three days upon a single hazel-nut, but who wore an oak-leaf hat, a spider-woven shirt, and hose and doublet of thistledown.[27]

Newbery began his project with quaint imitations of such periodicals as *The Tatler, The Spectator,* and *The Rambler.* These works, embodying the aims and methods of the English philosopher, John Locke, he published under the titles *The Little Pretty Pocket-Book* and the *Lilliputian Magazine.* Almost a half-century before, Locke had not only recommended the use of picture books as a study aid, but had also endorsed such works as *Æsop's Fables* as desirable reading for children. Locke thus proposed pleasure as a new element in reading and learning, since he declared that the fables which were "apt to delight and entertain a child may yet afford useful reflections to a grown man; and if his memory retain them all his life after, he will not repent to find them there amongst his manly thoughts and serious business."[28] Although Locke placed virtue as the first aim of juvenile reading, in contrast to the Puritanical "other-worldliness," he also sought to plant deeply in "infant minds" the seeds of absolute truth and common sense under the genial

sun of "innocent amusement."[29] His influence is clearly discernible in
the preface of the *Little Pretty Pocket-Book* which contains a letter to
parents and guardians laying down rules for making children strong,
healthy, virtuous, and happy.[30]

Benjamin Franklin, editor of the *Pennsylvania Gazette* in Philadelphia, recognized the genius of Newbery as early as 1750 by "importing
parcels of entertaining books for children," and by advertising them for
sale to the "little Masters and Misses" of the Colonies. One such allotment
included: *A New French Primer,* the *Royal Battledore,* the *Pretty Book
for Children,* and the *Museum or a Private Tutor.* Franklin may not
have been in full accord with the new technique of combining amusement and instruction in the training of the young, but he sold quantities
of the *Museum* at one shilling a copy, as prizes to "dutiful children for
excellence in scholarship."[31] The *Museum,* practically a library in itself,
was eminently suited to this purpose, for it contained not only directions
for reading with "eloquence and propriety," but also accounts of the
"ancient and present state of Great Britain," instructions on the solar
system, geography, rules of behavior, religion, and morality, admonitions
given by great men "just quitting the stage of life," and descriptions of
the Seven Wonders of the World.[32]

Hugh Gaines, publisher and patent medicine vendor, a decade later
was selling wholesale and retail many of Newbery's books at the Bible
and Crown Bookshop in New York. *Poems for Children Three Feet
High, Tommy Trapwit, Trip's Book of Pictures, The New Year's Gift,*
and the *Christmas Box* stocked his shelves and found their way to eager
little readers.[33]

In form and style, the *Little Pretty Pocket-Book* was typical of the
new attempt to "amuse" children by special books. Like most juvenile
texts of his design, it was in tiny format and in small type with embossed
gilt paper covers. Children were evidently expected to have good eyes,
for miniature volumes of this kind were common since it was thought
that they were most convenient for small readers to handle.[34] Although
the illustrations at the top of the pages were crude in quality and lacked
true perspective, in quantity they were numerous enough to please
eighteenth-century children whose treats of this kind were exceedingly
rare.

The "amusement" in this type of book is thinly scattered and all but
obscured by the poorly disguised morals attached to the fables. In keeping with the traditions of the times, the author employed little subtlety
but pinned his moral plainly in sight and pointed to it steadily. It was
natural that the first coating of entertainment should be spread rather

thin. One would think now that the section on good manners must have been discouraging. Cuts of polite children illustrated the product of the rules set down for direction of "juvenile conduct at home and abroad."[35] A well-bred child was cautioned: "Attend the Advice of the Old and the Wise." In the "alphabet of useful copies," he also found exhortations for the practice of self-control: "Be not angry nor fret, but forgive and forget."[36]

Isaiah Thomas of Worcester, Massachusetts, the American counterpart of Newbery, began in Revolutionary days to reprint pirated books to amuse children. In these publications Thomas reflected the new interest in child life that had begun to manifest itself in the colonies. Youngsters had been admonished to be good in order to escape by the narrowest margin the eternal pains of hell. Such precepts by 1776 gave way to counsels cautioning the young to be virtuous because such conduct made for a successful life in this world. Children glowing with a sense of righteousness and wide-eyed with interest heard how "Little King Pippin" reached his exalted state by an early application to his lessons; and how Giles, who had learned the alphabet from gingerbread letters, was rewarded by a fine gentleman for spelling "apple-pye" correctly.[37] Goody Twoshoes was also a shining example of learning and wisdom, and she was "set forth at large" for the benefit of those

> Who from a State of Rags and Care,
> And having shoes but half a Pair,
> Their Fortune and their Fame would fix,
> And gallop in their Coach and Six.[38]

Jack Dandy's Delight, a juvenile natural history written for Newbery by Oliver Goldsmith and pirated by Thomas for his American patrons, is another example of the new utilitarian attitude. The author, employing a new technique, pokes fun at children:

> The monkey mischievous
> Like a naughty boy looks;
> Who plagues all his friends,
> And regards not his books.[39]

Newbery and his disciple Thomas repeatedly protested that their books for children were always of a high moral order, but some of these works were more candid in tone than would be tolerated today; others were not only foolish, but their dull jokes transcended the child's understanding. An illustration of the failure to bring humor to the level of a child is found in *Be Merry and Wise; or, The Cream of Jests:*

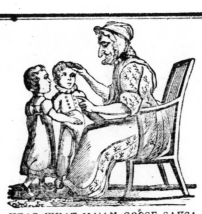

HEAR WHAT MA'AM GOOSE SAYS!

My dear little Blossoms, there are now in this world, and always will be, a great many grannies besides myself, both in petticoats and pantaloons, some a deal younger to be sure; but all monstrous wise, and of my own family name. These old women, who never had chick nor child of their own, but who always know how to bring up other people's children, will tell you with very long faces, that my enchanting, quieting, soothing volume, my all-sufficient anodyne for cross, peevish, won't-be-comforted little bairns, ought to be laid aside for more learned books, such as *they* could select and publish. Fudge! I tell you that all their batterings can't deface my beauties, nor their wise pratings equal my wiser prattlings; and all imitators of my refreshing songs might as well write a new Billy Shakespeare as another Mother Goose: we two great poets were born together, and we shall go out of the world together.

No, no, my Melodies will never die,
While nurses sing, or babies cry.

From THE TRUE MOTHER GOOSE, 1832

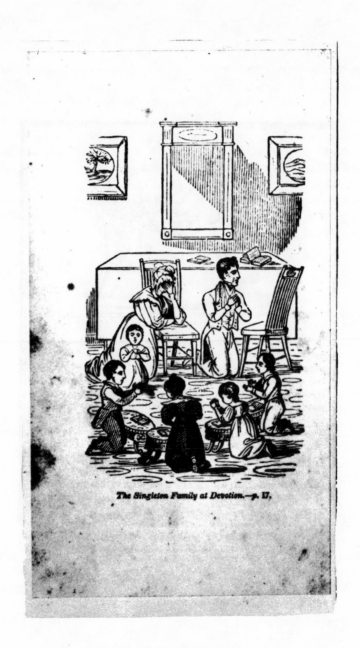

The Singleton Family at Devotion.—p. 17.

From EVENINGS AT HOME, ca. 1820

A certain doctor having raised a pretty fortune by irregular practice was desirous of purchasing a coat of arms to adorn his chariot, and accordingly asked a friend's advice, what he had best for them? "Oh! Doctor," said he, "nothing will suit you better than three ducks, and let the motto, if you please, be Quack, Quack, Quack."[40]

American children owe much to France for contributing Charles Perrault's *Histoires ou Contes du Temps passé*. This collection of well-loved nursery tales was first published in 1697 in a small volume whose frontispiece pictured an old woman with her distaff, seated by the fire, telling stories to a group of children. On a scroll in the background were the words *Contes de ma Mère l'Oye*.[41] In that form it was brought to England about 1729, where it was translated and reprinted as the *Tales of Mother Goose*.[42] This then was the first use of that renowned name; and it was not taken, as legend has it, from a Boston lady, Elizabeth Goose, the mother-in-law of the printer Thomas Fleet.[43]

The idea of editing these old nursery rhymes presumably originated with John Newbery about 1760, but he was no doubt assisted by Goldsmith, who was doing hackwork for him at that time, and whose favorite song, "There was an old Woman toss'd in a Blanket" was included in the preface for no apparent reason. This English version bore the title *Mother Goose's Melodies: or Sonnets for the Cradle;* and in the introduction Goldsmith clearly indicates that the melodies had long been in use among the British nurses:

The custom of singing these songs and lullabies to children is of great antiquity. It is even as old as the time of the ancient Druids. Charactatus, King of the Britons, was rocked in his cradle in the Isle of Mona, now called "Anglesea" and tuned to sleep by some of these soporiferous sonnets. We cannot conclude without observing, the great probability there is that the custom of making Nonsense Verses in our schools was borrowed from this practice among the old British nurses; they have, indeed, been always the first preceptors of the youth of this kingdom, and from them the rudiments of taste and learning are naturally derived. Let none therefore speak irreverently of this ancient maternity as they may be considered as the great grandmothers of science and knowledge.[44]

Perrault's contributions are simple in structure and universal in appeal; and as such they belong to the class of folklore which has parallels in nearly every language. Eight fairy tales have been particularly immortalized in the English collections. These, translated into English about 1729, are: *Cinderella, Red Riding Hood, Puss in Boots, Sleeping Beauty, Bluebeard, Diamonds and Toads, Tom Thumb,* and *Riquet with the Tuft.* Beginning about 1785, Isaiah Thomas gave American youth numerous editions of these tales of wonder and enchantment. Bound securely in gleaming covers, the story books were welcomed by children as the best reward for proficiency in their small tasks, or were prized as gifts from a beloved grown-up who understood the needs of young hearts.[45] No doubt the philosopher or the anthropologist can explain why the magical outlook on life expressed in these fairy tales continued to fascinate children at the very time it was being abandoned by their elders.

The American spirit began to pervade textbooks for the children of the new republic by 1790. But independence had to be asserted in the juvenile as well as in other literary forms. The schoolmaster had the particular duty of fashioning the mind and heart of the young, according to the ideals of the Founding Fathers, and it was he who set about revising the old British textbooks: Even the *New England Primer* gave up the couplet:

> Whales in the Sea
> God's voice obey.

and substituted for it:

> By Washington
> Great deeds were done.[46]

American writers prepared a number of small United States histories under the conviction that children must have their imaginations properly stirred to appreciate their country. These little works not only gave the spirit and atmosphere of Colonial and Revolutionary times, but also inspired an interest in a subject which had formerly been confined to chronology or to a study of the ancient and medieval periods. The authors of the new texts showed an enthusiasm for describing the beauties and resources of the various states and sections, with the result that these historical works also contained much geographical information. This novel compilation of native lore extended the mental horizons of boys and girls beyond the boundaries of their neighboring hills, and doubtless did much to awaken a spirit of national pride and stimulate hope in the future greatness of America.

Noah Webster's *Elements of Useful Knowledge, containing an Historical and Geographical Account of the United States* provided one of the first outlines of American history. Among the early biographies of our national heroes, *The Life of George Washington, Commander in Chief of the Army during the Late War, and Present President of the United States* was published in Philadelphia in 1794. It also contained selections on "The Vanity of Youthful Hopes," "'The Federal Prayer," and an "Epitaph on a Poor but Honest Man."[47]

Another work, *The History of America, abridged for the use of children of all denominations,* which appeared in Philadelphia in 1795, contained the woodcuts and accounts of discoverers and heroes, and of the various governors of the states.[48] An ingenuous combination of patriotism and obedience is found in *The Child's Instructor* written by John Ely, "a teacher of little children in Philadelphia," in 1791. Since the seat of government was located in that city at the time, a special story centered around the President and one Billy—a precocious child of five who remarked that "if you would be wise you must always attend to your vowels and consonants." When Washington took up his office in the city, Billy was requested by his mother to address some of her callers on the merits of the first President; he did so in these terms: "Americans! place constantly before your eyes, the deplorable scenes of your servitude and then the enchanting picture of your deliverance. Begin with the infant in the cradle; let the first word he lisps be Washington." The ladies, gratified at hearing Billy speak so well, predicted that eventually he would be a lawyer or even the president of the country; but the boy replied that he could be neither "unless his mamma gave him leave."[49]

The teaching of Jean Jacques Rousseau, that the chief aim of education was to develop the child according to the laws of nature, manifested itself toward the close of the eighteenth century in a new impetus given to child study. Juvenile literature as a result came under the control of the didactic school of writers. In England and subsequently in the United States, Rousseau's theories had even more effect on the actual life of the family than on books. As children were relieved of the old restrictions, they began to develop their individuality of action and powers of self-control; and parents, on their part, tended to make friends rather than philosophers of their boys and girls. This social progress was underscored in books by the make-believe accounts of impossible children and perfect parents. Most writers of juvenile books became theorists, who sought to make life fit their theories.[50]

Thomas Day, who wrote *The History of Sandford and Merton* in 1789, was one of the most widely read of the English didactic writers. His work emphasized the value of human life and the dignity of labor by denouncing artificial standards. Two six-year-old boys, Harry Sandford and Tommy Merton, exemplified the sharp contrast so familiar to eighteenth-century children. Harry, the "child of a plain, honest farmer," had a just sense of values; while Tommy, a horrible example of soft, effeminate rearing, was frivolously engrossed in worldly interests. In this ideal setting for moralizing, the tiresome remarks of Mr. Barlow, the tutor, covered a wide variety of subjects ranging from ghosts and toys to theology, geography, biology, astronomy, and political science. Despite its stilted language and priggish patterns, this work continued to have a wide circulation among American boys and girls for more than a century, and for years was considered one of the best books ever written for children.[51]

The evolution of children's books in England and America during the first half of the ninteenth century faithfully mirrors a change in the knowledge and aspirations of the social world. In the first two decades of the century, the utilitarian works of English female writers became immensely popular in the United States and threatened to eclipse the budding efforts of native authors.[52] From their experience as teachers or mothers these "well-informed" women definitely made a place for themselves in children's literature. As exponents of the didactic school, Anna Laetitia Barbauld, Martha Sherwood, Sarah K. Trimmer, and Maria Edgeworth soundly condemned fairy stories and all nonsense such as Mother Goose rhymes; while in the task of making children upright, generous, and resourceful, they confined themselves to staid tales of exact literal truth.[53] Their philosophy was clearly set forth in many prefaces like the following:

Such a creature as Jack Frost never existed, any more than old Santaclaw [sic] of whom so often little children hear such foolish stories; and once a year they are encouraged to hang their stockings in the chimney at night, and when they arise in the morning, they will find in them cakes, nuts, money, etc., placed there by some of the family, which they are told Old Santa-claw has come down the chimney and put in. Thus the little innocents are imposed on by those who are older than they, and improper ideas take possession which are not by any means profitable.[54]

One of these works entitled *The Seasons* takes advantage of the opportunity offered by "Gathering Apples, an Autumn Occupation" to deliver the following homily on drink:

Cider is a cheap, pleasant, and wholesome drink, much to be preferred to strong spirits, which are wonderful in their operations; for they will unroof barns, fill windows with old pillow cases, pull down fences, make cattle lean, children ragged and ignorant, break the hearts of tender mothers and affectionate wives, bring shame and disease, fill gaols and state prisons, and often bring men to the gallows: it is feared to eternal ruin.[55]

Mrs. Barbauld's most popular work, *Evening Tales,* is a good example of a juvenile miscellany that had a wide circulation in the United States in the early nineteenth century. Conversational in tone, it closely followed the Socratic method of teaching, for it was partly in the form of a dialogue between parents and children or tutor and child. These dialogues handled such topics as deportment, character traits, geography, natural sciences, and manufactures.[56] Besides the real loss in the banishment of fairies and elves, another disaster was a revival of the allegory in such works as Mrs. Barbauld's *Order and Disorder: A Fairy Tale.* The heroine of this story was assisted by the good fairy Order in repairing the damage caused by the bad fairy Disorder who had formerly been the girl's companion. Works describing the activities of such pseudo-fairies as Order plagued childhood for decades.[57]

This eviction of the fairies did not take place without protests from grown-ups as well as from children. *The Child's Annual,* published by Allen and Ticknor in Boston in 1834, gave "A Lament for the Fairies" in which the weakness of early nineteenth-century literature for children was ascribed to the absence of these fantastic folk:

> They meet no longer by the light
> Of moonbeams 'neath a tree;
> Why! one might walk abroad all night
> And not a fairy see!
> One would but catch a cold or fever
> Before the dawn of day;
> And these are things that happened never
> Till fairies went away.
>
> Farewell to all the pretty tales,
> Of merry elfins dining
> On mushroom tables, in the dales,
> Lit by the glow-worms shining;
> And tripping to the minstrel gnat,
> His jocund measure singing,
> While o'er their heads the lazy bat
> A silent flight was winging.
>
> Farewell! like theirs, my song is done:
> But yet once more I'll say—
> There never has been any fun,
> Since fairies went away.

Charles Dickens, decades later, deplored this literary tragedy which had struck childhood in the opening years of the century, and wrote to this effect in *Household Words* for October 1885:

It would be hard to estimate the amount of gentleness and mercy that has made its way among us through these slight channels [meaning fairy tales]. Forbearance, courtesy, consideration for the poor and aged, kind treatment of animals, the love of Nature, abhorrence of tyranny and brute force—many such good things have been nourished in the child's heart by this powerful aid. It has greatly helped to keep us ever young, by preserving through our worldly ways one slender track, not over-grown with weeds, where we may walk with children, sharing their delights.

Mrs. Sherwood, who was preoccupied with the thought of death, contributed the *Fairchild Family,* a collection of stories to prove the necessity of religious education. After a quarrel among his children, Mr. Fairchild illustrated the commandment "Thou shalt not kill" by taking the culprits for what he said would be a pleasant walk, and casually showing them a crossroad gibbet on which hung the body of a murderer. On another occasion the father took them to visit a dying farmer lad, who told the children his particular preparations for death had included a trip to the cemetery and an inspection of the family vault.[58]

Mrs. Trimmer made more agreeable contributions to child life in such works as her *Fabulous Histories, or, The Story of the Robins,* in which she represented Dicksy, Flapsy, and Pecksy, not as birds but as human beings capable of thinking and speaking. Written from a child's point of view, the story sought to inspire in thoughtless and even brutal children an idea of the kindness due birds and animals as a part of God's creation.[59]

Maria Edgeworth, the greatest of the moralists, was a friend of Thomas Day, the author of *Sandford and Merton,* and like him an admirer of Rousseau. In her work of educating the young, Miss Edgeworth was not dedicated to the idea of furnishing them informational material, but rather in improving their mode of living by a harmless and decidedly moral literature. Her treatise *Practical Education* embodied somewhat progressive ideas and methods for play and study. She recommended that those toys should be selected which would develop in the child a maximum of creative and constructive activity.[60] Opposed as she was to improbable fiction for children, Miss Edgeworth applied her genius to the production of the *Parent's Assistant,* a collection of realistic tales. Her father, in the preface, showed that the purpose of the book was to correct the weaknesses of the moralistic-didactic school of writing by the use of the suspense element: "To prevent the precepts of morality from tiring the ear and mind, it is necessary to make stories, in which they are introduced, in some measure dramatic; to keep alive hope, fear, and curiosity by some degree of intricacy."[61]

This "intricacy" diverted the child's attention from the moral of the story, and the result was a greater plot development than was usually found in such tales. The young reader could not predict so readily the ending of Miss Edgeworth's stories; hence the use of the new suspense device must have been intriguing. Another distinctive feature of her work was the realistic settings for her pictures of child life. Miss Edgeworth may thus be considered a pioneer in writing for the young. Such stories as "The Purple Jar," "Lazy Lawrence," "Waste Not, Want Not," "Simple Susan," and "The Orphan" gave to children, if not fairies, at least a host of benevolent noblemen, gracious ladies, and philanthropic merchants, who always appeared at the right moment to make awards or to point a moral.[62]

Juvenile poetry, produced by the English school of moralists and reprinted in this country at the turn of the century, reveals the low opinion many writers had of the child's appreciation of finer things. The purpose of this poetry approximated that of the didactic stories—to cultivate morals, to polish manners, and to communicate some useful knowledge to the young.[63] Ann and Jane Taylor, and Adelaide O'Keefe, the first of this group of British writers to devote themselves exclusively to juvenile verse, were forced by their convictions to disregard everything in their writings except the literal truth, moral ideas, and the elements of poetic form. They addressed children in endearing terms and kissed and caressed them, but there was plainly a lack of the genuine tenderness found in the cradle songs of "the good old nurses."[64]

In *Rhymes for the Nursery,* babies in the process of being put to bed were lectured about their well-being and allowed a smug acceptance of the good things of life. Their good parents, the joys of home, and play with a puppy were compared to the hard lot of poor children, but never with a suggestion of remedial measures that might lie within a child's reach. Instead of evoking compassion for the wretched, these works fostered in the fortunate child a complacent enjoyment of his comforts. Even more obnoxious than this smugness was the ghoulish advice to little children to learn of the uncertainty of life by a visit to a graveyard at twilight, there to read what "the grey mouldering stone tells of the mouldering dead." In the epitaphs pointed out by the Taylor sisters, one sees a revival of the Colonial attitude towards death, but with more emphasis on its repugnant physical aspects:

> You are not so healthy and gay
> So young, so active, and bright,
> That death cannot snatch you away,
> Or some dreadful accident smite.
>
> Here lie both the young and the old,
> Confined in the coffin so small,
> The earth covers over them cold,
> The grave-worms devour them all.[65]

Certainly in *Original Poems,* the infant horror stories of these women reached their zenith in depicting the little boy who fished for sticklebacks in his father's pond and met with swift and awful punishment for his crime :

> Many a little fish he caught,
> And pleased was he to look,
> To see them writhe in agony,
> And struggle on the hook.
>
> At last when having caught enough,
> And also tired himself,
> He hastened home intending there
> To put them on the shelf.
>
> But as he jumped to reach a dish,
> To put his fishes in,
> A large meat hook, that hung close by
> Did catch him by the chin.
>
> Poor Harry kicked and call'd aloud,
> And screamed and cried and roared,
> While from his wounds the crimson blood
> In dreadful torrents poured.[66]

The little fisherman was rescued by a maid, but he remained a dreadful example even to children whose fathers earned a livelihood at fishing. Justice never lagged in overtaking the culprit in these tales. Wicked children always came to grief; the good invariably escaped perils. Besides the danger of developing a false conscience, the constant repetition of the omnipresence of an avenging God was another emphasis which would now be viewed as harmful in its psychological effects:

> In every place by night and day
> He watches all you do and say.

With this conception persistently stressed, the child could have had no idea of God as a kind and loving father, but must have cringed under the all-seeing eye of the stern judge who spied on all his actions. In all these didactic precepts there was little to engender pity, hope, and love. By their incessant hammering on trivial faults, these stories offered children no opportunity to trace the effects of more serious sins on others, and then to make the proper application to their own lives.

Eliza Lee Follen, another English verse writer, unhappily attempted early in the century to reproduce the old Mother Goose tales without the nonsense. In the preface of her miniature book called *Little Songs for Little Boys and Girls,* Mrs. Follen gives enlightening insight into the prevailing opinions of adults about children's readings:

It has been my object . . . to catch something of that good humored pleasantry, that musical nonsense which makes Mother Goose so attractive to children of all ages. Indeed, I should not have thought of preparing a collection of new baby songs . . . if I had met with another book of this kind adapted to the capacity, taste, and moral sense of children, so I have attempted to imitate its beauties, and what is a far easier thing, to avoid the defects of Mother Goose melodies.[67]

Like every other attempt to supplant Mother Goose rhymes, this work failed miserably; the contrast between the enduring force of the old verses and the wretched weakness of the new ones shows the futility of this effort. Children loved the melodious language and pleasing sounds of a Mother Goose story which gave rise to tramping and clapping as well as happy mood:

> One misty, moisty morning
> When cloudy was the weather,
> I chanced to meet an old man
> Clothed all in leather.
>
> He began to compliment
> And I began to grin—
> 'How do you do?' and 'How do you do?'
> And 'How do you do?' again![68]

As a substitute for this jingle, Mrs. Follen presented one with the proper moral perquisites:

> The poor man is weak,
> How pale is his cheek!
> Perhaps he has met with some sorrow;
> Let us give him a bed,
> Where his poor weary head
> May rest, and feel better tomorrow.[69]

Fortunately this strict diet of moral tales was considered too heavy by some English writers, who made an attempt to amuse rather than instruct or preach to children. William Roscoe inspired a host of imitations by writing a sprightly poem, *The Butterfly's Ball and the Grasshopper's Feast,* for his little son's birthday in 1807. This tiny classic, one of the first in which the child's imagination plays with the life of the animal world, began with the words:

> Come take up your Hats and let us haste,
> To the Butterfly's Ball and the Grasshopper's Feast.[72]

Children in the company of other guests, such as the frog, the squirrel, and the dragonfly, could easily enjoy the hospitality of the "Land of Make-Believe," where they found fairylike preparations for the feast:

> A Mushroom their table, and on it was laid
> A Water-dock leaf, which a Table-cloth made.

This little poem not only set a vogue for fantastic verse in which animals and insects played the roles of human beings, but it also introduced the bright-colored pictures in which children took delight for the next thirty years. According to the advertisement on the back cover, the work sold for "one shilling plain and sixteen pence coloured." The tints were applied by a group of children working together, each armed with a brush and a pot of paint; and each child was responsible for applying his own color where it belonged on the humorous illustration. Thus the red, blue, and yellow patches appeared as the print passed from hand to hand.[71]

In 1822 Clement Moore, a New York educator, wrote for his own children the famous Christmas ballad, *'Twas the Night Before Christmas; A Visit from St. Nicholas*. He thus unwittingly produced what has been termed the first truly original story of lasting merit in the juvenile literature of America.[72] In this beloved tale, Santa Claus, the jolly patron of children, happily began his mission to the public of the United States. Mr. Moore's ballad was not only free from the restrictions of the moralists, but was brimming with spontaneous mirth, and in this respect was fifty years ahead of its time. It enchanted children from the very beginning by the extravagance of its expression and by the striking sound imitations in such lines as:

> Up on the house-top, click, click, click,
> Down through the chimney, good Saint Nick . . .

Ever since Dasher and Dancer brought good Saint Nick to celebrate Christmas as a national feast, children, excited by the tinkling bells and fragrant greens, have reveled in delightful anticipation of this holiday.

This survey shows that for the first quarter of the nineteenth century Americans followed their old tradition of reprinting English books exactly as they came to this country or at best with a few changes. Not only were stories with English settings published for American children, but descriptions of British flora and fauna, games and customs, almost excluded those of the United States. With the achievement of complete national independence and the growth of confidence in the improvement of the education system, demands were made for books emphasizing distinctly American characteristics.

Samuel Goodrich, whose pen name was "Peter Parley," was chiefly responsible for the elimination of the British background from most juvenile books used in America. Like the British moralists whom he supplanted, Goodrich violently denounced such stories as *Red Riding Hood* and such nonsense rhymes as "Hey Diddle Diddle" as being unchristian and unwholesome food for young minds. Beginning with the *Tales of Peter Parley about America* in 1827, he devoted thirty years of his life to writing over a hundred volumes of history, geography, science, and travel—all of which rivaled in interest the best English publications.[73] The appeal of these works was so great that Goodrich had many imitators at home; while spurious Peter Parleys sprang up even in England, where his simple factual stories had made him popular.

Besides the enthusiasm for perfecting the educational system by a better understanding of the child, other influences such as religion and the development of youthful aesthetic tastes and values were brought to bear on books for boys and girls. The steady decline of Puritanism, the gradual realization that the morbid tone and inartistic character of much of the old juvenile literature was harmful to the young, the revolt against the banishment of fairies, together with an increased regard for children and a more sympathetic understanding of their needs, combined by the sixties to form a new conception of child life that soon expressed itself in children's books. By this time the notion had crystallized in adult thinking that literature for the young was not only to be directed to moralistic or to utilitarian ends, but was also to afford the child happiness and entertainment. This change, which now seems sudden, was accelerated by a few remarkable books published after the Civil War. The first and greatest of these was an English work, Lewis Carroll's *Alice in Wonderland,* or what has been termed the "spiritual volcano of children's books." Its author made no apologies for the lack of moral preaching, and this enchanting tale permanently established the precedent that fun and nonsense were legitimate and desirable in juvenile literature.

Subsequently the natural child—with his faults as well as virtues—was to become the hero of juvenile literature. On this side of the Atlantic, before 1900, Aldrich gave us his *Story of a Bad Boy,* while in England E. Nesbit composed her delightful tales of healthy, imaginative English children.[74] In time it was found that young readers—and some old ones—delighted particularly in the very pranks and backslidings that had shocked the earlier generations. Both Mark Twain and Kipling made heroes of their "bad boys." Radio and television audiences today enjoy the accounts of the "fresh" hopeful who actually gets the best of his elders. So the pendulum of adult attitudes towards children seems to have swung from one extreme to the other in the decades between 1840 and 1970. But the latter phase is beyond the province of the present study.

[1]Rosalie V. Halsey, *Forgotten Books of the American Nursery*, p. 3.

[2]*Ibid.*, p. 8.

[3]Walter J. Homan, *Children and Quakerism*, p. 72.

[4]As quoted in *Friends Library*, XIV (1727), 12-13.

[5]As quoted in Sanford Fleming, *Children and Puritanism*, pp. 78, 79.

[6]As quoted in Alice M. Earle, *Child Life in Colonial Days*, p. 117.

[7]As quoted in Algernon Tassin, "Books for Children," *Cambridge History of American Literature*, II, 401.

[8]Charles Welsh, "Early History of Children's Books in New England," in *New England Magazine*, XX, 147.

[9]*Ibid.*, XX, 148.

[10]George Fisher, *The American Instructor*, Preface.

[11]Cotton Mather, *A Family Well-Ordered*, p. 11.

[12]*Ibid.*, pp. 17-18.

[13]As quoted in Welsh, *op. cit.*, 148.

[14]Benjamine Keach, *War with the Devil, or the Young Man's Conflict with the Powers of Darkness, in a Dialogue Discovering the Corruption and Vanity of Youth, the Horrible Nature of Sin, and the Deplorable Condition of Fallen Man*, p. 177.

[15]Douglas Campbell, *The Puritans in Holland, England and America*, I (1892), 440.

[16]*New England Primer, Further Improved with Various Additions. For the Attaining the True Reading of English. To which is added The Assembly of Divines Catechism*, pages unnumbered; See also Paul L. Ford, *The New England Primer*, p. 1.

[17]As quoted in Tassin, *loc. cit.*

[18]E. M. Field, *The Child and His Book*, p. 193.

[19]Welsh, *op. cit.*, p. 153.

[20]Halsey, *op. cit.*, p. 10.

[21]Welsh, *op. cit.*, p. 155.

[22]Field, *op. cit.*, p. 232.

[23]*Ibid.*, p. 239.

[24]Anon., *The Prodigal Daughter*, p. 1.

[25]Florence V. Barry, *A Century of Children's Books*, p. 63; See also Blanche E. Weekes, *Literature and the Child*, pp. 51, 52; Emelyn E. Gardner and Eloise Ramsey, *A Handbook of Children's Literature*, p. 173.

[26]Barry, *op. cit.*, pp. 38, 39.

[27]*Ibid.*, pp. 59, 60.

[28]*Ibid.*, p. 10.

[29]*Ibid.*, p. 9.

[30]*The Little Pretty Pocket-Book; Being a New Attempt to teach Children the Use of the English Alphabet by Way of Diversion*, Reprinted by Isaiah Thomas, pp. 7-14.

[31]Rosalie V. Halsey, *op. cit.*, pp. 60, 61.

[32]*Ibid.*, p. 62.

[33]*Ibid.*, p. 63.

[34]Quite the reverse of this opinion holds today, for the smaller the child the larger the book and the type provided for his use. Experiments have proved, moreover, that the diminutive volume does not appeal as strongly to a little boy or girl as a larger book; see Florence E. Bamberger, *Effects of the Physical Make-up of a Book upon Children's Selection*, p. 131.

[35]*The Little Pretty Pocket-Book*, p. 15.

[36]*Ibid.*, p. 75.

[37]Halsey, *op. cit.*, p. 110.

[38]Oliver Goldsmith, *The History of Little Goody Twoshoes*, reprinted by Isaiah Thomas, title page.

[39]Oliver Goldsmith, *Jack Dandy's Delight: or the History of Birds and Beasts; in Verse and Prose*, reprinted by Isaiah Thomas, p. 3.

[40]*Be Merry and Wise; or, the Cream of Jests and the Marrow of Maxims for the Conduct of Life. Published for the use of all Good Little Boys and Girls*, by Tommy Trapwit, Esq. Reprinted by Isaiah Thomas, p. 46.

[41]Halsey, *op cit.*, p. 219; Barry, *op. cit.*, pp. 41, 42.

[42]Charles Welsh, *op. cit.*, p. 159.

[43]Walter Taylor Field, *Fingerposts to Children's Reading*, pp. 216, 217.

[44]*Mother Goose's Melodies: or Sonnets for the Cradle*, reprinted by Isaiah Thomas, Preface, pp. v-x.

[45]Alice M. Jordan, "Early Children's Books," *Bulletin of the Boston Public Library*, XV (April 1940), p. 187.

[46]*The New England Primer*, pages unnumbered (Boston, 1749); *The New England Primer* (Hartford, 1800).

[47]Noah Webster, *Elements of Useful Knowledge. For the Use of Schools.*

[48]*History of America, abridged for the use of children of all denominations;* W. D. Cooper, *The History of North America* (Philadelphia, 1795).

[49]John Ely, *The Child's Instructor, consisting of easy lessons for children; on subjects familiar to them, in language adapted to their capacities*, p. 48.

[50]Barry, *op. cit.*, p. 105.

[51]Weekes, *op. cit.*, p. 55.

[52]Gardner and Ramsey, *op. cit.*, p. 184.

[53]Weekes, *op. cit.*, p. 56.

[54]*False Stories Corrected.* Preface.

[55]*The Seasons*, pages unnumbered.

[56]Anna Letitia Barbauld, *Evening Tales*, pp. 22-30.

[57]Annie E. Moore, *Literature Old and New for Children*, pp. 186, 187.

[58]*Ibid.*, pp. 205-9.

[59]Weekes, *op. cit.*, p. 56; See also Gardner and Ramsey, *op. cit.*, p. 176.

[60]Moore, *op. cit.*, pp. 195, 196.

[61]Maria Edgeworth (M. E.), *The Parent's Assistant; or Stories for Children*, 3 Vols. (1796), Preface. Reprinted many times in the United States.

[62]Barry, *op. cit.*, pp. 175-93; See also Moore, *op. cit.*, p. 199; Weekes, *op. cit.*, p. 59.

[63]Moore, *op. cit.*, p. 287.

[64]*Ibid.*, p. 71; See also Laurence Clay, "Mental and Moral Pabulum for Juveniles," *Manchester Quarterly* (January 1914), p. 71.

[65]Jane Taylor, *Select Rhymes for the Nursery*, p. 24.

[66]Adelaide O'Keefe, Ann and Jane Taylor, *Original Poems for Infant Minds. By several young persons*, pp. 32, 33.

[67]Eliza Lee Follen, *Little Songs for Little Boys and Girls*, Preface.

[68]C. S. Francis, *The True Mother Goose*, p. 96.

[69]Follen, *op. cit.*, p. 13.

[70]William Roscoe, *The Butterfly's Ball and the Grasshopper's Feast;* see also Barry, *op. cit.*, p. 218.

[71]A. S. W. Rosenbach, *Early American Children's Books*, p. 198; See also Kirkor Gumuchian, "From Piety to Entertainment in Children's Books," *The American Scholar* (Summer 1941), p. 348.

[72]Halsey, *op. cit.*, pp. 147, 148.

[75]Weekes, *op. cit.*, pp. 66, 67. See also Gardner and Ramsey, *op. cit.*, pp. 184, 185.

[74]*The Treasure Seekers, The Would-Be-Goods*, etc.

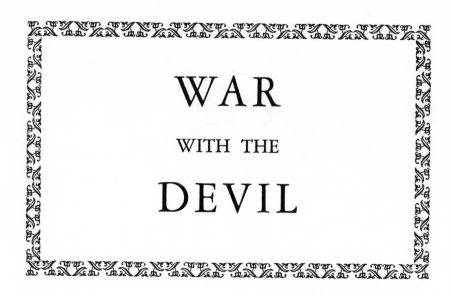

WAR
WITH THE
DEVIL

RELIGION was the precipitating factor in the establishment of the American Colonies, and its influence extended to every phase of child life. In the war with the devil against the allurements of the world and the weakness of the flesh, the young were instructed to turn in fear to the Word of God found in the Bible. As additional weapons of defense they were to utilize sermons, catechisms, primers, and the lives of holy children. Little ones were cautioned to appreciate this spiritual arsenal: "I am to regard with Reverence the awful Threatening contained therein, in order to deter me from sin and Vanity." Children of all creeds and sections were expected to "walk in the ways of the godly"; consequently the juvenile literature issued by any sect generally illustrated the religious attitudes common to all denominations.

The policy of the Mother Country at the beginning of the Colonial era in matters ecclesiastical had been to plant the Established Church in all sections except where dissenting sects predominated.[1] But the dissenting colonies might well have copied the pamphlet of the Virginia Council which declared that religion was the "maine and cheefe purpose" of the settlement.[2] The boundaries of the various colonies by 1700 not only set political limits, but also separated settlements of conflicting religious persuasions.[3] From the standpoint of creed alone the spiritual status of the young varied, for Puritanism dominated the religious experiences of the New England child just as Anglicanism did that of the youth of the Southern Colonies, while a variety of faiths including the Anglican, Lutheran, Presbyterian, and the pietist sects of Pennsylvania served to complicate religious life in the Middle Colonies. As a whole the picture was predominantly Protestant, for penal laws in all the Colonies made the open practice of Roman Catholicism practically impossible except among the Quakers of Pennsylvania and for a brief period in Maryland.[4] Hence this study will not include a consideration of the religious life of the few Catholic children, since for the most part that life has left no traces in the juvenile literary productions of the period.

The temper of the times set rigid theological standards as the norm for all children regardless of the type of Protestantism dominant in a particular colony. Children's books for the period 1700 to 1776 bear witness to the fact that the religious requirements of most Protestant sects throughout this country were consistently uniform in their stern demands for an exact adherence to definite beliefs and practices on the part of the young. The children of this era, as a result, grew up in an atmosphere of fear and repression. For example, William Penn, an affectionate father, thus admonished his children:

Fear God; That is to say have an holy Awe upon your minds to avoid that which is Evil and a Strict Care to embrace and do that which is Good. . . . Be of the number of his true self-denying Followers, to take up your Cross for his sake, that bore his for yours.[5]

The reason for the general severity of tone in addressing children is difficult to determine at this distance, but religion in all the Colonies was in a state of flux; because here, as in England, the ferment of the seventeenth century manifested itself in a perceptible relaxation of the old order—be it Episcopal, Quaker, or Independent. Although it is true that few deistic or skeptical works circulated in the Colonies during this period, yet the fiery religious enthusiasm of the first settlers had waned with their death. The generation of 1700 showed signs of a weakening faith in the old religious codes based on hopes of heaven and fears of hell. Writers, in desperation, sought in the most terrifying manner to warn "reprobates," however young, of the approaching "Day of Doom" with its attendant terrors for the depraved and unrepentant sinner. The prevailing apathy against which the spiritually minded shattered their lances is reflected in the nervous apprehension and the vehement language of children's books and sermons. A typical example of the exhortations addressed to those who had not been converted to God is seen in the following:

Believe it while you have no interest in Christ, while you do not love God, and delight in his Service, you are in Danger every Moment of falling into Hell. . . . Yes, the cold hand of Death may seize you, lively, gay, and merry as you are. And Oh! Where are you then?[6]

As little difference in tone or attitude is found in the various Protestant sources, the usual thesis that New England Puritanism exerted a preponderant influence on our national thought and development, particularly as it affected child life, is of doubtful validity. The evidence certainly shows that Colonial thought patterns were universally theocentric. The Anglican of Virginia and the Quaker or Presebyterian of Pennsylvania displayed the same courage and singleness of purpose as did the Puritan of New England. It is safe to say then that the variations of emphasis in minor points of dogma and practice were induced by a divergence of cultural heritage.

Most "godly" children pursuing the path of virtue began with the Bible and read it in its usual form from cover to cover. Less valiant souls perused the few juvenile versions,[7] "reduced to the tender capacities of little Readers . . . so as under God to make those excellent Books take such a firm hold of their young minds . . . as no Accidents of their future Lives will ever be able to blot out."[8] The authority of the Bible was upheld even in books of manners:

> The Scriptures of divine authority
> A perfect rule for all men to walk by,
> From them we learn the living God to know,
> And what the duty is to him we owe.[9]

Quaker children were given a concise explanation of the end for which the Scriptures were written: "All scripture given by the inspiration of God, is profitable for doctrine, for reproof, for correction, for instruction in righteousness, that the man of God may be perfect, thoroughly furnished unto all good works."[10] In the *Child Well-Instructed,* Colonial youth learned to appreciate the place of the Scriptures in his life: "I am to learn in them my Duty respecting God, My Neighbour, and my Self; together with what I must shun and avoid, with respect to each other."[11]

Dozens of catechisms prepared for the children of the various sects supplemented the study of the Bible. Foremost in this rank stood the *New England Primer,* designed to impress on the minds and hearts of youth the stern principles of Calvinism, since in its "Shorter Catechism of the Assembly of Divines" it mirrored the Puritan mood with absolute fidelity. A precise spiritual code was embodied in 107 questions which children could learn and accept as soon as they reached the age of discretion. This volume thus helped to forestall the threats to unity of belief that individualism admitted.

Cotton Mather counseled mothers to drill their children unsparingly in this catechism every day, and added: "You may be continually drop-

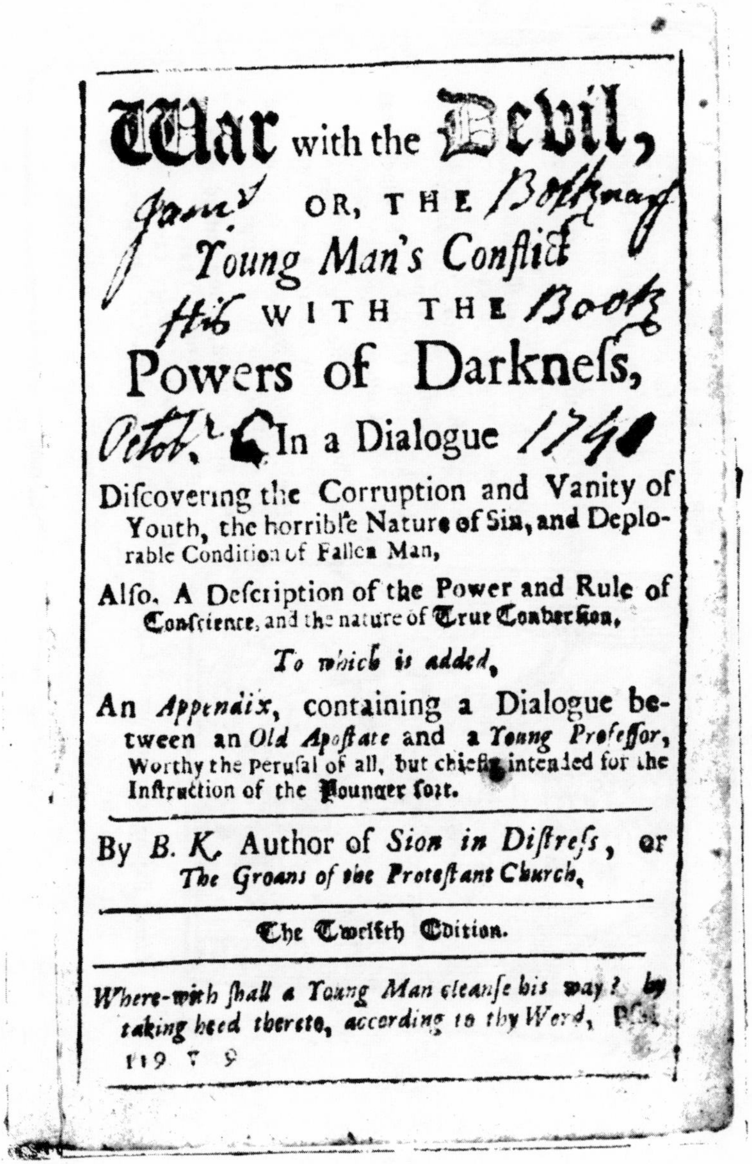

War with the Devil,

OR, THE

Young Man's Conflict

WITH THE

Powers of Darkness,

In a Dialogue

Difcovering the Corruption and Vanity of Youth, the horrible Nature of Sin, and Deplorable Condition of Fallen Man,

Alfo. A Defcription of the Power and Rule of Confcience, and the nature of True Converfion,

To which is added,

An *Appendix*, containing a Dialogue between an *Old Apoftate* and a *Young Profeffor*, Worthy the perufal of all, but chiefly intended for the Inftruction of the Younger fort.

By *B. K.* Author of *Sion in Diftrefs*, or *The Groans of the Proteftant Church*,

The Twelfth Edition.

Where-with fhall a Young Man cleanfe his way? by taking heed thereto, according to thy Word,

(handwritten annotations across the page: James, Bofhnay, His, Book, Octob.r, 1740, 119...)

A title page of 1707

But O to hear the awful Cries
    Of Mothers in Diſtreſs,
And *Rachel* mourn for her Firſt born
    Snatch'd from her tender Breaſt.

But ſoon the Monſter *Herod* dies,
    Then *Archelaus* doth reign ;
When *Jeſus* our moſt bleſſed Lord,
    To *Nazareth* he came.

From whence unto *Jeruſalem*,
    His Parents do repair
To keep the Paſchal Feaſt which was
    Their Cuſtom once a Year.

He then into the Temple goes
    Where many Learn'd and Wiſe
Great Doctors were, and doth diſpute
    With them to their Surpriſe.

Our lovely Lord, b'ing entred now
    Upon his thirtieth Year,
From *Galilee* to *Jordan* came,
    And *John* baptiz'd him there.   Now

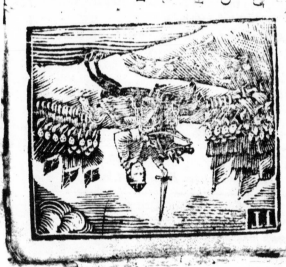

Herod ſlaying the innocent Children.
    But,

LII

ping something of the Catechism upon them: Some honey out of the Rock!" He described parental instruction as one of "the two Handles to be laid hold upon; the one is the proper Catechism and the other is the Public Ministry." On this twofold process he advised parents to "hear them say by rote the answers in their Catechism, question them very distinctly over again about every clause in the answers, and then what they hear in the Evangelical Ministry, do you apply it unto them after their coming home."[12]

Samuel Fuller, the Dublin Quaker, wrote in the preface of his catechism: "For good and early impressions on tender minds, often prove lasting means of preserving them in a religious life even to old age; and as they grow up, let us watch over them for good, and rule over them in the Fear of God, maintaining our authority in love. . . ."[13]

The Children's Catechism for the use of Scotch Presbyterians likewise exhorted parents to exert the utmost solicitude for the spiritual training of their children: "The Lord's language to Parents, with respect to every Child he gives them is, as the Daughter of Pharaoh said to the Mother of Moses, Exod.ii.9. 'Take this child and nurse it for me. For lo, Children are an Heritage of the Lord's.' "[14]

Thomas Vincent in his "Epistle to the Reader" began with the information that the "Popish Axiom"—"ignorance is the mother of devotion"—has long since been exploded, and he went on to say that "the world doth now see that without knowledge the mind is not good."[15] He counseled parents that the best way to conquer ignorance was to have the family in joint sessions commit the Catechism to memory in the following manner:

It is advisable that after the question in the Catechism is propounded, an Answer without the Book is returned by one of the Family, the same person or some other be called upon to read the explanation of it, the rest reading along with him in several books; by which means their thoughts (which are apt to wander) will be the more intent upon what they are about.[16]

Besides the wandering thoughts referred to here, the reader finds many other unintentional revelations of the normal frailties of Colonial children. Such a reference occurs in the sermon of Samuel Davies preached to the children of Hanover, Virginia, about whom he complained:

You are gay, merry, and thoughtless; and cannot bear to fix your thoughts on such disagreeable Subjects (Sic); and flatter yourselves it is time enough for you to submit to the Mortification of attending to them, as you advance into life. Your passions and appetites are strong and unruly: Your hopes warm and sanguine. And therefore I am afraid sundry of you will hardly allow me a serious hearing, tho' but for an hour. However, whether you hear or whether you forbear, I must endeavor to deliver my message to you in the name of God.[17]

Lest the impression be given that unruliness was confined to the South, we find this advice from Cotton Mather on the question of children's obedience: "Lay your charges upon your Children. Parents charge them to work about their own Salvation. To charge 'em vehemently, is to charm 'em wonderfully. Command your Children, *and it may be they will obey.*"[18]

Impelled by the fear that the numerous catechisms might eventually supplant the Scriptures in the religious education of children, Samuel Fuller wrote the following to urge a more assiduous use of the Bible in child-training:

Now tho' we of this generation in these protestant countries, are so signally favour'd with the free and undisturb'd use of this large and most excellent volume . . . yet seeing such incessant labours and pains are taken both early and late to propagate the pernicious doctrines of infidelity, deism, profaneness, and atheism; we esteem it both imprudent and dangerous to delay the first seasoning of the minds of our dear and tender offspring, with the fundamentals of the christian doctrine, till they are of a capacity and ability to collect and extract from thence the same for themselves.[19]

The author went on to explain that since his book was intended principally for the use of children, " 'Twas not thought convenient to amuse their tender minds, at first, with too many sublime and controverted points," which he said, "can be thoroughly assimilated only late in life."[20]

Sermons couched in graphic language and delivered in ringing tones were a device used by the ministers of the various denominations to plant salient truths deeply in the hearts of the young. Such subjects as the total depravity of youth, the fear of God's judgments, and the duty of obedience to parents were usually discussed. Sometimes, incidentally, pride in one's own province, or its neighbors, found expression in these theological exhortations. Thus Samuel Moodey thundered in Massachusetts: "Turn ye, turn ye, from your Evil ways, for why will ye die, O children of New England? Poor Hearts; You are going to Hell indeed: but will it not be a dreadful thing to go to Hell from New England, from this Land of Light to that Dungeon of Eternal Darkness?"[21]

Funeral elegies and "histories" of godly children were also mighty instruments employed by the ministry to illustrate the meaning of life and death to trembling young sinners. A typical example of the hundreds of this type was preached by Benjamin Colman in Boston in 1714. He reminded his young audience at the beginning of his discourse of the ravages disease had made in their numbers during the preceding year, and then added:

You have seen many of your own age buried in the Winter past; divers of whom died hopefully, and made a gracious End. You have been sick (most of you) your selves; and many of you remember the Religious Frames you were then in, and the holy Desires and Purposes you then had. Some have been so wrought upon by their Danger, that I hope truly they have been brought home to Christ. I wish the number of such were greater.[22]

By far the most popular history of pious children who died early deaths was the Janeway *Token,* an English work reprinted in the colonies. It began with the words:

You may now hear (my dear Lambs) what other good Children have done, and remember how they wept and prayed by themselves; how earnestly they cried out for an interest in the Lord Jesus Christ. . . . Would you be in the same condition as naughty Children? O Hell is a terrible place, that is a thousand times worse than Whipping. God's Anger is worse than your Father's Anger.[23]

A Legacy for Children, a collection of the "last expressions and dying sayings" of the little Quakeress, Hannah Hill of Philadelphia, was another morbid work, approximating the *Token* in tone. Among other things, the young reader learned that Hannah had an extraordinary "gift in reading the Holy Scriptures, and other good books, in which she took much delight; and if any Friend gave her a book, she would not seem satisfied until she read it through; and would sometimes get much of it by heart."[24]

In the early eighteenth century, memorizing of hymns was considered the most effective means of giving "children a relish for virtue and religion." Foremost among such works ranked *The Divine Songs* of Isaac Watts, for the author, like St. Paul, attempted to be "all things to all men." He stated in his preface: "As I have endeavour'd to sink the language to the level of a child's understanding . . . so I have designed [*sic*] to profit all (if possible) and offend none."[25]

In moments of temptation these songs—"this constant furniture of the mind"—were to be a buckler against the onslaughts of the Evil One because they gave children "something to think about when alone and to sing over to themselves." Since it was believed that "what was learnt in verse was longer retained in the memory and sooner recollected," the songs "by running through the mind" were an "effectual means of keeping off temptation, when a word of Scripture was not upon the thoughts."[26] By giving their thoughts a "divine turn" the songs might raise a "young meditation." As a result, children would not be made to seek relief for an "emptiness of mind out of the loose and dangerous sonnets of the age." As an integral part of the morning and evening family devotions, these hymns too played their role; and for the greater convenience in this respect the author confined the verse to the most useful of the Psalm tunes.[27] The proper attitude of humility desired in a child toward God is detected in the closing verse of the first hymn:

> My heart resolves, my tongue obeys,
> And Angels shall rejoice,
> To hear their Mighty Maker's praise
> Sound from a feeble voice.[28]

All denominations in the external observances of religion afforded the child practically the same status—that of an actual or potential member—but the performance of the spiritual duties involved by such membership varied with individuals in different sections of the country. In the first place, children everywhere were expected to attend public worship with the same regularity, attention, and devotion that marked the practice of their elders on the Lord's Day. In the South, where the population was purely agricultural and widely scattered, with the nearest chapel perhaps twenty or thirty miles from the child's home and the common mode of travel by horseback or in canoes, it is logical to suppose that few children actually attended public services with any degree of regularity. It does not necessarily follow from this fact, however, that the Anglican or Presbyterian child lacked instruction in his religious obligations, for this duty was usually performed by the mother or tutor in the home.[29]

In the New England and Middle Colonies, where churches were more numerous and at a reasonable distance, minor inconveniences were not sufficient to excuse a child from his obligation of attending Sunday services. This can be seen in the diary of Anna Green Winslow, a girl of twelve, who records for March 4, 1771: "We had the greatest fall of snow yesterday we have had this winter. Yet cousin Sally, miss Polly, & I rode to & from Meeting in Mr. Soley's chaise both forenoon and afternoon, & with a stove was very comfortable there."[30] A few weeks later she relates that the "snow is near gone in the street before us, & mud supplys the place thereof," and that on Sunday morning she "made shift to walk to Meeting" but fortunately was given a ride home in a chaise. She adds that her aunt walked over and "she sais thro' more difaculty than ever she did in her life before. Indeed had the stream get up from our meeting house as it did down, we might have taken boat as we have talk'd some times of doing to cross the street to our opposite neighbor Soley's chaise."[31]

The right of membership in all denominations brought with it an implied obligation for children to make a public profession of their faith or of their religious experiences as soon as possible after they had attained the use of reason or could distinguish between right and wrong. This manifestation could take the form of a "baptismal covenant," or the public avowal of a conversion of the heart and mind to God, or the more mature pledge of fidelity to a particular code of religious principles by the ceremony of confirmation. Hence it is that the "Short Baptismal Covenant" was subscribed to and kept by many children "for their use and comfort." This formula for a first profession of faith was composed for the use of Congregationalists, but since it contained only the broadest principles of Protestant theology, it was also used by other denominations in Colonial America:

I take God the Father to be my chiefest Good and highest End.
I take God the Son to be my Prince and Saviour.
I take God the Holy Ghost to be my Sanctifier, Teacher, and Comforter.
I take the Word of God to be my rule in all my actions.
And the people of God to be my people in all my conditions.
I do likewise devote and dedicate to the Lord, my whole self, all I am, all I
    have, and all I do.
And this I do deliberately, and as far as I know my own heart sincerely, freely,
    and for evermore; depending always on the sovereign Grace of God and
    the Merits of the Lord Jesus Christ alone, for assistance and acceptance.[32]

Puritan children were taught in their infancy that the "church is a Congregation of Saints joyned together in the bond of the Covenant to worship the Lord, and to edifie one another in all his holy Ordinances."[33] Since the Puritan ideal was a regenerate church, all of whose members had experienced particular operations of the divine grace, even children were required to give before their congregation a detailed account of their conversion experiences.[34]

For the pietist sects, particularly the Quakers, conversion meant not so much a sudden, emotional turning away from evil, but rather a growing appreciation of the "Light of Christ within" which would lead the child, they believed, to all truth and right living. With the help of his parents or elders, every child was to make an examination of conscience to see the possibilities of good and evil which lay before him. To do this he had to know the effects of sin in the soul of the individual, and also the power of the "Inner Light." As the child acquired this wisdom, he gradually became converted and reached the state of the inner or second birth.[35]

The Anglican infant shortly after birth was "born again" by baptism in which through his sponsors he vowed a life of faith and obedience to their creed, renounced Satan and all his works and pomps, and implored the inspiration and assistance of the Holy Trinity. Only later, after he was safely within the fold, did the child learn the fundamental truths of his spiritual rebirth—that man had lost his divine heritage by the sin of our first parents, but that he had been redeemed by Christ's passion and death. To gain the fruits of redemption, the child must become a member of Christ's mystical body by baptism, a sacrament which brought him a title to the grace of the Holy Spirit, the promise of resurrection and immortality, the acceptance of God's will, and pardon for sin.[36]

In the strictly spiritual matters pertaining to the inner life of the soul, the attention of children was concentrated primarily on three great conceptions: the nature and attributes of God, the duties of the child to his Creator, and the means to be employed for salvation.

It would seem that the Protestant child's conception of God was rather briefly stated, for in describing the nature and attributes of the Almighty he was given this summation: "God is a spirit, Infinite, Eternal, Unchangeable in His Being, Wisdom, Power, Holiness, Justice, Goodness, and Truth."[37] Although the Holy Trinity was a mystery or a truth which could not be clearly understood, the offices of the persons of the Holy Trinity were quite simply defined in the child's Catechism. This explained God the Father as the author of his being and the maker of all things, to whom the child as a member of the human family must submit his will in all cases.[38] Christ, the Son of God and the Redeemer of Souls, was to be the exemplar for holiness of life; for the child read that Jesus was "humble and meek, and contemned the vanities of the world; he was charitable and compassionate to men's souls and bodies; he was patient under afflictions and pious and devout towards his God and Father; he was obedient to his laws and resigned to his good pleasure in all things."[39] The Holy Ghost was described as the "Spirit of the Father and of the Son, the Comforter and Sanctifier of all God's people, and that which reproves the world of sin, and these Three, Father, Son, and Holy Ghost, are one God, blessed forever."[40]

In contemplating the omniscience and omnipotence of God, the attributes so frequently stressed in their little books, children received not only an incentive to a good life, but also a deterrent to evil. The confusion and humility of the childish soul under the searching eye of the

Creator is recorded in the verses of Dr. Watts entitled "The All-seeing God":

> Almighty God, thy piercing eye
> Strikes through the shades of night,
> And our most secret actions lie
> All open in thy sight.
>
> There's not a sin that we commit,
> Nor wicked word we say,
> But in thy dreadful book 'tis writ
> Against the judgment day.
>
> Lord at thy foot ashamed I lie,
> Upwards I dare not look;
> Pardon my sins before I die,
> And blot them from thy book.[41]

"The Compendious Body of Divinity," which Puritan children memorized a few lines at a time, contained, besides the general truths of Christianity, a résumé of the relation of the soul to God:

> God is Pure Spirit, Infinite,
> In Truth abundant, of great power and might . . . .
> We all do from polluted Parents spring
> And in our flesh there dwelleth no good thing.
> None righteous are, but all of every sort,
> Have sinn'd and of God's Glory are come short.
> But God so loved us that he did give,
> His only Son that thro' him we might live.[42]

The duties of the child to his Creator bound the youth to "honour God, to love him above all things, to fear him, to put his trust in him, to pray to him, to praise him, to give him thanks, to be obedient to his laws, and to resign himself to God's holy will in all things."[43] On further inquiry, the child discovered that by a faithful performance of these duties he could be happy and in God's favor; yet by reason of the fall of Adam and Eve, all men fail in the fulfillment of their duties: "God made man upright; but hearkening to the Sollicitations of the Old Serpent, which is the Devil, he quickly rebell'd against his Maker . . . whereupon ensued such a corrupt Principle, as disposed him to Rebellion ever after."[44]

If his faults were only involuntary, the child could plainly expect indulgence, but quite soon did he learn that no man is free from voluntary error, nor does anyone acquit himself perfectly of his duty to God. Such voluntary sins as might have been avoided certainly made him liable to punishment.[45]

On the question of forgiveness of sin and the means of salvation the greatest divergence of Protestant opinion lay. At one extreme, the Calvinists held that since forgiveness of sin was a gratuitous gift, far above the deserts of any, God was entirely free either to bestow it or withhold it. His grace was given only to a few of the elect, chosen from all eternity by His love and good pleasure.[46] These elect or children of God recognized their "effectual calling" by the conviction of their own sin and misery; then being enlightened in the knowledge of Christ, they freely embraced His will as revealed in the Gospel. The next step for them on the road to salvation was "Justification," or "an act of God's free grace, wherein He pardoned all their sins, and accepted them as righteous, through the merits of Christ received by faith alone."[47]

The subsequent operation of grace in the chosen soul was "Adoption," whereby "he was received into the number and enjoyed the right to all the privileges of the Sons of God."[48] Sanctification of the soul followed in which the "whole man was renewed after the image of God, and enabled more and more to die to sin, and to live unto righteousness."[49] The benefits to be enjoyed in this life from such a regeneration were the "assurance of God's love, peace of conscience, joy in the Holy Ghost, an increase of grace, and perseverance therein to the end of life." According to this doctrine, the souls of believers were at death made perfect in holiness and immediately passed to glory; while their bodies, being still united to Christ, rested in their graves to await the resurrection.[50]

The ultimate joy of this conversion after the trying ordeal of purification can be readily appreciated:

> Oh! Happy I, and blessed be the day,
> That unto Truth and Conscience I gave way,
> I would not be in my old state again,
> If I thereby some thousands might obtain.
> From Wrath and Hell, my Soul is now set free
> For I don't doubt that I converted be.
> The Word with power, so to me was brought,
> A glorious change within my Soul is wrought.[51]

Samuel Moodey explained the fate of the many unregenerate thus: "This doctrine of Predestination has an ungrateful sound in some Ears: Predestination does not make men guilty of death; does not force them to Sin, and throw them to Hell: No, impenitent Unbelievers precipitate themselves into the place of Torment. Tis therefore their own Place."[52] Hence it was that Puritans sought by "thoughts that breathe and words that burn" not only to prepare the tender hearts of youth for the work of conversion, but also to prevent the young from relapsing into the ways

of the ungodly. Since the doctrine of predestination was taught to a
large percentage of American children in Colonial times, juvenile books
stressed the element of fear. "Youth," in a very popular work, gave expression to his religious conviction in these words:

> But I am call'd of God and do obey
> The Voice of Truth and Conscience every day.
> God's called Ones, I'm sure you can't deny,
> But they are such whom he doth justifie:
> Therefore tis clear and very evident,
> That Grace alone hath made me penitent.
> My heart is sound, My Grace true also,
> My Confidence there's none shall overthrow.[53]

"Truth" then warned the boy that fear was the proof of conversion:

> Thou seemest too confident, 'tis a bad sign;
> For fears attend where saving grace doth shine.
> I tell thee (Youth) that many called be,
> But few are chosen for eternity.[54]

To inspire a salutary fear in youthful hearts, ministers posed such
frightening questions as: "What kind of place is hell, which sinners
are hastening to as their home?" The answer followed directly with
horrible precision: "It is for dimension a very large place . . . a bottom-
less pit. It is also large and wide for it must afford lodgings for many
Worlds of People, of all which tho' as the Sand of the Sea for Multitude,
a Remnant only will be saved . . . the Almighty King and Judge himself who hath and keeps the keys of hell, shuts and none can open, locks
the brazen gates upon his prisoners."[55] With this frightful image in
mind, children could find little spiritual security even in the performance
of the ordinary Christian virtues, for they were given repeated warnings
of their impending doom: " . . . though you pray and fast, deal justly
with all, and give liberally to the poor, yet if you know not the truth
as it is in Jesus, you can never get to Heaven. And till you discover
that you are in the Wrong Way you will not so much as Enquire the
Right."[56]

The beliefs of the Quakers and other pietist sects were diametrically
opposed to the Puritan theory of predestination and total depravity. The
Pietists held that the child was born neither good nor bad, but in an
unmoral state with capacities for future good or evil, so that in time
he must make a deliberate choice between right and wrong. This voluntary turning to God under the inspiration of his "Inner Light" was the
only conversion required of the young. It was simply a safeguard cast

about the child's original state of justice.[57] Accordingly, Quaker boys
and girls were taught that the saving grace of God is given to all men,
but that some are lost although the grace is sufficient, "because they do
not obey the blessed discoveries of light and truth; but turn from them
to wantonness like truants from this saving school of grace. . . . Such
who rebel against and quench the good spirit of God are the cause
of their own destruction."[58] It must have been a source of consolation
to these children to learn that their eternal happiness depended simply
on a sincere repentance for their sins induced by a deep love of God, and
accompanied by an honest endeavor to obey His holy laws.

Anglicans and Lutherans were among those denominations support-
ing a theory of salvation for the child at some point between the extremes
of the Puritan doctrine of total depravity on the one hand, and the
Quaker belief of infant amorality on the other. This more moderate
group recognized in the doctrine of original sin the sad effects of man's
fall, and saw in it also the evil that vexed the souls of children during
their earthly pilgrimage. This sin it was that darkened the childish
understanding, weakened the will, and inclined young hearts to evil.
Since these denominations were united in their purpose of blotting out
the stain of sin thus inherited from our first parents, and of restoring
the child as quickly as possible to his lost state of "original justice," they
made use of infant baptism. Thus little ones, by the saving grace received in this sacrament, were early armed with a powerful weapon
against the temptations that beset them even from childhood. It was
their belief that although the fall of mankind was a universal tragedy,
salvation is an individual responsibility. Each child must work out his
salvation for himself; for by the redemption the supernatural graces he
required were supplied him. Although faith was the prerequisite to
justification, the Church, the divinely appointed organism for the ad-
ministration of the sacraments, supplied the grace necessary for the young
ultimately to attain eternal life. Accordingly, through the redemption of
Christ and by the operation of grace in the soul, the way was opened
for these children to achieve heaven and eternal happiness with God.
Perhaps it was this spiritual security that has permitted the history of
these moderate denominations to be eclipsed by the graphic Puritan or
Quaker records of "juvenile conversions." In this regard, a missionary,
the Rev. Mr. Currie, wrote at Radnor, Pennsylvania, in 1741: "The people
of the Church of England gave themselves up to none of those wild
Notions and enthusiastic ravings, which some people practiced so much;
but by their very sobriety in such unsettled times increased their following."[59]

The Colonial child in his battle for righteousness was "duty-bound" to God, to his neighbor, and to himself by a stern religious code. This varied in emphasis in different localities, but everywhere it held the child to a high standard of theological observance. That not all children attained the desired degree of perfection was of course admitted as evidence of the depraved state of fallen men. In the face of occasional casualties, the war against evil was never relaxed, nor were the victories of the heroes left unsung.

His duty to God bound the child to obedience to the divine will as contained in the Ten Commandments, and to an exact knowledge of the Holy Scriptures.[60] Part of this duty demanded a stringent observance of the Sabbath. Even a cursory examination of juvenile literature indicates this, for verses intended to produce the proper Sabbath mood were among the first to be learned:

> This is the day when Christ arose
> So early from the dead:
> Why should I keep my eye-lids clos'd,
> And waste my hours in bed?

> Today with pleasure Christians meet,
> To pray and hear thy word,
> And I would go with cheerful feet,
> To learn thy will, O Lord.[61]

The Assembly of Divines set rigid rules for Sabbath observance when they decreed:

The Sabbath is to be sanctified by an holy resting all that Day, even from such worldly Employments and Recreations, as are lawful on the other Days, and spending the whole Time in publick and private Exercises of God's Worship, except so much as is to be taken up in the Works of Necessity and Mercy.[62]

Violators of this commandment were believed to meet with the summary judgment of God and man. This belief was supported by such accounts as the incident of "fourteen Young Persons who on a Lord's Day in the winter time would go to play at Football on the Ice, but that broke under them, and they were all drowned." It was further reported as a horrible example to wavering youth that "two Young Men, belonging to New England, would be so profane as to ride a race on the Lord's Day, but when they were on their Horses Backs, God smote 'em with a strange kind of palsey of which they both died, after they had been for several months in a very miserable condition." The report goes on to say that "Sabbath breakers expose themselves to that which is worse than any temporal judgments, viz., To Spiritual and Eternal Judgments."[63]

Another duty of children to God required the daily recitation of certain prayers both in union with the family and alone, an obligation which was expressed in such counsels as: "Sanctify God in your heart daily, make him your fear, your love and delight,"[64] and "Perform daily duties both in Family and Closet (especially these three of Prayer, Meditation, Reading) with serious intention, heat of affection, diligence, and delight."[65] The Quaker Catechism gave this advice about prayers: "They are to be fervent, short and sound, to proceed from the Spirit, and with good understanding, in deep humility, in the Name of our Lord Jesus Christ, with purity, charity, fervency, and constancy."[66]

Prayer was defined as "the offering up of our desires to God, for things agreeable to His will, in the name of Christ, with confession of our sins, and thankful acknowledgment of his Mercies." Although three parts of prayer were thus acknowledged—petition, confession, and thanksgiving—it was universally accepted by the various sects of this country that "prayer most properly doth consist in petition."[67]

The Lord's Prayer, divided into seven parts, was the chief devotion of all denominations; but other forms were also used. Samuel Fuller tells children that prayer is "speech or earnest breathing of the soul to the Almighty whether exprest in words or not."[68] This included then, on the part of the child, not only spontaneous ejaculations, but also such formal petitions as the "Morning and Evening Prayers" included in the catechisms and primers. A typical evening prayer of the times is found in the Thumb Bible, *Verbum Sempiternum:*

> Forgive me dearest Lord for Thy dear Son
> The many ills that I this day have done,
> Teach me to live that I may ever dread
> The Grave, as little as I do my Bed.
> Keep me this night, O keep me King of Kings
> Secure under thy own Almighty Wings.[69]

The love and respect that all children were bound to pay their parents or those whose "authority by nature or providence had a just claim to their submission such as guardians or tutors" was a sacred obligation next in importance to serving God. To these "superiors" children were required to be humble, submissive, and obedient at all times, and "to let their bodies be pliable and ready to manifest in due and becoming ceremonies the inward reverence they bore to those above them."[70] Catechisms told children how to honor their parents—"to love them, to obey their commands; to conceal their infirmities; to maintain them when old and in want; and to submit to their admonitions and corrections."[71] Little readers were not only counseled in the paths of filial reverence, but also were solemnly warned "of the heavy curse of God that would fall upon children who made light of their parents." In terrifying terms they read that "there is a secret Blast of God upon Undutiful Children; they are afflicted in their Estates, in their Bodies, they are followed by one plague after another. And if Undutiful Children ever live to have Children of their own, God pays 'em in their own coin."[72] To stamp this lesson clearly in the young mind, little boys and girls were taught the hymn:

Have we not heard what dreadful plagues
Are threatened by the Lord,
To him that breaks his Father's law
Or mocks his Mother's word?

What heavy guilt upon him lies!
How cursed is his name!
The ravens shall pick out his eyes,
And Eagles eat the same.[73]

Charity or love of neighbor was held to be the badge of a Christian, but one can gather from books and sermons that it was not practised to any heroic degree. Nevertheless little ones learned by heart the Saviour's words: "This is my commandement that ye love one another, as I have loved you." William Penn, on this point, advised his children: "Be natural; love one another and remember that to be void of natural affection is a mark of apostacy. . . . It is a great fault in families of this day."[74]

The practice of the Golden Rule was strongly recommended in most juvenile books. It was found in verse in all the primers:

Be you to others kind and true,
As you'd have others be to you:
And neither do nor say to Men,
Whate'er you would not take again.[75]

Children were also taught to retire for secret prayer and a diligent examination of conscience "every day that came over their heads." For this office they read such cheerless exhortations as: "Be sensible of thy Original Corruption daily, how it inclines thee to evil, and indisposeth thee to good; groan under it and bewail it as Paul did. Also take special notice of your actual sins, or daily infirmities in Thought, Word, Deed. Endeavour to make your peace with God for them before you go to bed."[76] In an Anglican catechism, the master or mistress was advised to instruct the child to "confess and bewail in particular every sin which may have been committed by him or her in the day past; whether Lying, Taking God's Name in Vain, Stealing, Quarrelling, Stubbornness, or any other."[77] An example of such introspection is seen in the case of Elizabeth Butcher, who was born in Boston in 1709. When she was about two-and-one-half years old, "as she lay in her cradle, she would ask herself the question, 'What is my corrupt Nature?' and would make answer again to herself, 'It is empty of Grace, bent unto Sin, and that continually.' She took great delight in learning her Catechism and would not willingly go to bed without saying some part of it."[78] Young Nathaniel Mather, in one of the "directories" which he drew up for himself, wistfully recorded the hope: "O that I might lead a spiritual Life, wherefore let me regulate my life by the Word of God."[79]

Cotton Mather in the preface of his *New England Token* made these searching inquiries of his young readers: "Do you do as these children did? Did you ever see your miserable state by Nature? Did you ever get by yourself and weep for sin and pray for grace and pardon?"[80] Children were thus obliged to search their hearts and by an earnest self-analysis to ascertain signs of their spiritual progress and to discover the extent of their submission to the will of God. Samuel Davies, after exhorting a group of school boys to do good, said: "You are now in your tender forming Age, most likely to receive good impressions. And now is the Time when God is wont to display His Grace in converting young Sinners. . . . Spend a little time this evening in Prayer, in examining whether you have come to Christ or not, in meditating on the condition of your souls."[81]

Whether one can explain or even justify the harsh theological code taught these Colonial children would seem to be a matter of opinion. It might be held that a people facing a hard world were aided, as a matter of morale, by stern religious teachings even in their youthful years; and if we are to believe the record, some children found joy in this code. On the other hand, it would seem to many a modern critic that the children of pious families were unnecessarily terrified. One is inclined to think that the emphasis upon a God of Wrath was such as to hide from the little ones that God of Love to whom modern Christians usually turn. This conclusion, of course, leads to a criticism of the Calvinistic tradition in general; but it may at least be suggested that the harsher elements in that tradition bore most heavily on such little ones as were inclined to heed them.

* * * * * *

The American Revolution not only changed some of the established churches of Colonial times, but also popularized such rationalistic philosophies as deism. This cult, repudiating revelation and the divine inspiration of the Scriptures, developed the idea of a benevolent God whom man served best by doing good to his fellow men. The Revolution also revived the old Unitarian concepts that denied the dogma of the Trinity, the deity of Christ, and endorsed the increasing interest in humanity. As a result of this ferment, a new "live and let live" spirit entered American thought at the close of the eighteenth century. This change was accelerated by ideas of liberty and the rights of man, and furthered by the spread of nationalism and the growth of religious lethargy.[82] To counteract this materialism, most writers of religious books for children not only advocated a spirit of toleration, but also blurred the sharp theological distinctions either by compromising with dissenters or by omitting supposedly minor points of dogma.

Another influential source of the new trend in child life from 1776 to 1835 was the gradual relaxation of the rigid Puritan standards. This mitigation of standards may be explained by the defection of the middle class from the doctrine of predestination. In the early days, Puritanism had provided the New Englanders with a theology that had apparently sustained them in their sufferings by supplying them with a moral basis for earthly success. As a social power in the new republic, it had fostered a morality for these people which allowed men to improve their spiritual standing by worshiping God on the Sabbath, and by serving Him the rest of the week through a shrewd management of their worldly estates. Although Puritanism is thus said to have idealized acquisitiveness as a Christian duty, it could not survive an era of commercial activity; for the "elect" Puritan could not successfully carry on business with "unregenerates" if he insisted on reminding them of their sinfulness.[83] Hence it was that the merchants of Puritan New England finally realized that toleration for other creeds was necessary to stimulate trade and commerce. This was to be the basis of their nineteenth-century prosperity.[84]

Once the barrier of intolerance was broken the main stronghold of Puritanism collapsed, for the doctrine of predestination then came under the attack of skeptics. Disbelief in the doctrine of election for the few and damnation for the masses was widespread at the opening of the nineteenth century. A humanized liberalism had introduced a new and more hopeful note into the religious life of Puritan New England.

In keeping with the new spirit of liberal Christianity which emphasized the fatherhood of God and the brotherhood of man, it is not surprising to find in a popular juvenile book of the times an account of a father advising his children to cultivate an "enlarged charity" for all mankind, however they might differ from others in religious opinions. Although he urged them to show respect to the ministers of every persuasion, he warned them never to seek direction of conscience from these ministers as that procedure might undermine their own faith. It is significant of the trend of the times to find that on the same page in which the father advocated toleration he also deplored the spiritual lethargy which had infected the rising generation—"the coldness and listlessness in whatever relates to religion."[85]

Two very different methods were at hand by which the churches could deal with the rapidly developing secularism of the late eighteenth century. The one was to meet it with the vigorous resistance employed by the early American Calvinists, a scheme that would have plainly proved self-defeating; the other was to compromise with the enemy by harmonizing the old theological standards with the current scientific knowledge, and thus to evolve a new code of ethics and politics based on reason. The latter process, which was eventually chosen by the liberal leaders of America, not only diluted theological tenets by blending them into the entire mass of cultural concepts, but also led directly to the growth of natural religion and deism.[86]

Under the more comfortable tenets of natural religion as conceived by liberal Anglicans, the Christian had no severity to fear, for the basis of ethics was changed from a sense of sin to a desire for happiness. Since this code held that a man from birth possessed the inclination to brotherhood and coöperation, his salvation did not require a conversion, but simply an ordering of his life according to the universal law which his reason would dictate. Quite logically, the doctrines of Calvinism were abhorrent to these new humanists, who denounced predestination as a perversion of the truth that all men were aided by the inner light of reason; and who argued that it was inconsistent with the benevolence of God to create a human being destined for an irretrievable hell. The general deduction reached by this reasoning was that a well-ordered inner life presupposed a well-ordered outer life, under the mild direction of such an organization as the Anglican Church.[87]

Although liberalism in America was thus originally a humanitarian and not a theological movement, natural religion under the name of deism tended to supplant Christianity instead of strengthening it as first proposed. Deism repudiated the idea of evil as a part of the natural order, for it held that since an all-wise and all-good God had created the universe, the creation must be a reflection of his goodness. The evils found in human society were therefore temporal and accidental, induced not by man's perverted will but by his ignorance. In this particular doctrine lay the germs of the Unitarian and Universalist theories, which likewise stressed the ideas of "the benevolence of the Deity and salvation for all men," thereby eliminating the dogma of hell from their creed.[88] Although it may be criticized as having overrated the inherent goodness of humanity, deism by Revolutionary days had become a far-reaching gospel of intellectual and spiritual importance. Nearly all the leaders of political liberation were deists with the possible exception of John Adams, Roger Sherman, and John Hay.[89]

By 1776, four of the colonies, Rhode Island, New Jersey, Pennsylvania, and Delaware—largely under the control of the Baptists or Quakers—were unhampered by the restrictions of an established church. In this respect they had for more than a century been the exceptions among the colonies. With the opening of the war, insistent demands for the separation of church and state, especially in Virginia and New England, eventually resulted in dissociating political and religious institutions throughout the country.[90]

The outcome of the Revolution necessitated certain changes in the Anglican Church in America. The first was to change the name to "Protestant Episcopal" in order to emphasize its relationship to other Protestant groups. The next change, of necessity, was that of transferring its allegiance from the King of England as its head to that of a governing body, the General Convention, which was analogous to Parliament. The Convention consisted of a House of Bishops, and a lower house of ministers and clergy elected in equal proportion from every diocese. In the case of the Prayer Book, alterations were made discarding the Athanasian Creed, and a prayer for the President replaced the prayer for the King, but the substitute was never widely used. Although the Episcopal Church, from the beginning of the Republic, was transformed into a decidedly American institution, its membership, which was confined mainly to the more comfortable classes, remained comparatively small.[91]

The Presbyterian Church in the United States was undeniably an American institution, but its Calvinistic doctrines of predestination and election were diametrically opposed to the optimism of the nineteenth century. In order to strengthen the position of their church the more conservative Presbyterians formed a "Plan of Union" with the Congregationalists in 1801, and thus in a common endeavor until 1837 carried on their missionary expansion in western New York and in the Old Northwest Territory. The body of conservative Presbyterians could never bring themselves to accept the conditions of Protestant success in evangelizing the frontier; namely, the subordination of dogma, the use of ministers not formally educated, and the excitement of revivalism. Standing firm, they preferred to lose their most flourishing western community, that of the Cumberland Presbyterians of Kentucky, rather than to concede what now seem to have been minor points of discipline and dogma. In prosecuting that decision they spent much vital energy in doctrinal quarrels that otherwise might have been devoted to spreading their beliefs in the West. As a result of this lost opportunity to dominate the religious scene on the expanding frontier, the Methodists and Baptists were given added scope for their missionary activities in that region.[92]

Roman Catholics, with the growth of tolerance that marked the close of the Revolution, were gradually freed from the civil disabilities which had harassed their existence and limited their numbers in the Colonial era. Consequently there was no effective opposition when the Holy See appointed John Carroll as the first Roman Catholic bishop with his residence in Baltimore.[93]

Bishop Carroll's diocese at the time of his induction included only thirty thousand Catholics, hence he readily recognized the fact that as a minority group his church would have to look to immigration for its growth and strength. Immigration was to prove a fruitful source of membership, since the attraction which the new country had for submerged laboring classes brought a steady stream of workmen from the Old World. Economic betterment impelled numbers of German Catholics to seek homes in this country; while religious oppression also intensified this movement by driving thousands of Irish to find refuge here in the decade after 1820. With the exception of occasional groups of French political refugees, Ireland and Germany furnished nearly all the Catholic immigrant population to the close of our era.[94]

Most of these newcomers were either destitute or had but small resources, and so were forced by lack of means to settle down in an American port instead of moving westward. As a result, eastern cities—Boston, New York, Philadelphia, and Baltimore—became the chief centers of Roman Catholic influence.[95]

The aftermath of the Revolution brought not only the wave of skepticism already noted, but also a decided decline in fervor among orthodox Christians. This indifference was indeed evident along the Atlantic seaboard but more particularly so in the almost creedless western frontier. There where men were free from the usual restraints of settled communities, fighting, gouging, intemperance, profanity, and general lawlessness were the order of the day. Even among the gentle Quakers of

Pennsylvania, irreligion seemed to lay hold of youth. A plaintive protest to this apathy was raised in a letter to the "children and youth of the Society of Friends," written in 1805 by Frederick Smith, in which he deplored the growing negligence of Quaker parents in regard to the religious education of their children. He pointed out that as a result of this carelessness the Society had lost much of the plainness which had distinguished their ancestors, and the rising generation had developed an alarming tendency to conform to the world. The indulgence of parents was blamed for the defection of the children, who were evidently fast acquiring a distaste for the religious duties of their faith and were gradually uniting with the more liberal Christians.[96]

This ebb in religious feeling did not last long, for the reaction to it in the hearts of many noteworthy religious leaders fired them with a burning missionary zeal. After 1795 Protestant home missionaries under the direction of such men as Bishop Asbury rode the circuit and aroused a new interest in religion. Catholic priests also, particularly the Dominicans under Bishop Flaget of Kentucky, traversed the states north of the Ohio River and kept alive the faith of Catholic families scattered on the frontier.[97]

In contrast to the quiet religious revival which was taking place in the eastern states, the awakening of the West was accompanied by such extraordinary manifestations as the country had never before witnessed. Camp meetings conducted by evangelists met not only the religious but also the social and emotional needs of the "saints and sinners of every age and of every grade" who dwelt on the fringe of settlement.[98]

* * * * * *

Although the fundamental principles of Christianity previously described as the basis of the child's religious life did not change perceptibly from 1776 to 1835, nevertheless a growing tendency towards a more benevolent attitude in the treatment of children is clearly discernible in the moderate type of religious instruction given American neophytes. Since the "greatest good for the greatest number" was the spiritual as well as the material goal of most Americans, little books for children contained numerous pleas for tolerance and also warnings to parents that "care should be taken not to press too closely upon children such non-essential points as form the distinguishing peculiarities of the various sects of Christians."[99] Not only were the differences in creeds to be overlooked in religious teaching, but the belief was definitely expressed that it was "better for the mind to be left in perfect freedom to choose its own creed; if the feelings are religious God will enlighten the understanding; he who loves what is good will perceive what is true."[100]

It is not to be supposed from these remarks that dogma was discarded by the various Protestant denominations under the pressure of rationalistic trends. Parents were often advised to strike a middle course by teaching their children the doctrinal points of theology which had been traditionally embraced by the family; but to allow the young to reason and examine and form opinions for themselves. This new liberal policy is reflected in the book, *Advice to Christian Parents:*

Do not teach them to be bigots: to believe that everyone that differs from them and their father is a heretic. . . . We do not wish to see either you or your children possessed of a wavering mind, and an unsettled judgment, and borne about by every wind of doctrine; but we do wish you to form their sentiments upon the foundation of God's word and reason.[101]

Among the first expressions of the new trend was a work published in 1788 by Isaiah Thomas, the famous printer of Worcester, which bears the title *A Curious Hieroglyphick Bible; represented with Emblematical Figures for the Amusement of Children: designed chiefly to familiarize tender Age, in a pleasing and diverting Manner, with early Ideas of the Holy Scriptures.* In the gloom of the Colonial period just past, the idea of amusing little Christians by any religious device would have been denounced as an inspiration of the devil. Children were expected to approach theological truths in the same spirit as their elders. No sugar-coating even with "emblematical figures" was ever applied to any morsel of dogma, however bitter it might have been to the childish taste. Hence the opening words of this miniature Bible must have struck a pleasant but surprising note for the younger members of post-Revolutionary society, since the author noted that there "appeared not to have been any work of this kind yet offered for their amusement." He proceeded to give parents the novel warning: "Do not compel Children to learn certain Tasks in certain measured Hours, for such Compulsion or Restraint is oftener an Obstacle than an Encouragement towards learning the necessary and useful sciences."[102]

Popular as this small Bible was, young readers were frequently exhorted in the new illustrated catechism to spend more time in a diligent study of the ordinary version of the Word of God—the mainspring of their spiritual life. That the book was easily accessible to children may be inferred from the following lines:

That sacred book inspir'd by God,
In our own tongue is spread abroad;
That book may little children read,
And learn the knowledge which they need.[103]

To counteract disobedience to authority, religious instructors used the Bible as a source of examples for filial obedience.[104] In one of the new juvenile treatises on the Bible, the story of Solomon's reverence for his mother, Bethsheba, was cited for the edification of American boys. The tone is quite different from the old admonition to the undutiful child which warned him that a "peculiar curse" pursued the disobedient child in this world and that eventually "ravens would pick out his eyes and eagles eat the same." After describing Solomon's cordial greeting to his mother and how he had caused a seat to be placed for her at his right hand, the following deduction was made from this "amiable example of one of the greatest and most accomplished men that ever lived":

A young man however high be his birth, who is habitually disrespectful to his mother, deserves to be ranked among ill-bred clowns: While on the other hand, there is scarcely any surer mark of good nature, good breeding, and good sense, in a young man, than his habitually behaving towards his mother with respectful attention.[105]

Parents on their part were urged to be diligent in religious instruction and circumspect in their example because children formed their sentiments and manners by an imitation of others. To support the theory that the young "not only discover their intellectual powers, but acquire many sentiments of good and evil in the early years of their life," the elders were given the example of St. Augustine, whose youth was described as "very loose and disorderly." It was pointed out, however, that the prayers of his pious mother, Monica, had wrought a miracle of grace; by her saintly example the profligate youth was changed from a "disgrace to society" to one of the "most eminent champions for evangelical truth."[106]

The failure of compulsion in dealing with children was tacitly acknowledged in another small book of the times, *Nurse Truelove's New Year Gift,* which actually counseled bribing the child to learn the New Testament by the gift of a little speller or a pretty gilt book. This delightful volume, in its very title, proclaimed the utilitarian philosophy that was subtly seeping into child-training. According to the new code, children were to practise virtue, not primarily to escape hell-fire or to gain heaven, but for the same reason that prompted the making of this little book—

to merit a temporal advantage. The book was to be presented "to every little Boy who would become a great Man, and ride upon a fine Horse; and to every little Girl who would become a fine woman, and ride in a Governor's gilt coach."[107]

The child was also told that he could promote the glory of God in three ways: first, by acknowledging Him as the author of his being; second, by loving his fellow creatures, and doing every possible good for their persons, characters, and spiritual interests; and thirdly, by living temperately with respect to eating and drinking, and by subduing his passions when he found them unruly.[108] In this manner the new optimism of the day provided for the peace and happiness of youth in their relations to God, to their fellow beings, and to themselves. Although the *New Year Gift* was in advance of its times, since the ideas that it contained were more common at the turn of the century, nevertheless it indicates the trend of adult thinking in matters of child discipline.

Another popular work of this type bore the title, *Take Your Choice: or The Difference between Virtue and Vice, Shown in Opposite Characters*. The very first comparison was made between "Industry" and "Idleness"; but in spite of the title, neither subject was considered from the point of view of vice or virtue and their respective connotations, but only from the standpoint of expediency. Industry was represented by a good little girl who had been educated in those principles which established all "the amiable properties in female character," such as affection for her nearest friends, respect for all mankind, a love of study, and "no small attention to useful industry." In glaring contrast, the girl Idleness, although endowed with "a beautiful face and form" and a quick mind, repeatedly shocked her friends by wasting her time and failing to learn her lessons, for which omission she was often "set in the corner of the classroom with the cane down her back and spurned by all her classmates as a great dunce."[109] These practical didactic tales increased in popularity because they filled so nicely the behavior patterns of the young nation engaged in a program of territorial development. Children's stories stressing the excellence of morality portrayed temporal success as the usual recompense of an industrious youth. The following "short sermon" on "How to Make Money" epitomized the philosophy that shaped the thinking of American children during the decades when busy brains and hands were exploiting the resources of the vast new country:

If he has good health and is industrious, even the poorest boy in our country has something to trade upon: and if he be besides well educated, and have skill in any kind of work, and add to this moral habits and religious principles, so that his employers may trust him and place confidence in him, he may then be said to set out in life with a handsome capital, and certainly he has a good chance of becoming independent and respectable, and perhaps rich, as any man in the country.[110]

One of the first distinctly American textbooks published at the close of the eighteenth century gave children an interpretation of the pleasures of a devout Christian life that was in sharp contrast to the spirit prevailing in 1700:

I have formerly (with the world) accounted the spirit of a Christian, to be a melancholy spirit: and the ways of holiness unpleasant paths, leading into the deserts of sad retiredness; but . . . now I see there is a heaven on the way to Heaven, and one look of faith yields more comfort and content than all the pleasures and delights the world can afford.[111]

Many of the female writers of children's books who began their activities early in the nineteenth century agreed on the necessity of cultivating the minds of the young in the things of the spirit. These women believed that the religious principles children imbibed, and the habits they contracted in their early years, were of the utmost importance; for proper training not only gave children's character a unique quality in the first years of life, but generally stamped the form of their whole later conduct and even their eternal state. Hundreds of volumes were produced to underscore the great lesson of child life—the capacity of knowing, loving, and serving God here, as a preparation for a blissful eternity. In driving home their great points, these authors sought to mold warily the

tender minds so susceptible of impression, to lead them imperceptibly to virtue by such methods as seemed rather to amuse than to instruct, to excite their attention with natural images, and to enlarge their ideas with such stories as were calculated for giving them delight, and at the same time were capable of imprinting on their tender minds sentiments of religion, justice and virtue.[112]

In contrast to the writers of an earlier period who overworked the proverb, "the fear of the Lord is the beginning of wisdom," or who warned children that "heaven and hell are no trifles," the new school renounced this Hebraic interpretation of man's relations to his Maker. It taught that true religion had "nothing to terrify its youthful votaries"; that its aspects were mild and placid, its sentiments pure, liberal, and enlivening, and that it forbade no innocent gratifications.[113] Children were gently advised to study the life of Christ in the New Testament, and thus to "avert that most alarming of all human miseries, a conscience at war with itself" by concentrating on the mercies of their Redeemer, and by trusting in the love of the Saviour whose precepts were to guide their lives.[114]

The new writings sought to impress on tender minds a sense of confidence in the ever present Deity and to show little ones that if dangers threatened, their Almighty Protector was always near. The love of God had been mentioned in most children's works prior to 1800, but this attribute of the Almighty was often eclipsed by the emphasis placed on His power and wrath. In contrast, a Catholic textbook of the later period gave this interpretation of the place of love and fear in the child's spiritual life:

If the greatness of God obliges us to fear and honour him with a profound respect, his goodness engages us as much to love him. We must fear God by reason of his greatness, which renders him infinitely adorable; and we must love him because of his goodness which makes him infinitely amiable; we must not separate these two virtues, love and fear. He that is without fear cannot be justified. He that loveth not abideth in death.[115]

To overcome the fear of being left alone, children were impressed with the necessity of living in the presence of God, and of being cautious of their words and actions. The habit of living under the immediate eye of Almighty God was believed to be an antidote for cruelty, lies, and stubborn temper—those common faults of early childhood so difficult to eradicate. This lesson of reverence for the presence of God, the certainty that "life meant looking up to Someone greater than himself," the idea of a state far above his own which yet encompassed his earthly existence, was later described by a child of the period:

The thought of God seemed as natural as the thought of my father and mother. That he should be invisible did not seem strange, for I could not with my eyes see through the skies beyond which I supposed he lived. But it was easy to believe that he could look down on me, and that he knew all about me. We were taught very early to say, "Thou, God seest me;" and it was one of my favorite texts. Heaven seemed nearer because someone I loved was up there looking down on me. A baby is not afraid of his father's eyes.[116]

Many adults by 1800 whose spiritual lessons had been "painfully learnt and darkly understood" advocated that religious education in early life should be addressed to the heart rather than to the mind. In keeping with this plan, the affections were to be filled with love and gratitude to God, but no attempt was to be made to introduce doctrinal opinions into the understanding. To that end, the child's ponderous "Compendium of Divinity" used in former days was much abridged and simplified. It was thought enough for the child to be told that God was his father, that everything in the world was formed by His wisdom and preserved by His love. No opportunity was lost of impressing on the child's mind that God loved the children He had made, that the wicked removed themselves from God, but that He never withdrew from them. An important point in the code was the teaching that since grace was always shedding its holy beams upon the human soul to purify and bless it, only the perversity of the individual could prevent the effective operation of that divine influence.[117]

The optimistic advocates of a "natural religion," or those who sought to find in nature the normal and only final answers to all philosophical problems, again and again warned parents that the prayers of children should be simple and suited to their understanding and state of mind; that the young in any event should not be expected to enter into the spirit of prayer with the feelings and reactions of adults. A love for the sublime and beautiful works of nature was to be cultivated early in childhood, not merely to afford a source of enjoyment, but to promote a devotional spirit, and to elevate the mind "by raising the views 'through things which are seen' to Him who is invisible."[118]

The attempt to reach a knowledge of God through a contemplation of His works led a number of early nineteenth-century writers, particularly women, to focus unusual interest on nature study. Impressed by the grandeur and order of nature, they arrived at the conviction that life is essentially good and that the universe is controlled by a benevolent God whom man may approach by various avenues of worship. Hence some of the juvenile aids for religious instruction written by these advocates of "sense-experience" used nature study to prove the transcendental, as in Emerson, and often incorporated pantheistic ideas in their lessons for boys and girls. One wonders what the reactions of young minds may have been, for example, to this suggestion in Mrs. Barbauld's *Hymns in Prose*:

Child of reason . . . what has thine eye observed and whither has thy foot been wandering?

I have been wandering along the meadows, in thick grass; the cattle were feeding around me. . . .

Didst thou see nothing more? Return again, child of reason, for there are greater things than these. God was among the fields; and didst thou not perceive him? His beauty was among the meadows; his smile enlivened the sunshine. God was amongst the trees, his voice sounded in the murmur of the water; his music warbled in the shade; and didst thou not attend? God was in the storm, and didst thou not perceive him? God is in every place; he speaks in every sound we hear; he is seen in all our eyes behold.[119]

A general recognition of the child as a distinct personality could not be effected by the exponents of the new school of spiritual thought until the nineteenth century was well on its way. The humanitarian Gallaudet, in his *Child's Book on the Soul,* counseled adults that the inquiries made, the difficulties stated, or the doubts expressed by the child should be treated with the greatest consideration, for he added, "They who would teach children well, must first learn a great deal from them."[120] This author, as late as 1831, expressed the opinion that there was a great deal too much complexity in the early religious instruction of children. To correct this evil he urged the teaching of but one simple truth—that the child possessed a soul, distinct from the body, which would survive it and live forever. He declared that this truth could be taught from an observation of natural phenomena such as animals, flowers, and pebbles. From this observation the child was to be made to feel that he was not a mere animal, for as an intellectual, moral, and accountable being destined to an endless existence beyond the grave, he had higher enjoyments than those which were sensual.[121]

Much of the theological instruction of the early nineteenth century did not register permanently in young minds, nor was it of a uniform character; nevertheless children in general were taught that certain deeds such as disobedience to parents, lying, and stealing were forbidden by a "Power" that was not to be challenged. Public opinion then rarely excused youth, thus morally equipped, who deliberately defied or even evaded these fundamental precepts.[122]

Juvenile authors reflected in their writings the unyielding attitude of the righteous towards the willful and unpardonable "crimes of youth." Stories abounded in which the punishment for disobedience swiftly overwhelmed the obdurate child. Whatever zeal may have inspired some of these writers, their works could hardly have failed to have disastrous effects not only on the minds of small readers, but also on their relations with their parents. For example, one such tale, utilizing the horrible-example technique in relation to the sin of disobedience, told the sad experiences of "Little Fanny," a child of an age to play with dolls. This child's criminal career began after she had been denied permission to stroll in the park in order to show off her own finery; she subsequently violated her parents' wishes by stealing out with her nurse. She was then kidnapped from her wicked maid for the sake of her fine clothes, became a "dirty beggar," and as such "dwelt with vice which doubled all her pain." Eventually Fanny became a street vendor and cried "Fish to sell!" but she soon turned to the milk and egg business as a cleaner occupation. The unfortunate girl kept the thought of her home and parents constantly in mind, and the childish reader must have been amazed to learn that all this time "her mother's watchful eye followed her close," but that "prudence withheld maternal love" from rescuing the daughter until a longer trial had proved Fanny's virtue. After a sufficient purgatorial process, Fanny was restored to her family by being sent to deliver butter and eggs at her mother's new home. The reader was assured that the prodigal was no longer idle, vain, and eager to maintain her own opinion, but a pious, modest child beloved by all.[123]

The ultimate value of fictitious reading for children was widely debated. "To tell a story" was the common expression for lying, and for the lovers of absolute truth the term embraced not only actual falsehood but the delightful old fables, fairy stories, and poetic legends as well.[124] What now seems a source of much pleasure and profit for children was, as a result of this rationalization, bound up by a fine-spun theological thread and withheld from the enjoyment of the young. Advocates of literal truth deplored the fact that "stories of fairies, hobgoblins, and the like must fill the mind with improper ideas."[125]

To underscore this interpretation of truth, the child was given the "histories" of good children who had "died and gone to heaven" in which the little reader could learn that such chosen souls had always preferred tales of truth. For example, "Little Edward," who was born in Philadelphia in 1831, had found books his chief source of amusement from his fourth year. The point was made that although he had read a great deal for one so young, nevertheless if he "knew a story was not all true, he did not care about reading it."[126]

In regard to the external observances of piety, there was still a universal agreement on the fitness of silence, self-abnegation, and a serious deportment both at family and at public worship. The idea was steadily gaining ground, however, that little ones should not be compelled to attend church services until they were capable of behaving in a proper manner.[127] Fear was expressed that children might develop a dislike for the Sabbath, and a want of reverence for its sacred character. There is no question that those who still clung to the old traditions of the Sabbath restrained children from what now seems a natural and innocent expression of gayety on that day. If boys and girls laughed or jumped or touched their playthings, they were told that it was wicked to do because it was the Lord's Day. There is evidence that the day indeed became hateful to certain children, for they learned to consider it a period of gloom and privation and thus to associate the Bible and attendance at church with other distasteful experiences.[128]

An increasing number of adults also realized that, since small children could not sit still and read all day, they should not be bound to the adult code of Sabbath observance—which on the part of many children was naturally resisted as a state of bondage. Religious observance was to be made as pleasant as possible and oppressive rules and prohibitions avoided. Theodore Dwight dared to write the following advice to fathers about the "Sabbath going" of their offspring:

Children should be made as comfortable as possible at church. They cannot comfortably sit long in one position, especially in seats made for persons four times their size. We should never forget what "church going" is to them. Let us be set at a table five feet high and four feet wide, with high walls before and behind us, for three or four hours for time is longer to them, without permission to see or ability to understand; certainly it would be poor comfort to tell us, after unspeakable fatigue and endurance, that we were so good we might go again in the afternoon. Children cannot keep from restlessness or slumber in such circumstances and they should be lifted up and laid down, and always kindly treated. If quite small a few sugar plums may be taken to guard against a turn of crying. If they cannot be seated on a little high and narrow bench as to look a little about them, they may be allowed to stand up on the seat for a short time, and occasionally be held up to see a baptism, the organ, or the choir.[129]

Although medical authorities had warned against terrifying children, some juvenile works still exploited the easily aroused emotion of fear by a surfeit of horrifying tales. As long as the frightful physical phases of death were stressed in children's books there was naturally an interest in the "histories of godly children" of the Janeway variety, which had been so popular in the previous century. One such book, *A Memorial for Children, Designed as a Continuation of Janeway's Token,* frankly admitted this influence in its title; but the fact that most of the accounts were of recent occurrence seemed to justify its publication. The section addressed to living children might easily have had the effect of driving young readers into ways of wickedness in order to escape an untimely death—since the good always seemed to die young! After listing the virtues practised by the youthful paragons of perfection who had happily passed so soon to their reward, the author posed tremendous questions for his young readers: "Don't you wish to be like them, and to die as they did? That it may be so, you must do as they did: you must pray that the Lord would make you his children."[130]

Mary Pilkington wrote biographies of pious boys and girls in the same strain of spirituality as the work just described; and not only enumerated for children the blessings of an early death but also offered the virtuous youth but small hope for longevity. Her "moral and instructive examples for the female sex" contain a disturbing warning to the girlish reader:

> Beauty, nor wit, nor sense can save,
> From death's imperial dart:
> 'Tis virtue makes an early grave,
> Gives comfort to the heart.[131]

Boys could also draw alarming inference from an epitaph by this same writer which formed the closing chapter of a devout boy's life:

> Struck by stern death's unerring dart,
> When every virtue bloomed;
> When rich perfection graced his brest [sic]
> Then was his heart entombed.[132]

George Burder, in his *Early Piety: or Memoirs of Children Eminently Pious,* obliquely questioned the influence that descriptions of the edifying deaths of youths might have on the behavior patterns of normal children still attracted to the pleasures of this life. In referring to the models of early sanctity depicted in his work, Burder cautiously remarked:

Many of them died very young, (not that they died the sooner because they were good; but being good, they were the sooner fit to die); now, you yourself may die young too, therefore, pray earnestly to the Lord, for the pardon of all your sins, and beg for grace to make you fit to live, and then you will be fit to die.[133]

The fact that the author himself doubted the value of these disquieting "histories" doubtless accounts for their contrast to those of the Janeway school. Much of the vigor and fire of the old "memoirs" of godly Colonial children engrossed in the analysis of their "corrupt nature" is wanting in the new work, while the villain of the piece, "a sad and miserable child, Jack Perverse," is far from convincing. His history reveals that by 1812 the fear of the master's rod had supplanted the dread of a wrathful God—even among the "eminently serious":

Though his parents sent him to a very good school, yet he was such a dunce that he could not learn a single verse in the Testament without blundering; and when he was reproved, used to answer again with impertinence; and was so sulky and obstinate, that correction only made him worse. When any mischief was going forward at school, he was sure to be found at the head of it; by which means his task was left undone, and then to avoid punishment, he would play truant, the consequence of which was that he was not only well flogged, but a heavy log was fastened to his leg, and a great fool's cap was put on his head; so that he became the sport and derision of all that beheld him.[134]

The Lilliputian Masquerade "lashed the follies of the age" and reproduced the "dance of death" motif—a skeleton with an arrow in one hand and a letter of summons in the other. This work warned the child that however grim the mask might appear, death ought to be esteemed as a friend, for by thinking of it often he might pass his life profitably and at last be "relieved from a troublesome world to partake of the pleasures of one where sorrow is not known."[135]

The Taylor sisters, however, put the last ghoulish touch to the solemn picture of a small child's contemplation of death. In their verses "About Dying" and in "Lines on a Snowdrop," instead of dwelling on joys of holy souls in the presence of their God, these writers stressed the revolting physical aspects of death—those most likely to have disastrous effects on the youthful imagination. In "Lines on a Snowdrop," the fate of the poor little child, doomed forever to the "pithole," must have left weird impressions upon sensitive young readers. Witness, for example, the following dialogue:

> *Child*
> Tell me, Mamma, if I must die,
> One day as little baby died,
> And look so very pale and lie
> Down in the pit-hole by its side.
>
> *Mamma*
> 'Tis true, my love, that you must die,
> The God who made you says you must
> And every one of us shall lie,
> Like the dear baby in the dust.
>
> These hands and feet and busy head,
> Shall waste and crumble quite away;
> But though your body shall be dead,
> There is a part which can't decay.[136]

Gradually a benign attitude on the part of other adults mercifully spared the child the more revolting details of his dissolution. After he had been impressed with an idea of God's love he was led by degrees to know about the final trial of life.[137] More humane writers took children in spirit beyond the grave and gave them a foretaste of the delights awaiting those who loved God. A new note of hope was found in the contemplation of millions of their fellow creatures who had finally reached that haven of "everlasting rest, at which all have it in their power to arrive."[138]

The horrors of death were sometimes softened in children's works to foster the faith "that looked beyond the tomb"; nevertheless the solemnity of the subject was still emphasized. Children were urged to meditate frequently on death to forestall any terror that a casual reference to the subject might bring.[139] Since associations of grief were common in the frequent deaths of large families, a forthright acceptance of the facts of life and death was regarded as a much-desired virtue. Parents were exhorted to speak of the departed as being alive and waiting for the rest of the family to join them in an endless eternity of love.[140]

The Sunday school in the United States was of English origin and had for its primary aim the instruction of the poor in the rudiments of secular knowledge. By the opening of the nineteenth century this institution had been adapted to the American scene with a slight change of objective—"to perfect the children of the Congregation, or others, in the knowledge of the Catechism of the Church; to promote the reading of the Holy Scripture; and to teach those to read who were not otherwise taught." In this statement made by the Episcopal Church of Hudson, New York, in 1822, one notes in the words "or others" the growing "live and let live" spirit of American churches. In the rest of the declaration one may recognize the shift in the responsibility for the religious instruction of the young from the home to church institutions.

The literature of the Sunday school during this age of declining theological zeal further reflects the change not only in the spiritual status of the child but also in the general Protestant tendency to lower denominational barriers in the decades after 1825. Each church early in the century had its own apologists and publications which expounded with a lively zeal a definite code of doctrine acceptable to young aspirants of that particular creed. The American Sunday School Union had been formed in 1824 by merging the resources of various denominations, and thus provisions were made for a confederated system of religious instruction.[141] To execute this program of consolidated religious education on a nation-wide scale, auxiliary branches of the Union soon sprang into existence in almost every state and territory. In 1830 the Union resolved to establish a Sunday school in every neighborhood in the western states that was without one, and in 1833 it adopted a similar resolution with respect to the southern states. For this purpose it employed about 350 missionaries, many of whom were students in theological seminaries, to traverse the country and to revitalize decaying schools or to establish new ones.[142]

The object of the Society was twofold: to provide the young with oral instruction, and to furnish suitable juvenile reading material to be used in the schools and at home. The Union consequently published hundreds of volumes for its libraries, exclusive of an infinite variety of educational works, magazines, and journals.[143]

These publications were compelled to drop their distinct sectarian teachings, and the best sellers became either those that inculcated only broad religious principles agreeable to all Protestants, or those entirely devoid of dogma.[144] Accounts of conversions, directions for the observance of the Lord's Day, temperance propaganda, stories stressing the duty of charity to the poor and kindness to animals, and warnings against idleness and frivolous play were the subjects most commonly treated. Many of the publications reflected the new note of cheerful hope that characterized this era, as the following reveals: "Do remember that religion is so far from being gloomy, that it renders its possessors cheerful in hours of great trial. Surely it is far more pleasant to walk in the light of truth than in the darkness of sin."[145]

Under the revivalist influence, innumerable accounts of "hopeful conversions" formed an important part of this literature, as manifestations of grace were recorded for the general edification. In speaking of the "good fruits," the report for 1826 read as follows:

In one of the Sunday School Unions, more than thirty scholars have become pious during the past year. One little girl, ten years old, who thinks she has found grace to choose the good part which shall not be taken from her, has often retired, in the time between school hours, with her little companions, into some silent place in the woods, to kneel down and pray—to speak to Jesus the friend of little children.[146]

Much of the temperance literature lacked subtlety and conviction because the most commonplace occurrences of life or even the ordinary pleasures of childhood were made to serve propaganda purposes. Minor human frailties such as spending pennies at the confectioner's, thrilling to the wonders of a spring circus, or holding a spoonful of brandy in the mouth for toothache, after sweeping condemnations, were used as springboards from which an unwary youth plunged into a drunkard's grave. Statistics with their peculiar persuasive powers were brought to bear on the situation: and the young were told that in the Mad River district of Ohio alone more than four million gallons of whiskey were manufactured in a single year, or enough for two gallons for every man, woman, and child of that state! After admitting that much of the liquor was destined for exportation, the writer warned the "whole world to avoid Ohio Whiskey as they would the pestilence!"[147] The fact that more than thirty thousand people died every year "of strong drinks" in this country, and that the Bible said such would not inherit the kingdom of God, was considered sufficient grounds for a prolonged warfare against the "vice that most disgraced mortal man."[148]

The spirit of reform in Sunday school literature further manifested itself in hundreds of horrible examples of the unhappy fate reserved for those merciless children who were cruel to animals. The punishment, which was always swift in overtaking the youthful culprits, was frequently of an immoderate severity, out of all proportion to the malice intended. In most cases the retribution meted out made no provisions for the mischievous nature of normal children. For example, in a story prefaced by the remark, "Children are very apt to be cruel," an account was given of a small boy who during a ride in a cart with other children yielded to the temptation of "pricking the poor horse on the back to make him go faster." With lightning speed his punishment came; for "the poor animal plunged with pain, and darting suddenly around a corner, the boy was thrown out and crushed to death!" The author concluded this grim tale with the moral: "He had gone out from his parents' house in health and spirits. He was now returned a stiff cold corpse. And cruelty to an animal caused his sad death."[149]

With the old Colonial theological code of the child's religious life disrupted by a variety of influences—social and religious—the trend of the times was plainly sketched in books for children and in the manuals used by their parents as guides for spiritual instruction. Theological concepts were gradually displaced in religious training either by examples and rules for good conduct or by moral stories calculated to preserve the peace and prosperity of American society by a timely cultivation of the natural virtues. Even the prayers for little children took on a new tone and strikingly contrasted to those early petitions filled with terrifying allusions to a God of Wrath and the tortures of the damned:

> Give us a humble active mind,
> From sloth and folly free;
> Give us a cheerful heart, inclin'd
> To useful industry.

> A faithful memory bestow,
> With solid learning store;
> And still, O Lord, as more we know,
> Let us obey thee more.[150]

---

[1]William W. Manross, *A History of the American Episcopal Church*, p. 40.
[2]As quoted by William Warren Sweet, *The Story of Religions in America*, p. 44.
[3]Thomas C. Hall, *The Religious Background of American Culture*, p. 44.
[4]Theodore Maynard, *The History of American Catholicism*, p. 91.
[5]William Penn, *Fruits of a Fathers Love. Being the Advice of William Penn to His Children Relating to Their Civil and Religious Conduct*, p. 2.
[6]Samuel Davies, *Little Children Invited to Jesus Christ, A Sermon Preached in Hanover County, Virginia, May 8, 1758*, p. 11. Davies succeeded Jonathan Edwards as president of Princeton College. For infant minds such passionate proddings sounded the approach of the "Great Awakening," a movement which transcended political as well as religious boundaries.

[7]Anon., *The Children's Bible, or an History of the Holy Scriptures,* Title Page.

[8]*Ibid.,* Preface. Besides the Thumb Bibles containing scriptural verses and prayers, so popular with the children of this country, there were also other works such as the tiny book called *The History of the Holy Jesus* which gave naïve interpretations of the New Testament and closed with the solemn admonition:

> Keep close to his most just Commands,
> In all things please him well;
> Then happy it will be with you
> When thousands go to Hell.

A Lover of their Precious Souls, *The History of the Holy Jesus,* pages unnumbered.

[9]Eleazer Moodey, *The School of Good Manners, Containing Principles of the Christian Religion,* fifth edition, p. 72. This was an American variation of a British work, *English Exercises* by J. Garretson, first published in London in 1685; see A. S. W. Rosenbach, *Early American Children's Books,* p. 22.

[10]Samuel Fuller, *Some Principles and Precepts of the Christian Religion by One of the People called Quakers,* pp. 24, 25 (Quoting II Tim. 3: 16-17).

[11]Samuel Phillips, *The Orthodox Christian: or, A Child-Well-Instructed in the Principles of the Christian Religion,* p. 79.

[12]Cotton Mather, *A Family Well-Ordered,* pp. 19, 20.

[13]Samuel Fuller, *op. cit., Dedication,* pp. iii-v.

[14]John Muckarsie, *The Children's Catechism,* p. 23.

[15]Thomas Vincent, *An Explicatory Catechism: or, an Explanation of the Assemblies Shorter Catechism,* Preface, p. i.

[16]*Ibid.,* p. ii.

[17]Davies, *op. cit.,* p. 4.

[18]Mather, *op. cit.,* pp. 25, 26 (author's italics).

[19]Fuller, *op. cit.,* Introduction, pp. vi-xi.

[20]*Ibid.*

[21]Samuel Moody, *Judas the Traitor Hung up in Chains. To give Warning to Professors that they Beware of Worldlymindedness, and Hypocrisy; Preached at York in New-England,* p. 3.

[22]Benjamin Colman, *A Devout Contemplation of the Meaning of Divine Providence, in the Early Death of Pious and Lovely Children. Preached Upon the Sudden and Lamented Death of Mrs. Elizabeth Wainwright, Who departed this Life, April 8, 1714. Having just completed the Fourteenth Year of Her Age,* Preface, p. iv.

[23]James Janeway, *A Token for Children, Being an Exact Account of the Conversion, Holy and Exemplary Lives and Joyful Deaths of Several Young Children.* Preface to the original English edition. Cotton Mather added the *Token for the Children of New England.*

[24]*A Legacy for Children, being some of the Last Expressions and Dying Sayings. of Hannah Hill, Jurn. of the City of Philadelphia, in the Province OF Pennsylvania, in America, Aged Eleven Years and near Three Months,* p. 32.

[25]Watts, *op. cit.,* Preface, p. ii.

[26]*Ibid.,* pp. iii, iv.

[27]*Ibid.,* p. iv.

[28]*Ibid.,* p. v.

[29]S. D. McConnell, *History of the American Episcopal Church,* p. 87.

[30]Alice M. Earle, *Diary of Anna Green Winslow, A Boston Girl of 1771,* p. 39.

[31]*Ibid.,* pp. 54, 55.

[32]Eleazer Moodey, *The School of Good Manners,* pp. 32, 33.

[33]John Cotton, *Spiritual Milk for Boston Babes,* p. 10.

[34]Cotton Mather, *Magnalia Christi Americana,* pp. 11, 56-62.

[35]Walter J. Homan, *Children and Quakerism,* pp. 40, 41.

[36]Clifton H. Brewer, *A History of the Religious Education in the Episcopal Church to 1835*, p. 77.

[37]*The Reverend Assembly of Divines, A Shorter Catechism*, p. 2.

[38]Henry Heywood, *Two Catechisms by Way of Question and Answer: Designed for the Instruction of the Children of the Christian Brethren . . . who are commonly known and distinguished by the name of Baptists*, p. 67.

[39]*Ibid.*, p. 33.

[40]Samuel Fuller, *op. cit.*, pp. 30, 31.

[41]Isaac Watts, *op. cit.*, pp. 13-14.

[42]Eleazer Moodey, *op. cit.*, pp. 72-76.

[43]Henry Heywood, *op. cit.*, pp. 20, 21.

[44]Samuel Phillips, *op. cit.*, p. 20.

[45]Henry Heywood, *op. cit.*, p. 23.

[46]John Mackarsie, *The Children's Catechism* (Presbyterian), p. 11.

[47]*The Reverend Assembly of Divines, Shorter Catechism*, pp. 13-15.

[48]*Ibid.*, p. 15.

[49]*Ibid.*, p. 16.

[50]*The Reverend Assembly of Divines, Shorter Catechism*, p. 15.

[51]Benjamin Keach, *War with the Devil*, pp. 38, 39.

[52]Samuel Moodey, *op. cit.*, p. 10.

[53]Benjamin Keach, *op. cit.*, p. 45.

[54]*Ibid.*, p. 46.

[55]Samuel Moodey, *op. cit.*, pp. 26, 27.

[56]*Ibid.*, p. 60.

[57]Walter J. Homan, *Children and Quakerism*, p. 32.

[58]Samuel Fuller, *op. cit.*, pp. 21, 23.

[59]As quoted in Clifton H. Brewer, *A History of the Religious Education in the Espicopal Church to 1835*, p. 60.

[60]Isaac Watts, *op. cit.*, pages unnumbered.

[61]Watts, *op. cit.*, p. 30.

[62]*The Reverend Assembly of Divines, The Shorter Catechism*, p. 26; Early in the eighteenth century, the Puritans in America developed a trend towards individualism which was implicit in all dissent and especially in Congregationalism. Alarmed by the diversity of belief and by the indifference displayed by many parents in catechising their children, the General Court of Massachusetts adopted the longer and shorter catechisms that were drawn up in London about the middle of the century by the great Westminister Assembly of Divines. Although these works had been compiled by Presbyterians, the Congregationalists of this country seized them as the only escape from the schism that threatened to split each congregation into small factions. See Paul L. Ford, *The New England Primer*, pp. 10-12.

[63]Eleazer Moodey, *op. cit.*, p. 42.

[64]*The Rule of the New Creature*, p. 12.

[65]*Ibid.*, p. 4.

[66]Fuller, *op. cit.*, pp. 52, 53.

[67]Thomas Vincent, *An Explicatory Catechism*, p. 296.

[68]Fuller, *op. cit.*, p. 53.

[69]John Taylor, *Verbum Sempiternum, The Third Edition with Amendments*, pages unnumbered.

[70]Eleazer Moodey, *op. cit.*, p. 27.

[71]Henry Heywood, *op. cit.*, p. 47.

[72]Cotton Mather, *op. cit.*, pp. 41-43.

[73]Isaac Watts, *op. cit.*, p. 27.

[74]William Penn, *op. cit.*, p. 27.

[75]*The New England Primer*, pages unnumbered.

[76]Anon., *The Rule of the New Creature*, p. 3.

[77]John Lewis, *The Church Catechism Explained by Way of Question and Answer and Confirmed by Scripture Proofs, 35th edition*, p. 105.

[78]James Janeway, *op. cit.*, p. 132.

[79]*Ibid.*, p. 87.

[80]*Ibid.*, Preface.

[81]Samuel Davies, *op. cit.*, p. 24.

[82]Thomas C. Hall, *The Religious Background of American Culture*, pp. 126-46. See also Herbert M. Moraid, *Deism in Eighteenth Century America;* Edwin A. Burtt, *Types of Religious Philosophy;* John H. Hough, *The Christian Criticism of Life*, pp. 84-94.

[83]In the catechism, *Spiritual Milk for Boston Babes*, children were taught in regard to the Commandment "Thou shalt not steal" that they were to "get their goods honestly, to keep them safely, and to spend them thriftily"; John Cotton, *Spiritual Milk for Boston Babes*, p. 5.

[84]Joseph Haroutunian, *Piety Versus Moralism, The Passing of New England Theology*, Introduction, pp. xiv-xviii.

[85]John Gregory, *A Father's Legacy to his Daughters*, pp. 13, 14.

[86]Ernest S. Bates, *American Faith, Its Religious, Political and Economic Foundations*, pp. 218-20.

[87]Ernest S. Bates, *op. cit.*, pp. 222-23.

[88]Joseph Haroutunian, *op. cit.*, pp. 181-87.

[89]Ernest Bates, *op. cit.*, p. 226.

[90]*Ibid.*, p. 283.

[91]William W. Sweet, *The Story of Religions in America*, pp. 283-88.

[92]*Ibid.*, pp. 305-8.

[93]*Ibid.*, p. 293

[94]James A. Burns, *The Growth and Development of the Catholic School System in the United States*, pp. 11, 12.

[95]William W. Sweet, *op. cit.*, p. 390.

Since the Catholic Church in this country, especially beyond the Alleghenies, was in its formative stage before 1835, the status of the Catholic child will not figure prominently in this study; even at the close of this era few distinctly Catholic books had been published in this country. Parents and teachers made use of European publications, especially those from Germany and England, although a few American publishers made reprints of the textbooks prepared by the Brothers of the Christian Schools in Ireland. In this respect it is worth noting that the shift in the basis of the child's spirituality from a theological to a moral emphasis did not hold true for the Catholic child. In the few Catholic textbooks of the 1820's now available, at least three-fourths of the material presented rested on a foundation of theology. Although the contents of these books were milder in tone, they were quite as dogmatic in theory as similar Protestant texts of the preceding century. James A. Burns, *op. cit.*, pp. 136-40.

[96]Frederick Smith, *A Letter to the Children and Youth of the Society of Friends*, pp. 3, 4; William W. Sweet, *op. cit.*, pp. 322-31.

[97]*Ibid.*, pp. 321-26.

[98]*Ibid.*, p. 332.

[99]Hoare, *op. cit.*, p. 151.

[100]Child, *op. cit.*, p. 74.

[101]John Hersey, *Advice to Christian Parents*, p. 46.

[102]*A Curious Hieroglyphic Bible*, Preface, pp. vii-viii.

[103]Phillip Doddridge, *The Principles of the Christian Religion: Divided into Lessons, and adapted to the Capacities of Children*, p. 6.

[104]*Ibid.*, p. 11. See also, *Wisdom in Miniature or The Young Gentleman and Lady's Magazine. Being a Collection of Sentences Divine and Moral*, pp. 7-10; J. G., *A Small Help Offered to Heads of Families for Instructing Children and Servants*.

[105]Ezra Sampson, *Beauties of the Bible, being a selection from the Old and New Testaments with various remarks and brief dissertations, designed for the use of Christians in general, and particularly for the use of schools, and for the improvement of youth*, Preface, p. iii.

[106]John Witherspoon, *A Sermon on the Religious Education of Children, Preached in the old Presbyterian Church in New York to a very numerous audience*, pp. 2-4.

[107]*Nurse Truelove's New Year Gift: or, The Book of Books for Children, Adorned with cuts*, Preface.

[108]*Ibid.*

[109]*Take Your Choice: or, The Difference between Virtue and Vice, Shown in Opposite Characters*, pages unnumbered.

[110]*The Youth's Friend*, XL (1838), p. 19.

[111]Enos Weed, *The American Orthographer, in three books by a Physician and Surgeon in difficult Cases*, p. 43.

[112]Mrs. Richard Griffith, *Letters Addressed to Young Married Women*, p. 65.

[113]Mrs. Bonhote, *The Parental Monitor*, p. 121; William Mason, *The Closet Companion, or an Help to Serious Persons*, p. 45.

[114]Mrs. Bonhote, *op. cit.*, p. 124. See also Bielby Porteus (Bishop of London), *A Summary of the Principal Evidences for the Truth and Divine Origin of the Christian Revelation Designed for the Use of Young Persons*, pp. 47-56.

[115]W. E. Andrews, *The Catholic School Book, containing easy and familiar lessons for the instruction of youth of both sexes, in the English language and the paths of true religion and virtue*, p. 173.

[116]Lucy Larcom, *A New England Girlhood*, p. 63.

[117]Lydia Maria Child, *The Mother's Book*, p. 73; see also Sunday and Adult School Union, *Milk for Babes or a Catechism in verse for the use of Sunday Schools*, p. 17.

[118]Mrs. Louisa Hoare, *Hints for the Improvement of Early Education and Nursery Discipline*, p. 142.

[119]Anna Letitia Barbauld, *Hymns in Prose for the Use of Children*, pp. 18-19.

[120]Thomas H. Gallaudet, *The Child's Book of the Soul*, Preface, p. vii.

[121]*Ibid.*

[122]*The History of Little Dick*, Preface.

[123]*The History of Little Fanny, exemplified in a series of figures*, pp. 7-15.

[124]Lucy Larcom, *op. cit.*, pp. 74-78.

[125]*The Seasons*, Preface; *False Stories Corrected*, Preface; *Garden Amusements*, Preface.

[126]Committee of Publication, American Sunday School Union, *Memoir of an Infant Scholar*, p. 17.

[127]Child, *op. cit.*, p. 64; Hoare, *op. cit.*, p. 148.

[128]Child, *op. cit.*, pp. 64, 65. There is an interesting account in this connection of a small girl who after much coaxing was unwisely permitted to attend a performance of *Der Freyschutz*, a German play in which wizards, devils, and flames predominated. The child's terror increased until her loud sobs compelled her parents to take her home. When asked by her grandmother if she did not like to go to the theatre, she replied, "Oh, no Grandmother, it is a great deal worse than going to meeting!" Hoare, *op. cit.*, p. 64.

[129]Theodore Dwight, Jr., *The Father's Book: or, Suggestions for the Government and Instruction of Young Children on Principles Appropriate to a Christian Country*, p. 93.

[130]George Hendley, *A Memorial for Children: being an authentic account of the*

Conversion, Experience, and Happy Deaths of Eighteen Children. Designed as a Continuation of Janeway's Token, pp. 65-66.

[131]Mary Pilkington, *Biography for Girls: or Moral and Instructive Examples for the Female Sex,* p. 21.

[132]Mary Pilkington, *Biography for Boys; or Characteristic Histories, calculated to impress the youthful mind with an admiration of virtuous Principles, and a Detestation of Vicious Ones,* p. 23.

[133]George Burder, *Early Piety: or Memoirs of Children Eminently Serious, Interspersed with familiar Dialogues, Prayers, Graces, and Hymns,* Preface, p. iv.

[134]Burder, *op. cit.,* pp. 32, 33.

[135]*The Lilliputian Masquerade, Occasioned by the Conclusion of Peace between those potent Nations, the Lilliputians and the Tommythumbians,* p. 60.

[136]Ann and Jane Taylor, *op. cit.,* p. 24.

[137]Mrs. Richard Griffith, *op. cit.,* p. 101.

[138]Mrs. Bonhote, *op. cit.,* p. 124.

[139]Lydia Huntley Sigourney, *Letters to Mothers,* p. 285.

[140]*A Father to His Daughter, The Daughter's Own Book, or Practical Hints,* p. 237.

[141]*New Jersey Sunday School Journal,* I (1827), p. 8.

[142]*Ibid.,* p. 29.

[143]Mrs. Isabelle Mayo, *The Aspects of Religion in the United States of America,* p. 172.

[144]American Sunday School Union, *First Lessons on the Great Principles of Religion, Designed to be used in Infant Sabbath Schools and Private Homes,* p. 56.

[145]American Sunday School Union, *The Youth's Friend,* XXXIII (1826), p. 84.

[146]*Ibid.,* p. 90.

[147]Committee of Publication for the American Sunday School Union, *The Glass of Whiskey* (1885), p. 8; *The Six-Penny Glass of Wine* (1833), p. 24; Youth's Penny Gazette, III (1845), p. 33; Philadelphia Publications.

[148]John S. Abbott, *The Child at Home; or the Principles of Filial Duty Familiarly Illustrated,* p. 71.

[149]*The Youth's Friend,* XXXIII (1826), p. 131.

[150]The American Tract Society, *A New Picture Book,* p. 13.

The Art

OF

DECENT BEHAVIOUR

The manners of American children were basically conditioned by the grim determination of Colonial parents to pass on to coming generations the habits and customs of their European ancestors. These colonists, banded together on the fringe of forests inhabited by savages, were beset by a very real fear of seeing their society lapse into barbarism. Despite limited contacts with their former European culture, early Americans used every available means of developing the "art of decent behaviour" to perpetuate their traditional social amenities. This was true whether one considers the English of Virginia and New England, the Dutch of New York, or the Germans of Pennsylvania.

The Colonies boasted few wealthy families, hence social betterment here meant incessant toil, thrift, and saving, for children as well as for adults. The dangers and privations of those early days required health, courage, and unlimited endurance. Harsh conditions of life fostered a peculiar social code under which the individual American uniformly abhorred weakness in himself or in his neighbor. Springing from the rigors of this Colonial "proving period," a new dynamic force entered the character of the people, and was reflected through succeeding generations in the manners and customs of American child life.[1]

The Bible, in every colony, served as a basis for a rigid code of manners and morals that was intended to preserve for children the sacred traditions of their forbears. Europe, too, set standards for a patriarchal family government based on the Old Testament. The family with the father as the guiding spirit early became the basic unit of American life and the focal point of moral training.[2] The Colonial father exercised supreme authority over his wife and children, and from all accounts took his administrative duties seriously. It was the father who propounded the law of the home with the inflexible strictness of a judge. He dealt with his children as he expected God to deal with him—with less of mercy than of justice. Paternal discipline, reinforced by the Bible and strengthened by threats of damnation for undutiful children, made a great point of unhesitating, explicit obedience.[3]

That children should "mind" was generally a foregone conclusion. Technically at least, there was no parleying, no giving excuses, no revocation of command; but the father's will, once expressed, implied obedience at all costs. Against the autocracy of that will, even the mother might set herself futilely, and the children weep and plead in vain. The father's exercise of highest authority in the family was everywhere accepted as part of the religious faith of the times. Fatherhood was regarded as a sacred, God-appointed trust, for the discharge of which the head of the family owed a strict accountability to the source of his authority.[4]

The influence of the mother in the Colonial family was passive, but was generally more immediately attractive to the children than the father's tyrannical sway. Although the law failed pitifully to protect her rights, and customs relegated her to an inferior position in the home circle, the mother seems to have left deep impressions on the character of society. Consciously, by precept and word, and unconsciously, by manner and example, she established herself as the resistless influence which shaped the laws of childhood.[5]

This mode of family government, which seems harsh today, was considered by many even in 1700 as too severe. It was a rule in which affection held no place against decrees of stern justice. There was something, however, to be said for this code, since children trained under it were taught to fear God, to reverence authority, to respect old age, and to honor virtue.

The starched models of Colonial childhood drilled in the school of good manners were often not only formal and precise in their relations at home and abroad, but unnatural even in the company of those of their own age. Frequently, too, they were pinched and narrow in their ideas of what constituted a good life. Most children, nevertheless, imbibed certain sterling qualities from this rigorous home training; for boys and girls accustomed to its instant obedience usually became law-abiding and self-respecting citizens.[6]

This position of the child, which demanded him to pay respect and "civility" to his elders and betters, was defined by Christopher Dock, the gentle master of the Skippack school in Pennsylvania, who wrote in his "One Hundred Rules of Conduct":

Thy love for thy parents cannot be better expressed than by a willing obedience, doing their bidding, accepting their punishments, bearing their weaknesses with patience, and never intentionally offending them. . . . All this thou owest to thy grand-parents, step-parents, guardians, and other superiors.[7]

Even with child life dominated by adult authority and moral precept, the lot of Colonial youth was ameliorated in some degree by the innate tenderness of most grown-ups. This fact is sometimes disregarded in our reconstruction of an era which was generally bleak and cheerless for the young. Although the spontaneity of childhood must have been suppressed to some degree, as the very names "Submit," "Content," and "Patience" carefully stitched into early samplers might suggest, actual brutality was uncommon in Colonial homes.[8]

Cotton Mather warned parents on this score: "Our authority should be tempered with kindness and meekness and loving tenderness, that our children may fear us with delight, and feel that we love them with as much delight."[9] Parents were given a precise method of correction to be employed as the first resort when children "do amiss." He counseled: "Call them aside; set before them the precepts of God which they have broken, and the threatenings of God which they provoked. Demand of them to profess their sorrow for their fault, and resolve that they will be no more so faulty."[10]

When this procedure actually failed, another more drastic was conveniently at hand. Then it was that the "plentiful supply of warm birches" was to be used in accordance with the biblical injunction: "Withhold not correction from the child; for if thou beateth him with the rod, he shall not dy; thou shall beat him with the rod and shalt deliver his soul from hell."[11] This action was to be the last resource of the father, who was cautioned: "Never to give a blow in a passion. Stay till your passion is over and let the offenders plainly see that you deal with them out of pure obedience."[12]

William Penn, in the matter of family discipline, likewise admonished his married sons and daughters against a coarse and clamorous method of enforcing obedience, which he denounced as a vulgarity that should never disgrace the behavior of parents. Although those responsible for good order were told to make their children feel the power they had over them, he earnestly advised parents to try all the milder methods first:

If God give you children, love them with wisdom, correct them with affection; never strike in passion and suit the correction to their age as well as fault. . . . I know the methods of some are severe corrections for faults, and artificial praises when they do well, and sometimes rewards; but this course awakens passions worse than their faults; for one begets base fear if not hatred; the other pride and vain glory, both which should be avoided.[13]

Curiously enough, even under the rigid disciplinary code of the day, children contrived to be "spoiled"; and the variety of "humours" recorded for the Colonial "infant" has an amazingly familiar ring to the modern reader. One author asked, for example: "How comes it that the most sprightly talkative child cannot be prevailed upon to shew its tongue to the doctor; yet the moment his back is turned he will loll it out twenty times?"[14] The writer's litany of despair included a child who would not sleep but on a lap; another who gave no peace to the household unless rocked in a cradle; a third cried when the cradle was taken away, and to show why it cried was quiet the minute it was brought back; a fourth "swilled tea or some other improper liquid out of all measure and time"; and the last unhappy culprit "ate trash until he could eat nothing else, nor that itself." To the recorder, the reason for this infantile criminality was plainly evident—"Parents do not teach their children to obey. Instead of compulsion or reason they use flattery, bribes, and deceit."[15]

It is in the light of the foregoing discussions that the rules for good manners must be read. Beneath the formality and stilted language was the earnest desire on the part of parents to follow literally the biblical injunction so frequently seen in books of the period—"Train up a child in the way he should go, and when he is old he will not depart from it." The preface of the widely circulated *School of Good Manners,* compiled by Eleazer Moodey, a Boston schoolmaster, opened with the sentence: "It is acknowledged by (almost) every One, That a good Carriage in Children is an Ornament, not only to themselves, But to those Whom they descend from."[16] On the other hand, the editor remarked: "Children of but mean, careless or ill Breeding, brings Disgrace on their Parents, as well as Contempt on Themselves." Colonial social standards scathingly denounced a "clownish and unmannerly" child as the saddest sight of the times. The following exhortations explain the ideal sought in juvenile conduct:

1. Let thy Thoughts be Divine, Awful, and Godly.
2. Let thy Talk be Little, Honest, and True.
3. Let thy Works be Profitable, Holy, and Charitable.
4. Let thy Manners be Grave, Courteous, and Chearful.
5. Let thy Diet be Temperate, Convenient, and Frugal.
6. Let thy Apparel be Sober, Neat, and Comely.
7. Let thy Will be Compliant, Obedient, and Ready.
8. Let thy Sleep be Moderate, Quiet, and Seasonable.
9. Let thy Prayers be Devout, Often and Fervent.

THE
SCHOOL
OF
Good Manners.

Compofed for the Help of Parents
in Teaching their Children how
to carry it in their Places during their Minority.

BOSTON:
Re-Printed and Sold by T. & J. FLEET,
at the *Heart* & *Crown* in Cornhill, 1772.

Title page of the guide to "decent behaviour"
first edited by Eleazer Moodey in 1754

Who coaxed me, physic for to take,
Giving me sugar plums and cake,
If I would drink it for his sake?
                    My Father

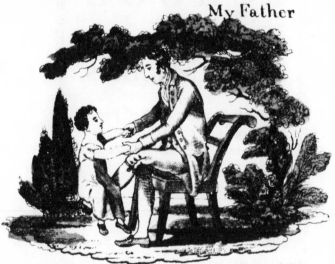

Who placed me on his foot to ride
While anxiosly my Mother cried,
To hold her Boy lest he should slide
                    My Father.

From MY FATHER

10. Let thy Recreations be Lawful, Brief, and Seldom.
11. Let thy Meditations be of Death, Judgment, and Eternity.[17]

The solemnity with which adults had surrounded childhood was mainly responsible for much conduct that was unchildlike or precocious. The gloomy pall of severity that hung over many Colonial homes was unfortunately sanctioned by such writings as those which Lord Chesterfield, in 1738, addressed to his little son: "I do not recommend upon all occasions a solemn countenance. A man may smile, but if he would be thought a man of sense, he would by no means laugh."[18] Not only was laughter thus summarily banished from the life of the well-bred boy, but he was also reminded that "romping, punning, joking, mimicry and waggery" would render any one contemptible in spite of his knowledge or merit.[19]

For generations the shocking example of a little girl who smiled in Midway Church was presented to children by grown-ups as the antics of one possessed of "hoofs and horns."[20] To acquire the gravity desired by genteel Christians, children were occasionally advised to strike a happy medium: "Let thy Countenance be moderately chearful, neither Laughing nor Frowning. Laugh not aloud, but silently smile upon occasion."[21] Keen-witted children doubtless felt the effects of such ill-advised efforts to suppress unseemly mirth. Boys and girls must have wearied also under the attempts adults made to develop in them the "certain dignity of manner" which was supposed to mark the refined "little men and women whose one solid pleasure in life was duty."[22]

Boys and girls were inevitably prepared for their social responsibilities by a variety of "Don'ts" and "Musts" found in little manuals of conduct so popular in the eighteenth century. The task of fitting children for their places in society rested primarily with the parents whose example and precept taught their little ones to accept these principles of right and wrong, and to appreciate the fact that ill-breeding, as well as bad conduct, brought unpleasant consequences. The method used in drilling children in their lessons frequently stifled not only bad habits—rudeness, untidiness, or lack of courtesy to strangers—but often warped the personality of the young. Despite the fact that the code of manners was depressingly negative and all-embracing in its treatment of child life, it illuminates for us today many interesting crannies of the Colonial child's apparently tedious existence.

Books on children's behavior invariably gave first place to proper religious decorum at the "Meeting House." One of the most widely studied manuals admonished the little Christian "to sit where thou art ordered by thy Superiors," and to "lend thy place for the easing of anyone that stands near," and in the meantime to listen to the words of the minister "that thou mayest remember." The first and last rules of this section tell a tale of patient endurance, and obliquely reveal glimpses of a normal childish reaction to boredom:

1. Decently walk to thy Seat or Pew; run not nor go wantonly.
9. Be not hasty to run out of the Meeting-House when the Worship is ended, as if thou wer't weary of being there.[23]

Such formal rules of behavior presumed that the child should be solemn and sober in the presence of older persons; for even in domestic life, the laws of courtesy were intimately blended with religious obligations. The resulting attitudes and conventions were of great importance in shaping the social standards of the nation at a time when neighborhood life comprised for most people the whole of their outside world. Without these precise customs, life in the sparsely settled Colonies would undoubtedly have degenerated, as many feared, into a semi-barbarous state. The dignified religious tone and the prim polish of a Colonial boy's correspondence to his parents can be seen in this model letter of the time:

Honoured Father and Mother.
Your Kindness calls for my Dutiful Acknowledgement: I wish I could better answer your Love to me, and your Cost upon me: The increase of my Learning is by me endeavoured, and in some measure pressed after, I hope I shall have the constant assistance of your Prayers, for the Accomplishment thereof; in the confidence of which I humbly take my leave, and rest,
Your Dutiful Son,
T. R.
Cambridge, May 1
1708.[24]

Further illustrations of the "awful respect" for his elders and of the stiff, ceremonious relations between parents and children can be found in such advice as the following: "Never sit in the Presence of thy Parents without bidding, tho' no Stranger be present. Never speak to thy Parents without some Title of Respect, Sir, Madam, etc. according to their quality." The child was also told to bear without murmuring or sullenness his parent's reproofs, "even though they might be causeless and undeserved."[25]

Although rather primitive forms of serving and eating meals prevailed for the most part in the Colonies, considerable formality in this family ritual was required of children. Since some homes did not have a sufficient supply of wooden or pewter trenchers or of drinking cups, the joint use of these articles by the junior members of the family was common. In many homes all the children could not be conveniently seated on the ordinary narrow bench or form, but were compelled to stand at a side table during their entire meal, from which, with trenchers in hand, they returned to the great table for additional helpings. The custom that seems still worse and that prevailed among people of low social standards demanded that children stand behind their parents, and receive, like privileged paupers, the food handed back to them.[26]

The ideal in table manners for children was apparently to eat in silence at the greatest convenient speed and to depart from the table the minute the last mouthful had been swallowed. At these joyless repasts the little ones were never permitted to take their seats until a blessing had been invoked, and their parents had requested them to be seated. Even then they were not to ask for anything on the table, but were to "tarry" until it was offered to them.[27] Their youthful sense of justice must have been outraged too. They were told not "to murmur or frown" if their parents or strangers were served special dishes in which the children did not share.[28]

Some of the more detailed rules for table manners throw light on the lack of furnishings, as well as on some of the interesting customs which called forth such singular admonitions. One rule was as follows:

Bite not thy Bread but break it; but not with slovingly Fingers, nor with the same wherewith thou takest up thy Meat. Gnaw not Bones at the Table but Clean them with thy knife (unless they be very small ones) hold them not with a whole hand, but with two Fingers. Drink not nor speak with anything in thy mouth.[29]

The child was told to keep his food to his own side of the trencher, and not to take salt with a greasy knife, not to "rake" his mouth with his fingers, nor to throw bones or rinds under the table. The need for refrigeration was reflected in the admonition: "Smell not thy meat, nor put it to thy Nose: turn it not the other side upward to view it upon thy Plate or Trencher."[30] The status of the child in the home is clearly established by a final word of advice on table manners:

As soon as thou shalt be moderately satisfied; or whensover thy Parents think meet to bid thee, rise up from the table, tho' others thy Superiors sit still.

When thou risest from the Table, take away thy Plate; and having made a Bow at the side of the Table where thou sattest, withdraw, removing also thy seat (if removable).

When thanks are to be returned after eating, return to thy Place, and stand reverently till it be done; then with a Bow withdraw out of the Room, leaving thy Superiors to themselves (unless thou art bidden to stay.)[31]

In his relations abroad, respect for a superior was demanded with the greatest firmness, for courtesy required that the child walking in the garden or on the street with an older person must give him the right hand. The youth was also cautioned, "Walk not even with him, Cheek-by-jole; but a little behind him." Just how much was exacted in this matter of respect, or how far the child's patience was tried, is painfully indicated in the rules on discourse:

If thy Superior speak anything wherein thou knowest he is mistaken, correct not nor contradict him, or grin at the hearing of it. If thy Superior be relating a Story, say not I have heard it before, but attend to it as if it were to thee altogether new; Seem not to question the truth of it; If he tell it not right, snigger not, nor endeavour to help him or to add to his Relation.[32]

In all sections of the country, children were well grounded in personal consideration for the old and afflicted members of society. Hence to be courteous to the meanest and poorest was considered the true index of a great and generous mind—an attitude which functioned in the place of modern organized charity.[33]

Conduct at school and among other children was naturally given special attention in the training of the Colonial child, whose social contacts were so narrowly restricted. Among the more reasonable instructions for the amenities of school life were injunctions "not to run hastily in the street, or to go too slowly; wag not to and fro or use any antick or wanton posture either of thy Head, Hands, Feet or Body. Throw not anything in the Street as Dirt or Stones." To regulate his actions within the school, the boy was counseled "to bow at coming in pulling off thy Hat, at no time to quarrel or talk in school, or to bawl aloud in making complaints." Provisions were also made for receiving the inevitable school visitor: "If a stranger speak to thee in school, stand up and answer with respect and ceremony, both of word and gesture, as if thou spakest to thy Master."[34] While due allowance was granted for human frailties, they were limited to certain bounds as indicated by the warnings: "Spit not in the Room but in the Corner or rather go out and do it abroad. If thou canst not avoid yawning, shut thy Mouth with thine Hand or Handkerchief before it, turning thy face aside."[35]

As undue levity was always frowned upon, it is not surprising to find boys enjoined not to go "Singing, Whistling, nor Hollowing along the Street." The existence of a spirit of school rivalry is implied in the warning not "to jeer nor affront the scholars of another school, but to show them love and respect, and to let them pass quietly along." In speaking of the deadly feuds of schoolboys in 1771, for instance, Samuel Breck recounts the many bloody battles fought on Beacon Hill between the boys of the north and south ends of the town of Boston during which "slings and stones were very skillfully used."[36] Protected by the sanctity of his office, the teacher was not involved in this warfare. Among the ironclad rules for juvenile deportment, the diplomatic treatment advocated for the master of a rival school was classic: "Especially not affront the Master of another School, but rather, if thou knowest him, or if he live either near thine House or School, uncover thy Head to Him, & bowing pass by him."[37]

Having discharged this salvo of admonitions at defenseless youth, the author assured them that the observance of these rules would deliver them from the disgraceful titles of "sordid and clownish," and would moreover "intail upon the mention of their names, the honour of Genteel and Well-bred Children." In parting he warned them: "Be always obsequious and respectful, never bold, insolent or sawcy either in Words or Gestures."[38]

Colonial children were consistently denied the right of self-expression, but no amount of repression ever succeeded in stiflling completely their spirit. If, in defiance of public opinion and propriety, he could not give vocal expression to his emotions and sentiments, his smoldering passions often found escape in the leaves of his diary. The personal record of little Sally Fairfax of Virginia vehemently testifies to this fact:

On Friday the 3d of Jan. that vile man Adam at night killed a poor cat of rage, because she eat a bit of meat out of his hand & scratched it. A vile wretch of New Negrows, if he was mine I would cut him in pieces, a son of a gun, a nice negrow, he should be killed himself by rites.[39]

Another diary, that of Nathaniel Ames, a student at Harvard in 1761, gives an account of the temporary suspension of one Joseph Cabot and shows the heights to which youthful fury could rise when sufficiently provoked. Nathaniel wrote of his friend: "As soon as the President said he was rusticated, he took his hat and went out of the Chapel without staying to hear the President's speech out. After Prayers he bulrags the Tutors at high Rate & leaves College his Mother faints at the news."[40]

The opposite pages in the diary or "Monitor" of Mary Osgood Sumner were headed, "White Leaf" for her good deeds, and "Black Leaf" for her faults. On a "Black Leaf," she recorded this confession of childish wrongdoings: "I left my staise on the bed. Spoke in haste to my little Sister. Spilt cream on the floor in the closet. I got vexed because Sister was a-going to cut my frock. Was not diligent at learning at school. Part of this day I did not improve my time well."[41] Fortunately the good deeds listed in this "Monitor" far outnumbered the bad; and the

"White Leaf" began with a typical entry: "I went and said my Catechism to-day. Came home and wrote down the questions and answers, then dressed and went to the dance, endeavored to behave myself decent."[42]

When youthful piety and vanity made their respective impacts on the heart of Anna Green Winslow of Boston, she faithfully kept the record of her conflict in a diary which she sent by installments to her parents in Nova Scotia. While she admitted that a "Miss of 12 could not possible do justice to nice Subjects in Divinity," she proceeded to sermonize her parents at long range in the following manner:

I must tell you, how cource soever it may sound to your delicacy, that while you are without holiness, your beauty is deformity—you are all over black, & defiled, ugly and loathsome to all holy beigns, the wrath of the great God lie's upon you, & if you die in this condition, you will be turn'd into hell, with ugly devils, to eternity.[43]

Ten days later Anna had fully recovered from her preoccupation with "ugly devils" and was afraid she might be mistaken for a peddler. With all the vanity natural to a girlish heart, the child wrote in nervous anxiety to her mother:

I hope aunt wont let me wear the black hatt with the red Dominie—for the People will ask me what I have got to sell if I do, or, how the folk at New guinie do? Dear Mamma, you dont know the fation here—I beg to look like other folk.[44]

With the limited means of communication and travel the average child had but little knowledge or contact with the world beyond his family circle or the village boundary. Foreign news in the scantiest measure, and usually about some European catastrophe, filtered into the Colonies months after the events had happened. Hence no effort was made in the children's books to include world maps or descriptions of foreign peoples. The best informed were those youth who lived in the seaport towns, where they were regaled by the sailors at the wharves with colorful tales of adventure among strange peoples. Ordinarily the home, the church, the school, and the residences of close relatives and friends comprised the narrow orbit in which Colonial child life revolved.[45]

Masculine rights and interests predominated the circumscribed life in which children moved. The lot of the girl was usually confined to commonplace domestic duties as a preparation for the fulfillment of her future obligations as wife and mother. A comparison of the sexes in 1755 may be found in an earnest injunction addressed to a small boy: "Wrangling and quarrelling are the characteristics of a weak mind, leave that to the women, be you always above it."[46]

Girls repeatedly heard the lesson that the "virtues which make a figure in the world" do not fall to the lot of women. It was pointed out that "feminine virtues are of a simple and peaceable nature; but the great virtues are for men."[47] Since women were allowed nothing but the single merit of being obscure, they were thought to have a particular need for the support and consolations of religion. To underscore this point, a father wrote to his daughters: "Your whole life is often a life of suffering. You must bear your sorrows in silence. You must often put a face of serenity and cheerfulness when your hearts are torn with anguish."[48] It was deemed especially desirable for the young girl to be pious; for she was told that "men considered her religion as one of the principal securities for that female virtue in which they were most interested."[49] It was in reaction to this one-sided moral theory that a mother wrote plaintively to her young daughter:

The virtues of women are difficult, because they have no help from glory to practice them. To live at home; to meddle with nothing but one's own self and the family, to be simple, just, and modest are painful virtues because they are obscure. One must have a great deal of merit to shun making a figure, and a great deal of courage to bring one's self to be virtuous only to one's own eyes.[50]

The girl, in the process of acquiring womanly accomplishments, was expected to maintain a certain dignified restraint which has been defined in a child's book as "one of the chief beauties in a female character, that modest reserve, that retiring delicacy, which avoids the public eye, and is disconcerted even at the gaze of admiration."[51] Since the existence of "reasoning and good sense" in feminine mental equipment was a moot question with male authors, girls were duly warned: "Be cautious in displaying your good sense. . . . But if you happen to have any learning keep it a profound secret from the men who generally look with jealous and malignant eye on a woman of cultivated understanding." Wit was thought to be the most dangerous talent a girl could possess, since it was considered so flattering to vanity that those who possessed it usually became "intoxicated and lost all self-command." Although it was conceded that "humor" in a girl would make her company much solicited, the young maiden was primly warned that since this gift was a great enemy to "delicacy," and a still greater one to dignity of character, it might sometimes gain its possessor applause but never respect.[52]

Good health was counted among the greatest blessings of life, but the absurd delicacy imposed on the female world directed the girl never "to boast of it, but to enjoy it in grateful silence." The idea of female "softness and delicacy" was so naturally associated with a corresponding delicacy of constitution, that when "a girl spoke of her great strength, her good appetite, or her ability to bear excessive fatigue, the male world recoiled in disgust."[53]

The desire for attention and the love of power at times caused Colonial children to vex one another and to tease even those they loved, in spite of the fact that such tendencies were summarily checked. The list of social evils usually included the childish yearning for notice and his indulgence of bad temper, both branded as deeds of darkest dye. One such display of temper on the part of his young son was recorded by Judge Sewall in his diary: "Joseph threw a knop of Brass and hit his Sister Betty on the forehead so as to make it bleed and swell; upon which, and for playing at Prayertime, and eating when Return Thanks, I whip'd him pretty smartly."[54] Although a generous amount of civility to the "feminine sex" had from the earliest days characterized American manhood, evidence shows that good breeding and the cultivation of polite manners in this respect was frequently a painful process for the normal boy. In an account of the activities of a village school, it was recorded that high-spirited boys not only beat and kicked one another, or administered an occasional bloody nose, but so far forgot the traditions of their fathers as to kick some little girls who were picking "daisies and butter-flowers in the meadow, in order to make them pipe."[55]

While the ideals of "decent behaviour" were high during this period, the average child was not, in spite of some evidence to the contrary, inordinately hampered in his joy of living or in the normal pursuit of happiness. In a society as deeply imbued with a love of freedom as this, junior members were as clever as their elders in devising techniques for escaping insupportable restrictions in their daily routine. Pithy notations from the diary of Nathaniel Ames, a Harvard boy, verify this statement: "Fit with the Sophomores about Customs. Did not go to Prayers. President sick, wherefore much Deviltry carried on in College."[56] Richard Hall, who was attending a school in Boston, left a record testifying to his boundless energy and ill-tempered behavior. Not only was he perpetually at play in the streets; but he grieved his thrifty aunt most by knotting up his good linen handkerchiefs into cudgels to beat his companions. After they had served that purpose he had heedlessly discarded them. Finally, in desperation, the long-suffering lady wrote to his father:

Richard wears out nigh 12 pairs of shoes a year. He brought 12 hankers with him and they have all been lost long ago; and I have bought him 3 or 4 more at a time. His way is to tie knottys at one end & beat ye Boys with them and then to lose them & he cares not a bit what I shall say to him.[57]

Notwithstanding the fact that youth of Colonial days generally fulfilled to the letter such restraining injunctions as: "Among Superiors speak not till thou art spoken to, and bid to speak,"[58] nevertheless these children, in spite of their dull, drab "company manners," were not always models of propriety. Records tell of the noisy disorder of the boys' gallery or the boys' pew in the meeting-house, of young culprits playing ball or flying kites in the streets and thereby frightening horses, of "wicked boys" robbing bird nests and orchards, or throwing stones and snowballs at people in the streets. It follows that rules really did not bear too heavily on youthful consciences, for boys could readily rationalize such as the following:

Quarrel not with any Body thou meetest or overtake; abuse not thy Companions by word or deed, if thy Companion be a little too gross or sarcastical in speaking, yet strive not to take notice of it; deal justly among Boys thy equals, as solicitously as if thou wert a Man and about Business of higher importance.[59]

Like modern maidens, little girls of that gloomy era were often overcome by attacks of giggling. This weakness is evident in the diary of Anna Winslow, who was "suddenly shaken by a fit of unruly mirth during a futile attempt to spell wednessday." Of this she wrote: "My aunt says, that till I come out of an egregious fit of laughterre that is apt to sieze me & the violence of which I am at this present under, neither English sence, nor any thing rational may be expected of me."[60]

Regardless of his motives, Cotton Mather excused some mischievous lads who had broken windows of King's Chapel during their play:

All the mischief done is the breaking of a few Quarrels of Glass by Idle Boys, who if discove'd had been chastis'd by their own Parents. They have built their Chapel in a Publick burying place, next adjoining a great Free School, where the Boyes (having gotten to play) may, some by Accident, some in Frolick, and some perhaps in revenge for disturbing their Relatives' Graves by the Foundation of that Building, have broken a few Quarrels of the Windows.[61]

The Colonial interpretation of "decent behaviour" presupposed on the part of the child the recognition of just authority by a meek submission to "superiors," and a thorough training in all the rules that it behooved him to know. In addition, habits of self-control and the practice of self-renunciation in the fulfillment of a duty were considered everywhere as the earmarks of good breeding for boys and girls. This moral discipline was not easily acquired by children, for it was the outgrowth of a habit—the result of repeated acts of virtue. Parents therefore used their acknowledged authority as the most effective means of securing good order and the observance of duty.

Many who were responsible for shaping the customs and characters of American children recognized by 1776 the predominant weakness of the traditional training in the "art of decent behaviour." These believed that the old method of rearing and ruling the child by the rod was an act of great injustice, because the element of fear in this procedure engendered cunning and deceit, and accustomed the child to control his senses rather than to use his reason. The new dispensation of the *School of Good Manners* made nice distinctions in courteous conduct by telling the young that politeness was the expression of natural refinement, and good breeding the form of artificial civility. Good breeding restrained the child from giving offense; politeness empowered him to receive and give pleasure.[62]

*   *   *   *   *   *

A study of the manners and customs of American youth during the transition period from 1776 to 1835 embraces the ideas of two opposing schools of thought. As there was a divergence of opinion on the status of the child, the author of juvenile books were divided between those conservatives who would literally have the child "seen but not heard," and their opponents, the humanitarians, who sought to give youth opportunities for self-expression. Although the stern standards of Colonial child-training still had many supporters in the early nineteenth century, this era also marked the growth of a special interest in the peculiar rights of childhood. There was an increasing tendency on the part of many progressive adults to regard the child not as an inferior but as an equal. As a distinct personality in the family or community he was to be accorded certain rights and privileges demanded by his immaturity and lack of worldly wisdom.

In the turmoil of conflicting theories on child-training that stirred social thought in the early days of the Republic, the ideas of such reform writers as James Burgh steadily rose to dominance in our behavior patterns. Boldly and frankly, this group, who borrowed many of their ideas from Rousseau, deplored the "unhappy restraint" imposed by adults on the Colonial child. Even such details as the chiding lectures read to little boys and girls about holding up their heads, putting back their shoulders, turning out their toes, and making bows and curtsies were roundly condemned as factors in "disgusting the poor children against what is called behaviour."[63] It was pointed out to parents that even in grown people gracefulness consisted in "an easy and natural motion and gesture, and in an expression denoting kindness and good-will to those with whom they conversed." It was also claimed that if a child's heart and temper were formed to civility, the outward expression of it would appear in due time.[64]

As a result of this philosophy, much of the form found in the old "art of decent behaviour" gave way to moral suasion and to the practice of concealing the child's rules of conduct in didactic tales. Instead of the formal precepts that called for "courtesies and leg twenty times in a quarter of an hour,"[65] the child of the nineteenth century found his guide for social amenities in the *Juvenile Biographies* and in ubiquitous tales of "good children" which gave closer attention to shaping the mind and heart of the young.

Discipline and rules of conduct were less frequently enforced by the rod. It was demonstrated that the spirit of contradiction so strong in those children who had been irritated by harsh control led them to seize the first opportunity to oppose their elders regardless of the consequences. Some parents still persisted in the rigorous management of their offspring on the grounds that such discipline fortified the spirit against the unavoidable trials of life; others held that wisdom, common sense, and honesty forbade those in authority to do evil that good might result. The reformers of child-training urged that adults make allowances for "puerile incapacities," and on this point wrote: "We have never been able to make ourselves just such as we wish to be, and shall we require an infant to surpass us in exertion and self-command? By demanding too much we shall disgust or discourage him from performing what he might find practicable under more cheering influence."[66] It was suggested that the denial of pleasure might have a more permanent effect than the use of the rod.

A more independent development of American behavior patterns kept pace with the growth of the new republic, and gradually there came to be less slavish imitation of European manners and morals. It was commonly believed that juvenile politeness, either of feeling or of manner, could never be taught by set maxims; but that everyday influence, unconsciously exerted, was the all-important factor in forming the character and manners of children. Little ones were no longer required to memorize the exacting rules in the *School of Good Manners*, for the onus of responsibility was shifted to grown-ups. Parents were now told that if they were habitually polite, their children would become so by mere force of imitation without any specific directions on the subject.[67]

Naturalness of manner was now desired in preference to the pompous formalities of the early days, and parents were urged to practise in the home such manners as they wished their children to have in company, in order that the young could apply their training with ease and grace.[68] As a result of this early training in resourcefulness and independence, American children were often misjudged by Europeans who, mistaking their disarming fearlessness for impudence, charged our youth with a want of courtesy and fine feelings.[69]

Native prophets of woe also chanted their jeremiads for the spoiled children of the early nineteenth century, and vehemently blamed the new standards of family government for the "depravity, luxury, and corruption" of the age. Parents were often charged with starting too late with the course of instruction and discipline that would insure a willing obedience to their authority. Among the opponents of the new order was John Hersey, a disciple of John Wesley, who exhorted parents to return to the old methods of child training:

Break their wills betimes. Begin this work before they can run alone, before they can speak plainly, or speak at all. Whatever pain it cost, conquer their stubbornness; break their wills if you would not damn the child. . . . Therefore let a child from a year old be taught to fear the rod, and cry softly. At all events at that age make him do as he is bid, if you whip him ten times running to do it; let none persuade you it is cruel to do this. . . .[70]

This same author lamented the great amount of vice found in the streets of towns and cities, which necessarily tainted and corrupted young minds that came within its influence. Listed in the variety of snares laid for youthful morals, we find included not only the influence of dissolute, lazy children, but such "sinks of iniquity" as "tippling shops," oyster houses, billiard and gambling rooms, and the most alluring of all—confectionery shops! Bitterly he complained that by some strange but culpable derangement of municipal law, the confectioner could with impunity keep his door half or entirely open on the Sabbath. Since his "plums, sweetmeats," and various other delicacies were eagerly sought by youth, the temptation to steal their parents' or employers' money to satisfy that taste was thought to be an ever-present evil. Without reservations, Hersey sweepingly condemned all such "houses of traffic" as the source of that stream of vice that overflowed the country, and left its sediment in the jails and almshouses. Parents were accordingly warned that if they did not wish to murder their children morally, they must keep them out of the streets except when they were "on their way to or from business."[71]

At the opposite pole of thought on disciplinary measures were those romanticists who believed that a child's feelings were as sensitive as a man's, but that the little one's powers of discretion and self-defense were much weaker. Hence this school upheld the theory that a child would gradually learn to correct his own impoliteness, whereas the interference of an adult might permanently injure his character. As it was believed that if a child were let alone he would correct many faults out of self-respect, adults were to help the young acquire this quality by being respectful to them. That there was no better way to teach a child good manners than to practise politeness towards him became a new social axiom in the United States. A Moravian work stressing this idea gave the following analysis of the new status of the child:

A great deal is said of the necessity of breaking a child's will. Why need a child's will be broken? He will have use for it all. The difference between strength of will and weakness of will is often the difference between efficiency and in-efficiency. Train a child to self-control, so that his will may be his strong point, but do not break his will. . . . While essential obedience should be secured, wide margin should be granted for the expansion of a child's own individuality, for his peculiar mental action and for the cultivation and the gratification of his tastes.[72]

While the advocates of this system realized that such approach to child-training might easily lapse into a weak and vicious indulgence, even that state was considered no worse than the arrogant and tyrannical exercise of power characteristic of the previous century. No cognizance of the child's individuality had been taken by adult authority which, by making itself felt alike in great and small matters, had exacted from the young perhaps at best only a grudging service. The more enlightened parents of the new era avoided both extremes, and recognized that neither license nor slavery, but liberty, was a good thing for children as well as for adults.[73]

In reply to complaints about juvenile delinquency, the humanitarians asserted that many of the young went astray, not because there was a want of prayer or virtue at home, but because the home lacked sufficient gayety and affection. On the grounds that children required smiles as much as flowers needed sunshine, the reformers accounted for the "crime in the city streets" by explaining that since the young were little given to analyzing a situation, they simply avoided what displeased them if they did not find home congenial. According to the new code, then, it was the sour faces, harsh words, and continual fault-finding in the home that drove youth into the city streets. Not the wiles of the infamous confectioner, but the lingering shadows of Colonial gloom and the old ideas of childish depravity were perverting the young people of our growing republic.[74]

The most important publisher of moral tales for molding youthful manners was Isaiah Thomas of Worcester, whose "books to amuse" were printed late in the eighteenth century. These little gilt volumes were mainly responsible for changing the tone of children's reading from the religious to the didactic. In one of his first works, *Be Merry and Wise; or the Cream of Jests, and the Marrow of Maxims for the Conduct of Life,* he endorsed the new techniques to be applied in the moral training of youth: "Mould your arguments into questions rather than dogmatical assertions: seem as if you were putting people in mind of what they had forgot, not as teaching them what they knew not. Many are willing to be informed that hate to be excelled."[75]

In the preface to the *Little Pretty Pocket-Book,* the author called upon indulgent parents to "subdue their children's passions" by curbing their tempers. This was not to be done by chiding, by whipping, or by severe treatment, but by reasoning and mild discipline. When parents saw a child's temper aroused, they were advised to take him aside, to point out to him the evils that befell passionate people, and to show him that although their love as parents might make them overlook his faults, nevertheless giving way to an unruly temper "was so heinous a sin that they could no longer bear the sight of him." The little culprit was then to be shut off from all company for five or six hours; and after he had asked pardon for his offense and had promised amendment they were to forgive him. This method, regularly pursued, was believed to conquer the child's temper and to subdue it to reason.[76]

Enticing children to perform their little duties by bribes—a habit roundly condemned in previous decades—was approved by some of the new juvenile books. The theory was advanced that whatever stimulated children to a love of virtue or to learning ought always to be applied. An analogy was drawn, that the experienced physician "gilded the pill not only to attract the eye, but to take the nauseous taste away." Since "coaches and horses, sugarplums and baubles" were the things that attracted the attention of children, and were the only "blessings the infant understanding was capable of comprehending," if it were an evil to promise these things, it could be only a partial evil, which would wear away as the judgment of the child became better informed.[77]

As certain little individuals were not to be won by promises, their parents were advised to make use of threats suited to the childish understanding—only those, however, that would excite "tremendous ideas, and would make an impression on the mind." It was evident to the new moralists that the period for giving children serious threats was brief; for no matter how solemn the adult might be, little ones in a short time would scornfully regard all that might be held over them as "bugbears to frighten babies." Unusual punishments were advocated for children to produce a lasting impression and to stimulate an appreciation of sublime truths and good conduct in later life.[78]

Some of "Mr. Crop's" stories of bad boys reveal the subtleties of the new trend toward moral suasion in the training of children. He told his young readers that after the holidays certain boys had been "very unwilling" to return to school, and that someone had to excuse them to the master for not doing their home assignments during the vacation. This procedure taught the boys bad habits.[79] By such practices, these boys would eventually lose not only three months out of twelve, and thus be "looked upon as great dunces," but they would also let younger boys get ahead of them. What was worst of all, they would be obliged to go to school until they were fifteen or sixteen years old, and this was regarded in 1786 as a "very sad thought indeed!"[80] Since the purely theological aspects of such sins as sloth were almost lost sight of in this era, the punishment for idlers was just as materialistic as was the rationalization of their offense:

> Those who love to loiter and play,
> And good advice will throw away;
> They must without a supper go,
> And lose their share of plum-cakes too.[81]

The famous juvenile Goody Twoshoes denounced tales of ghosts, witches, and fairies as the "frolicks of a distempered brain," and assured children that good sense and a good conscience were the inevitable cures of these imaginary evils. Little boys or girls who were "good and loved Almighty God" and kept his commandments could sleep as safely in a churchyard as anywhere else (if they took care not to get cold); for Goody was sure there were no ghosts to frighten such children.[82] On the irresistible subject of death, Goody gave sage advice: "Therefore, play, my dear children, and be merry; but be innocent and good. The good man sets death at defiance, for its darts are only dreadful to the wicked."[83] Having delivered this brief homily, the author permitted the children to bury a little dormouse. When Goody asked them to write his epitaph, she received the following pious result:

> Ye sons of verse,
> While I rehearse,
> Attend instructive rhyme:
> No sins had Dor
> To answer for;
> Repent of yours in time.[84]

The *Juvenile Biographer* of this later period, in contrast to the *New England Token* of the early part of the century, further reflected the changing status of the child. By 1787, the awesome pious "histories" of the "godly youths" had vanished; but so too had much of the vitality and conviction of the older volumes.[85] Among the new models offered for childish imitation or for a horrible example were such obvious characters as Miss Betsey Allgood, a pretty little miss of seven, "who worked at her needle to admiration"; Master Billy Bad-enough, who robbed orchards and went birdnesting; and Master Dickie Sprightly, noted for his politeness, learning, and affability. The story of Miss Betsey Pert rather thinly veiled the current disrepute of boarding schools by dire warnings to the proud young females who came forth from those institutions. Betsey's case revealed that she had received a boarding-school education, in the course of which she had become so "puffed up" that she had no idea of any kind of industry because she had left that to those whom she considered poor and ignorant.[86]

Wisdom in Miniature, one of the most serious juvenile books published by Isaiah Thomas, contained selections from the writings of "many ingenious and learned authors both ancient and modern," and was consequently intended not only for the use of schools but also as a "pocket companion for the youth of both sexes."[87] In a section of "Time, Business, and Recreation," the child found sage advice on subjects dear to the American heart:

Time is the most precious, and yet the most brittle jewel we have; It is what everyone bids largely for, when he wants it, but squanders it away most lavishly when he has it.

Rise early to your business, learn good things, and oblige good men; these are three things you shall never repent of.

It is the great art and philosophy of life to make the best of the present, whether it be good or bad; and to bear the one with resignation and patience, and enjoy the other with thankfulness and moderation.

Let your recreation be manly, moderate, seasonable, and lawful: the use of recreation is to strengthen your labour and to sweeten your rest.[88]

Isaiah Thomas also printed for American children one of their first books of nonsense verses—*Mother Goose's Melody*—those songs that belong to the realm of folklore. Although the rhymes were nonsense, the satirical maxims and notes appended to them were perhaps the extenuating features of the book in the judgment of most American parents; thus the work was admitted to a permanent place in the juvenile library.[89] The following verse and moral, for example, contained the lesson of silence which the adult world had long required of the child:

> Ride a Cock Horse
> To Banbury Cross,
> To see what Tommy can buy;
> A Penny white Loaf
> A Penny white Cake,
> And a Two penny Apple Pye.

There's a good Boy, eat up your Pye and hold your Tongue; for Silence is the first sign of Wisdom.[90]

Among the other lessons in nonsense form, the song "Hush-a-bye-Baby" served as a "warning to the proud and ambitious, who climb so high that they generally fall at last." The story of the "little pig who went to market," proved to the child by some vague reasoning that if he did not "govern his passions, his passions would govern him."[91] The verse, "Dickery, Dickery, Dock, The Mouse Ran up the Clock," plainly pointed to the old maxim that "Time and Tide stay for no Man."[92] To the children of the towns, such as New York and Philadelphia, who frequently heard such cries in their own streets, the "Seasonable Song" must have had a peculiar appeal:

> Piping hot, smoking hot,
> What I've got,
> You know not,
> Hot, hot Pease, hot, hot
> Hot are my Pease, hot.

There is more Musick in this Song on a cold frosty Night, than ever the Syrens were possessed of, who captivated Ulysses; And the Effects stick closer to the ribs.

Huggleford on Hunger.[93]

Jacky Dandy's Delight: or the History of Birds and Beasts promised truthful little boys and girls "plumbpudding or hot apple pye," while it reserved a whip for naughty children who told false tales. The birds and beasts in this tiny volume had much to say about the manners and morals of youth.[94] Since the dog was undoubtedly the favorite pet of most little ones, it was readily accepted by them as a pattern for the faithful performance of their duties, as these lines might indicate:

> The Dog that's trusty in his kind,
> With gratitude should fire your mind;
> Mark well his service, his faithful way,
> And in your service copy Tray.[95]

On the other hand, the parrot was held up to ridicule along with many silly boys and girls, because he talked without thinking; and thus he "knew not why or wherefore he prattled":

> The chattering Parrot prates away,
> Or cries, "Poll's sick, alack aday!"
> Resembling those who when at school,
> Delight like him to play the fool.[96]

Respect for the advice of experienced older persons was still the theme of many stories; hence the *Sugar Plumb,* published by Thomas in 1787, included a delightful tale to underscore the child's lesson of reverence for the aged. An old mouse, at the point of death, assembled her "numerous family" and told them how to escape the dangers of the big house in which they all lived. Scarcely had this wise old mouse breathed her last, when her young family congratulated one another on being rid of the "Old Dotard," as they disrespectfully called her. Despising the good advice she had given them, they made their way to the pantry where they soon devoured a "pot of sweetmeats," and then began to celebrate their escape from the dangers of which they had been warned. But their mirth was short-lived, because a cat and two traps were posted in the pantry, and in less than a week not a mouse was left of those who has despised the experience and wise instruction of their grandmother.[97]

One of the best instances of the new "horrible example" technique used to impress certain precepts of manners on the youthful mind was found in a Worcester publication, *Vice in Its Proper Shape.* This work was based on the ancient Brahmin proverb, "Example is more powerful than precept." It invited young ladies and gentlemen into the author's little apartment to be "eye witnesses to the mortifying consequences of an ill-spent and vicious life, even to those who had not yet arrived at the age of manhood."[98] Among the wonders of this tiny volume were the surprising tales of the transmigration of "Jacky Idle into the body of an Ass," and of "Master Greedyguts into a pig"; while among the minor allusions were accounts of Jacky Fidget and of Polly Giddybrains.[99]

Little girls must have found in the fate of Miss Dorothy Chatterfast a powerful antidote for tale-bearing and common sins of the tongue. The body of a multi-colored, loquacious magpie was shown to them as the involuntary residence of the "late" Dorothy, who had been a notorious little gossip. Indeed, it was said that before she was three years old she could lisp out a tale in very intelligible language. Later she was equally attentive to every trifle at the school where she was sent "to learn the art of reading and the use of her needle." The moment she came home and before she had entered the parlor to make her curtsy, her little tongue began to "rattle like a mill clack." The author predicted that his little readers would turn away in disgust from this small bird who wagged her tail with surprising agility and clattered so rapidly as to frighten them.[100]

In contrast to the early rules for good conduct, with their forthright appeal to authority, one finds in the new order obscure gems of politeness hidden in dull verses of the following type:

> Good little boys should never say,
> "I will," and "Give me these;"
> O, no! that never is the way,
> But, "Mother, if you please."
>
> And "If you please," to sister Ann
> Good boys to say are ready;
> And "Yes, Sir," to a gentleman,
> And "Yes, Ma'am," to a lady.[101]

In the first decade of the nineteenth century, books of model letters were published which served to "encourage children at their first attempts in this pleasing and important art," and to give the modern reader intimate pictures of the era. Since the letters were supposed to have been written by the members of the families who were traveling or away at school, they contain interesting commentaries on the life and customs of the times. One of the most informative of these books was that compiled by Caleb Bingham, entitled *Juvenile Letters, being a correspondence between children from eight to fifteen years of age.*

For example, Miss Sophronia Bellmont of Boston, in 1801, kept a travelogue for her friend, Miss Caroline Courtland. Sophronia gave an account of her first day's travel, which consisted of a ride in a stagecoach from Boston to Providence, "a handsome town in Rhode Island," containing about seven thousand inhabitants, a college "commodiously situated on a hill," and some elegant churches with the handsomest steeples she had even seen.[102]

Having left Providence, Sophronia passed through many pleasant towns such as Norwich, New London, and Saybrook. At New Haven she made a "short tarry" to visit Yale College and the Library of that "delightful place." From that city her party took a packet for New York, and the girl gave an account of the fortitude with which she battled her first attack of seasickness. This unpleasant experience was soon forgotten in the five days she spent "rambling about the city, and spying out the curiostities." She was highly delighted with New York because she found the buildings far superior to those of Boston, while the streets were wider and better paved, and the people distinguished by great kindness.[103]

After a journey by stage to Philadelphia, Sophronia spent six days enjoying the sights of that town, which was larger and more regularly built than New York. Among the attractive features for her were the Franklin Library and Mr. Peale's Museum; but she was most impressed by the character of the "sect of Quakers or Friends," whom she judged to be "some of the excellent of the earth." Before sunrise she was taken to see the market, the largest in the country, which was quite full, as it was fashionable for the ladies to do their own marketing.[104]

By stage and packet the young girl proceeded to Baltimore, "the resort of strangers," and thence to Washington, the capital of the United States. Two days' residence there made her homesick, for it was "really a dull place," though what "length of years might make it," she granted, was not for a miss just entering her teens to predict. The public buildings were superb, and the rooms in the Capitol magnificent. She found Alexandria a "very pleasant place," and declared that had it "lain with her," she would have built the federal city there. Mount Vernon failed completely to arouse her enthusiasm, and she dismissed the historic spot with the remark that "whatever nature had wrought in its favor," it appeared to her gloomy in the extreme. After she had walked pensively for an hour or two over the solitary grounds, and had "dropped a tear on the patriot's tomb," she silently took her leave.[105]

To compensate her little friend for the "information and entertainment" of the travelogue, Caroline Courtland kept a diary and faithfully recorded the local news of Boston. One such item concerned the ideas expressed "in a circle of ladies" when the conversation turned to the subject of books suitable for children. The observations of a "respectable mother of a large family" are of particular interest for this study:

We all wish that our young folks should love reading; and the fondness for books is a mark of sense, and may be conducive to improvement. But how few books are fit for the perusal of the very persons for whom they are designed! Even of the few people, whose sentiments one would be willing they should imbibe, who will be at the pains to print? Those who do have no children of their own, either do not concern themselves about their principles or conduct, or have no knowledge of the avenues to their little hearts. They know not how very simple a tale ought to be; how very plain and short a moral; nor indeed are aware of the importance of supplying children with food for their curiosity, which will not vitiate their minds. And the married have but little time to make books.[106]

One of the best descriptions of city life was found in a little book published in 1825, called the *Picture of New York*. The frontispiece of this work gave a "distant view of the city," and described the "houses as packed together and as thick as trees in the forest," although none of the buildings in the picture was over three stories high, and only an occasional church steeple broke the low skyline. The author, in friendly fashion, told his little readers that if he had some good little girl and boy by the hand, he could show them the museum with its wonderful collections of animals and curiosities from different parts of the world. He could also point out the great City Hall that cost a half million dollars; or he might lead them through the beautiful Park to Broadway to see the splendid shops displaying a variety of "fancy goods, tastefully dressed off in the windows tempting people to buy." The little reader was warned that walking through the "extensive streets where many objects constantly presented themselves to view" would soon tire young people.[107]

Peter Parley also marveled at the sights of Broadway, where crowds of people, old and young, of all countries and all conditions, speaking English, French, Dutch, and even Chinese, bewildered visitors from the small towns and isolated farms. Class distinctions were sketched with surprising sharpness. Peter Parley remarked that there were by contrast "ladies covered with silks and ribbons, and barefooted girls whose parents could not provide them with shoes"; also "gay young men carrying their heads aloft with pride, and poor chimney sweeps covered with soot and wrapped in miserable blankets."[108] American children could thus early trace the lights and shadows of the new urbanization.

Little books of *Cries*, of which those of New York and Philadelphia were the most revealing, were equally suggestive of the status of city children. Accompanied by short homilies encouraging small peddlers "in the laudable example of application and industry," these *Cries* covered a wide range of juvenile activities. In them were sketches of little girls with baskets on their arms or heads, busy at different times of the day calling from door to door to see who would buy their radishes, cherries, tea-rusks, or matches. Boys also went through the streets calling, "Hot Muffins!" or "Spiced Gin-ger-bread!" either of which, accompanied by "a moderate dish of tea," was a common supper of the citizens.[109]

One of the most interesting cries in the New York version was represented by a cut of a young girl with a dish of corn on her head passing along the streets crying, "Hot corn! hot corn!" A note to the reader explained that in the fall of the year this cry "was abundantly heard" all over the city from children whose business it was to gather pennies by distributing corn to those "disposed to regale themselves with an ear." Another commentary stated that this corn, boiled in the husks while green and seasoned with a little salt which the girls carried with them, made "very pleasant eating."[110]

At the end of a description of a little match girl and her cry, "Do you want any matches? O buy my matches!" the Philadelphia book humanely recommended that "all good children" should remember that every comfort they enjoyed was produced in part by the labor of the poor, who "were entitled to much humanity and no ill nature."[111] The *Cries* also deplored the sight and sound of the young chimney sweeps as a reproach to civic pride and humanity. Both works expressed pity for these suffering children exposed to cold and hardship and compelled to spend their childhood in the most debasing work; but they declared that the "unnecessary bawling of these sooty boys grated on the ears of the citizens." Indeed, the wonder was expressed that in "such noisy places," where every needless sound should have been "hushed" such disagreeable ones were carelessly permitted.[112]

The development of a distinctive mode of dress for boys and girls marked the gradual emancipation of American childhood through the decades to 1835. As children of Colonial times were expected to behave like adults, they quite logically wore clothes appropriate for the role. Little ones of the upper classes, in particular, were dressed like miniature adults and allowed little freedom of movement. Fashion decreed that the small boy should wear a wig, a tricorn hat, a flowered waistcoat, tight knee-breeches, and high-heeled shoes; that the little girl, like her mother, should be encumbered with ankle-length skirts, voluminous cloaks, and heavy bonnets, as well as massive head-rolls.[113] A child's diary thus describes a little girl of twelve as she was clothed for one of the decorous "routs" of that time: "I was dressed in my yellow coat, my black bib and apron, my pompedore shoes, the cap with ribbons on it and a very handsome loket in the shape of a hart—the past pin my Hon. Papa presented me with in my cap, My new cloak and bonnet on, and my pompedore gloves."[114]

The reaction to these unsuitable fashions came after the Revolution, when enlightened parents began to dress their little ones more like children. Short hair became the vogue both for boys and girls. Boys were put into rather loose long trousers, and short coats and shirts with low necks; but girls retained for some years their mother's models, although in a somewhat simpler form.[115]

Children's books joined the crusade against the prevailing "pride and affectation in dress," and little girls in particular were regaled with alarming examples to prove that "prettiness is an injury to a young lady, if her behaviour is not pretty likewise." The finger of scorn was pointed at such foolish young creatures as "Miss Fanny Fiddle Faddle, a very pretty, gentle child about seven years of age, who did not want a tolerable share of good sense," but whose vanity was revealed in the *Juvenile Biographer:*

Miss Fiddle Faddle would not be seen in the morning with a Night-cap on, however decent it might be, no not for the World. All the Forenoon is spent at her glass, which she is sometimes ready to break in anger, because she cannot put her Cap on to her mind; and she has already been near an hour picking upon the proper Part of her Face to stick that Pach on. When she is in the Company of little Females of her Acquaintance, her whole Discourse turns upon the prevailing Fashion of Headdress.[116]

The French Revolution brought a change in the fabrics used for children's clothing; printed calicoes and loosely woven cottons took the place of the heavy silks and velvets of previous years. Since dress designs had to change to suit the materials, skirts slowly became shorter and less full, and dainty cotton fabrics—lawns, organdies, and percales—were woven with interesting sprig designs and dotted patterns to relieve the simplicity of the cloth. Colors became less vivid than they had been; and children in their "company clothes" were dressed in white or pastel shades, although coats and cloaks were usually made in darker colors.[117] The traditional long-skirted dress for little girls was replaced by the shorter Empire frock of childish simplicity. As the girl's feet and ankles were then visible for the first time in the century, the square-toed buckled shoes gave way to a lighter type of slippers similar to modern pumps.[118]

Fashions for small boys also changed slightly. Their coats were usually worn open down the front to show the white frilled shirt, and the long trousers were buttoned onto a blouse just under the arms. Older boys wore tailcoats of the same cut as their fathers', with flowered waistcoats and cravats, and either knee breeches or long trousers.[119]

A new epoch in the history of children's clothing was ushered in after 1825 by a return to the burdensome fashions of former years. This craze reached its peak of absurdity by 1830. The filmy materials of the first quarter of the century were replaced by heavier fabrics; the charming simplicity of the clinging skirt was no longer possible, and all trace of the Empire costume disappeared. Skirts became fuller and shorter and were braided and tucked; the normal waistline was once more emphasized by a tight belt. Well-dressed girls wore ruffled or lace-trimmed pantalettes flapping over the tops of their shoes, cart-wheel hats laden with ribbons and flowers, tight bodices, leg-o'-mutton sleeves, and high-plaited collars standing around the face. Although hoops were not generally used, skirts were held out by four or five corded petticoats starched to crinoline stiffness.[120]

The dress of small boys, in the medley of incongruous fashions, became more and more feminine, a trend clearly indicated by the long curls that replaced the short manly haircut of the previous decades. The full tunic reached to the knees, and the tight belt at the waist gave the boy a new silhouette. The trousers underneath the tunic were ruffled and tucked as much as those worn by the girls, while a ridiculously large tam-o'-shanter hat or peaked cap with a tassel, and the starched frill of cambric around his neck must have been constant annoyances to a normal boy.[121]

Little girls sat for hours, like martyrs of old, strapped to wooden backboards with their feet in stocks to develop a straight posture. The modern reader learns from those condemned to such extremes in fashion that when these genteel females in their "company clothes," burdened with layers of petticoats, encompassed with stays, and balanced on spike-heeled shoes, attempted to pay their respects to "superiors," they could bob their bodies in a curtsey, but by no means bend them, just as they might walk a little, but never run.[122] Oliver Wendell Holmes has left us a description of the torture inflicted on the children of that age in the efforts made to develop a stately bearing:

> They braced my aunt against a board
> To make her straight and tall,
> They laced her up, and starved her down,
> To make her light and small.
> They pinched her feet, they singed her hair,
> They screwed it up on pins:—
> Oh, never mortal suffered more
> In penance for her sins.[123]

Not all youthful Americans followed the fashions just described, for as the population pushed westward the pioneers adopted from the Indians those fashions best suited for boys and girls in the wild country. The women and older girls made the tough hides of forest creatures into jackets, trousers, and shoes, or cut coarse homespun "linsey-woolsey" into plain serviceable garments that were utterly devoid of style.[124]

In the early nineteenth century children of both sexes worked at canning tables, in the pitheads, or before the blazing furnaces. These boys and girls were clad alike in short trousers and little else, or in a shift—a straight shirt-like garment. Others, lightly garbed, bent over cotton rows, hoed vegetable gardens, or gathered fruits on the farms. All these poor young workers had no need for fancy frocks, coats, and hats, or even shoes and stockings. Their very nudity was the badge of poverty; for the more voluminous and ornate clothes were, the higher their wearers were supposed to be on the social ladder.[125] Elisha S. Horace has left a pen picture of an old-fashioned apprentice that exemplifies this simplicity in the dress of the poor:

Only figure to yourselves a young man of good proportions, handsome face, blooming beauty, dressed in a pair of deerskin breeches coming hardly down to his knees, which before they could be made fit to come into the presence of the ladies at meeting on the sabbath, were regularly blacked upon the preceding Saturday night at the dye-kettle of Deacon Holman, in order to give them a clean and fresh appearance for the Sunday. Imagine his legs covered up to the knees with a pair of blue woolen-yarn stockings, his feet encased with a thick and substantial pair of shoes, well greased and ornamented with a pair of small brass buckles, a present from his master for his good behaviour. Imagine that he wore a speckled shirt all the week, and a white one on Sunday, which was always carefully taken off as soon as he returned from meeting, folded up and laid by for the next sabbath.[126]

The upper classes in the United States copied French and English fashions as faithfully as conditions in this country and the meager transportation facilities would permit. The clothes of the wealthy usually served as models for middle and lower class imitation; but many Americans had ideas of their own on this point, and developed various theories on appropriate dress. Manuals of juvenile behavior discussed the subject of clothing, and counseled both parents and children that their clothes should be "decent, so as to answer the first end of dress"; garments were to be convenient, and their price was never to exceed the family income. Not only was "tawdry and fantastic" dress condemned, but children were shown the injustice of demanding costly apparel and of "laying out money for the moths to eat."[127]

*　　*　　*　　*　　*　　*

The Christian duty of employing time to the best advantage was one of the first moral lessons taught the children of this period. As idleness was considered the source of most evils, so industry was believed to turn the powers of the mind to good account. To train children in habits of industry, and to make them appreciate the value of time was highly important. An apt illustration of this philosophy was found in the story of "Tommy True," who, despising the "sluggard's bed," arose early, "ate his breakfast thankfully," and thus prepared himself for the day:

Then straight he takes his little hat,
And off to school he jogs away,
And let him meet with whom he will,
He seldoms stops to chat or play.

"This is my time to learn," says he,
"I never shall be young but once;
And if I throw this time away,
I must grow a silly dunce."[128]

Even the liberal and progressive Moravian educator, Christopher Dock, frowned upon his pupils' wasting the precious moments of their noon hour in play, and soon found an effective spiritual device to curb their spirits. Witness the directions in his *Schul-Ordnung:*

As the children carry their dinner, an hour's liberty is given them after dinner. But as they are usually inclined to misapply their time if one is not constantly with them one or two of them must read a story of the Old Testament, while I write copies for them. This exercise continues during the whole noon hour.[129]

Industry was not confined to lesson hours, or to the time assigned for the little stints about the home; on the assumption that children might be as idle at play as at work or over their books, the time devoted to relaxation had to be "properly and happily employed."[130] To drive youthful energies into active, vigorous pursuits, parents were advised to supply their children with "pleasurable objects"—varied, but not too numerous toys. Boys and girls were encouraged to buy and collect books for themselves, so that each child might enjoy a little library of his own.[131] As an antidote for quarreling and mischief on rainy days and winter evenings, mothers were urged to amuse and instruct their children by providing them with paper, pencils, and little pictures to cut out and to paste into scrapbooks. Thus the children of this era who were trained in domestic habits had many of their dull tasks brightened by some wholesome, simple pleasures disallowed in Colonial days.[132]

Time was generally considered the greatest blessing children could enjoy on earth, hence those who had acquired the art of managing this precious treasure properly had attained the highest wisdom. As a stimulus to lagging spirits, copybooks set before youth such pithy model sentences as: "Youth is the flower of age, the May of Time; then catch occasion in its proper clime," or "Rather depend upon your finger ends, than fix expectations on your friends."[133] The moral in the following verse was more pointed:

May we this important truth
Observe and ever hold,
"All those who're idle in their youth,
Will suffer when they're old."[134]

The maxims of "Poor Richard" repeated the copybook lessons; the almanac year after year set forth those fundamental ideas of industry that have left their mark on the American character. Any child could read at will the native logic: "If time be of all things the most precious, wasting time must be the greatest prodigality"; or, again, the exhortation: "Let us then be up and doing, and doing to the purpose: so by diligence we shall do more with less perplexity. What does it signify wishing for better times? We may make these times better if we bestir ourselves. Industry need not wish; and he who lives upon hope will die fasting!" The young boy was constantly assured that "he that hath a trade hath an estate; and he that hath a calling hath an office of profit and honour." Penniless young Americans were stimulated by the proverb, "Diligence is the mother of good luck, and God gives all things to industry"; and also by the assurance to "plow deep while sluggards sleep, and you will have corn to sell and keep."[135]

Habits of thrift were also cultivated, for most American children learned how to earn and use money. Many parents contrived a way for money to be fairly earned, provided a safe place for depositing it, and then gave the little financiers some pleasant plan for its use. For example, one father assembled his children every Saturday night, and gave each one a little pocket money in exact proportion to the child's good conduct during the week—the best child got the most, and the worst got none. The good deeds of this family were recorded in a pink book, and the bad ones in a black book. Any marks of bad temper, selfishness, or greediness, and fibbing or want of honesty, were faults that deprived these boys and girls of their reward. Although the children were allowed to spend the money as they pleased, each child was provided with an account book in which he had to put down every penny spent and on Saturday cast up the sum and show it to his father.[136]

Poorer children were pressed into service at home almost as soon as they could walk alone, for workmen were scarce in early America, and labor-saving devices unknown. Their religious beliefs quite appropriately extolled hard work as a virtue by teaching little ones such maxims as "Idleness is the devil's workshop." A variety of occupations, as a result, filled the daylight hours of these early American children with ample protection against the "Old Deluder Satan." The diary of a young Connecticut girl reveals at a glance how fully occupied was her day and how broad was the scope of her activities:

Fix'd gown for Prude,—Spun linen,—Work'd on cheese-basket,—Hatchelled flax with Hannah. We did 51 lbs. apiece,—Pleated and iron,—Read a sermon of Doddridge's,—Milked the cows,—Made a broom of Guinea wheat straw,— Set a Red Dye,—Had two scholars from Mrs. Taylor's,—Carded two pounds of wool and felt,—Spun harness of twine,—Scoured the Pewter.[137]

The missionaries David and John Brainerd have left a description of the active, busy life led by a boy in this same state; but the account also gives a fair picture of boyhood in any other section:

The boy was taught that laziness was the worst form of original sin. Hence he must rise early and make himself useful before he went to school, must be diligent there in study, and promptly home to do "chores" at evening. His whole time out of school must be filled up with some service, such as bringing fuel for the day, cutting potatoes for the sheep, feeding the swine, watering the horses, picking the berries, gathering the vegetables, spooling the yarn. He was expected never to be reluctant and not often tired.[138]

Indoor boys manufactured with their jackknives a number of wooden articles for farm and domestic use, while the making of birch brooms for the country store was an important industry. The lads did not grow rich, however, on broom-making, as the regular price paid was but six cents, and it took three evenings to make one broom. Although such tasks as splitting shoe pegs, setting card teeth, tying onions, and gathering nuts were also poorly paid, the gathering and marketing of wild cherries was a more profitable industry. Since this fruit was widely used in making cherry rum or cherry bounce, it usually netted about a dollar a bushel, and a large tree would yield about six bushels.[139]

American girls had been taught rules for sewing for more than a century, but it was not until 1817 that they were set down in book form. According to these directions, after the girls were first shown how to turn a hem on a piece of waste paper, they were to make a variety of stitches in a fixed order. Industrious maids practised how to sew and fell a seam, to draw threads and hemstitch, to gather a ruffle or skirt, to make buttonholes and buttons, to do herringbone stitch, to darn and to mark clothing, and to whip and sew on a frill.[140]

Even in the homes of the upper classes, where there were servants to attend to the needs of the family, girls usually helped with the cooking, and there was indeed much of it to do. The careful housewife of the period considered it a disgrace if her larder was not well stocked with pies, cakes, and breads of various kinds. Besides this cooking, there were two annual activities in which young girls of every household usually participated. In the spring came the task of candle-dipping; and in the autumn, soap-making, a tedious work, but a necessary duty to provide the soft soap which was used in the huge monthly washings typical of every household in those early days.[141]

Most Americans believed that coarseness and vulgarity were the effects of habit, and not inherent in the nature of the child. It was recommended in the early 1800's that parents should accustom their children to meet strangers with poise and dignity, and that boys and girls should be allowed to make social visits with grown-ups to dispel any tendency to a "painful and unbecoming bashfulness." But in this practice children were not to be encouraged in "showing-off, or constantly habituated to hearing themselves talked about."[142] Much as the failing had been ridiculed, it was remarked that it was still common "for mothers to talk a great deal about their children." The weariness with which strangers listened to such domestic accounts was considered a slight evil compared to the harm done children who were encouraged to think themselves important.[143] In defining the social status of the child in 1835, these lines of an old work may be invoked:

Methinks a little good Breeding may do the Children some Good! They should be taught the Rules of Behaviour; Good Manners do well become the Children of Good Christians. Our Children should be Taught how to address their Superiors with Modesty, their Inferiors with Gentleness, their Equals with Decency, and Inoffensiveness. . . . Unmannerly Children are but a Reproach to their Feeders and proclaim that they are better Fed than Taught.[144]

---

[1]Willystine Goodsell, *A History of the Family as a Social and Educational Institution*, pp. 395-404.

[2]Ruth Reed, *The Modern Family*, p. 51.

[3]John F. Ware, *Home Life: What It Is, and What It Needs*, p. 155.

[4]Calhoun, *op. cit.*, p. 83; see also Ware, *op. cit.*, p. 155.

[5]*Ibid.*, p. 72.

[6]*Ibid.*, p. 158.

[7]As quoted in Martin G. Brambaugh, *The Life and Works of Christopher Dock*, p. 218.

[8]Ethel S. Bolton and Eva J. Coe, *American Samplers*, p. 25.

[9]Cotton Mather, *op. cit.*, p. 22.

[10]*Ibid.*, p. 24.

[11]Mather, *op. cit.*, p. 25.

[12]*Ibid.*

[13]William Penn, *Fruits of a Father's Love*, pp. 33, 34.

[14]James Nelson (Apothecary), *An Essay on the Government of Children, Under Three General Heads, viz. Health, Manners and Education*, (New York, 1753), p. 171.

[15]*Ibid.*

[16] Eleazer Moodey, *The School of Good Manners*, Preface.

[17] *Ibid.*, pp. 69, 70.

[18] Philip D. S. Chesterfield, *Principles of Politeness and of Knowing the World*, p. 82.

[19] *Ibid.*, p. 113.

[20] Quoted by Alice M. Earle in *Child Life in Colonial Days*, p. 166.

[21] Eleazer Moodey, *op. cit.*, pp. 13-15.

[22] Dr. Gregory, *A Father's Legacy to His Daughters*, p. 111.

[23] Eleazer Moodey, *op. cit.*, pp. 2-3.

[24] *A Useful and Necessary Companion in Two Parts*, p. 82.

[25] Eleazer Moodey, *op. cit.*, pp. 4-6.

[26] Alice M. Earle, *Home Life in Colonial Days*, pp. 102-105; see also Earle, *Child Life in Colonial Days*, p. 216.

[27] Eleazer Moodey, *op. cit.*, p. 6. On this point Benjamin Franklin wrote: "Little or no notice was ever taken of the food on the table. If is was well or poorly prepared, in season or out of season, of good or bad flavour . . . we did not discuss it. I was brought up to pay so little attention to these things, that I cared little what kind of food was set before me." Albert B. Hart, *Source Readers in American History*, No. 1, p. 216.

[28] Eleazer Moodey, *op. cit.*, p. 6.

[29] *Ibid.*, pp. 6-7.

[30] *Ibid.*, pp. 7-9.

[31] *Ibid.*, pp. 10-11.

[32] Eleazer Moodey, *op. cit.*, pp. 15, 16.

[33] *Ibid.*, p. 28.

[34] *Ibid.*, pp. 17-19.

[35] *Ibid.*, pp. 6-9.

[36] Albert Hart, *op. cit.*, No. 2, p. 211. Whether it was remnant of the fighting practices of their British ancestors, or the result of the emotional disturbances of the times, this undeclared war of youth went on for years in spite of the whippings of schoolmasters and the scoldings of parents.

[37] Eleazer Moodey, *op. cit.*, pp. 19-22.

[38] *Ibid.*, pp. 26, 27.

[39] As quoted in Lothrop Stoddard, *The Story of Youth*, p. 283.

[40] Stoddard, *op. cit.*, p. 278.

[41] As quoted by Alice M. Earle, *Child Life in Colonial Days*, p. 167.

[42] *Ibid.*, p. 7.

[43] Alice M. Earle, *Diary of Anna Green Winslow, A Boston Girl of 1771*, p. 3.

[44] *Ibid.*, p. 7.

[45] *Ibid.*, pp. 213, 214.

[46] Chesterfield, *op. cit.*, p. 67.

[47] Dr. Gregory, *op. cit.*, p. 15.

[48] Anon., *Young Lady's Parental Monitor*, p. 127.

[49] Gregory, *op. cit.*, p. 22.

[50] *Young Lady's Parental Monitor*, p. 127.

[51] Gregory, *op. cit.*, p. 25.

[52] *Ibid.*, p. 28.

[53] *Ibid.*, p. 40.

[54] Samuel Sewall, *Diary 1674-1729*, Coll. of Mass. Hist. Soc., vols. V-VII (1878), vol. I (of series), p. 369.

[55] As quoted in Alice M. Earle, *op. cit.*, p. 226.

[56] As quoted in Lothrop Stoddard, *Story of Youth*, pp. 277, 278.

[57] As quoted in Alice M. Earle, *op. cit.*, p. 88.

[58] Eleazer Moodey, *op. cit.*, p. 14.

[59]*Ibid.*, p. 19.
[60]Alice M. Earle, *Diary of Anna Green Winslow*, p. 9.
[61]As quoted in Alice M. Earle, *op. cit.*, pp. 225, 226.
[62]John Potter, *The Words of the Wise*, p. 56.
[63]James Burgh, *Rules for the Conduct of Life* (Reprint of a London publication of 1767), p. 124.
[64]Mrs. Grant, *Sketches on Intellectual Education and Hints in Domestic Economy Addressed to Mothers*, pp. 20, 21.
[65]James Burgh, *op. cit.*, p. 124.
[66]Mrs. Grant, *op. cit.*, p. 21.
[67]Lydia Maria Child, *Letters to Mothers*, p. 110.
[68]*Ibid.*, p. 111.
[69]Arthur W. Calhoun, *op. cit.*, 54, 55.
[70]John Hersey, *op. cit.*, p. 26.
[71]*Ibid.*, p. 83.
[72]Jacob Smedley, *Hints for the Training of Youth; A Scrapbook for Mothers*, p. 51. This scrapbook contained articles like this written earlier in the century.
[73]Godham D. Abbott, *The Family at Home, or Familiar Illustrations of the Various Domestic Virtues*, pp. 144-54.
[74]Mrs. Richard Griffith, *Letters Addressed to Young Married Women*, p. 94; Rev. Charles Cooper, *Blossoms of Morality Intended for the Amusement and Instruction of Young Ladies and Gentlemen*, p. 156.
[75]*Be Merry and Wise or the Cream of Jests, and the Marrow of Maxims, for the Conduct of Life*, p. 78.
[76]*A Little Pretty Pocket-Book*, Preface.
[77]Anon., *The Wisdom of Crop the Conjuror exemplified in several Characters of Good and Bad Boys, with an impartial account of the celebrated Tom Trot who rode before all the Boys in the Kingdom till he arrived at the Top of the Hill called Learning, Written for the Imitation of those who love themselves*, Preface.
[78]*Ibid.*
[79]*Ibid.*
[80]*Ibid.*, pp. 30-32.
[81]*Ibid.*, p. 42.
[82]*The History of Little Goody Twoshoes; otherwise called Mrs. Margery Twoshoes. With the Means by which she acquired her Learning and Wisdom, and in consequence thereof her Estate*, p. 57.
[83]*Ibid.*, p. 58.
[84]*Ibid.*, pp. 115, 116.
[85]*The Juvenile Biographer; Containing the Lives of Little Masters and Misses; including a Variety of Good and Bad Characters. By a little Biographer*, First Edition, p. 114.
[86]*Ibid.*, p. 49.
[87]*Wisdom in Miniature; or the Young Gentleman and Lady's Pleasing Instructor, Being a Collection of Sentences, Divine Moral, and Historical*, Preface.
[88]*Wisdom in Miniature*, pp. 137-44.
[89]*Mother Goose's Melody: or Sonnets for the Cradle; Illustrated with notes and Maxims, Historical, Philsophical, and Critical*, The Second Worcester Edition, p. 33.
[90]*Ibid.*, p. 33.
[91]*Ibid.*, p. 54.
[92]*Ibid.*, p. 73.
[93]*Ibid.*, p. 72.
[94]*Jacky Dandy's Delight: or the History of Birds and Beasts; in Verse and Prose*, The First Worcester Edition, Isaiah Thomas, Preface.
[95]*Ibid.*, p. 16.

[96]*Ibid.*, p. 29.

[97]*The Sugar Plumb; or Sweet Amusements for Leisure Hours being an Entertaining and Instructive Collection of Stories embellished with curious cuts,* the First Worcester Edition, Isaiah Thomas, pp. 88-94.

[98]*Vice in Its Proper Shape; or, the Wonderful and Melancholy Transformations of Several Naughty Masters and Misses into those Contemptible Animals which they most resembled in Disposition. Printed for the Benefit of All Good Boys and Girls.* Preface.

[99]*Ibid.*, pp. 1-47.

[100]*Ibid.*, pp. 47-50.

[101]*The Daisy; or Cautionary Stories in Verse. Adapted to the Ideas of Children from four to eight years old. Part 1.* (1808), pages unnumbered.

[102]*Caleb Bingham, Juvenile Letters, Being a Correspondence between Children eight to fifteen years of age,* pp. 17, 18.

[103]*Ibid.*, pp. 18, 19.

[104]*Ibid.*, pp. 20-22.

[105]*Ibid.*, pp. 23-27.

[106]*Ibid.*, p. 45.

[107]*The Picture of New York,* p. 15.

[108]Samuel G. Goodrich, *Peter Parley's Tale about the State and City of New York, Illustrated by a map and many engravings. For the use of schools,* p. 25.

[109]*The Cries of Philadelphia; Ornamented with elegant woodcuts,* John Bouvier for Johnson and Warner, pp. 15-21. *The Cries of New York, Printed and sold by Samuel Wood at the Juvenile Book-Store,* pp. 1-20.

[110]*The Cries of Philadelphia,* p. 21.

[111]*Ibid.*, p. 22.

[112]*The Cries of New York,* p. 38. As a result of the annoying sight and sound of the young chimney sweeps, when an invention was patented in Washington in 1814 that cleaned chimneys as well as and more quickly than by the cruel method of sending up the little boys, people everywhere, prompted both by humanity and conscience, eagerly adopted the new device.

A comparison of the New York and Philadelphia *Cries* suggests interesting contrasts in the manners and morals of the two cities. For example, in the watermelon cry for New York City, the editor introduced a sermon on thieving: " 'Here's your fine ripe Water-melyons!' Watermelons are raised in great plenty and with ease, but the difficulty lies in preserving them from thieves. Strange, indeed, to tell, but it is so, there are many who would by no means take a cent from a neighbor's drawer, and yet steal watermelons!" On the other hand, the Philadelphia description contained no reference to stealing, but was short and informative, "The melons brought to this market are from the state of New Jersey." *Cries of New York,* p. 13; *Cries of Philadelphia,* p. 12.

[113]Elisha S. Horace, *Men and Manners in America One Hundred Years Ago,* pp. 233-37. An interesting description of these head-rolls is found in the diary of Anna G. Winslow of Boston, who wrote in 1771: "I had my HEDDUS ROLL on. . . . It makes my head itch, & ach, & burn like anything Mamma. This famous roll is not made *wholly* of a red *Cow Tail,* but is a mixture of that, & horsehair (Very course) & a little human hair of yellow hue, that I suppose was taken out of the back part of an old wig. But D– made it (our head) all carded together and twisted up. When it first came home, aunt put it on, & my new cap on it, then she took her apron & measured me, and from the roots of my hair on my forehead to the top of my notions, I measured above an inch longer than I did downwards from the roots of my hair to the end of my chin. Nothing renders a person more amiable than virtue & Modesty without the help of fals hair, red *Cow Tail,* or D— (the barber)." Alice M. Earle, ed., *Diary of Anna Green Winslow,* p. 71.

[114]Alice M. Earle, *Diary of Anna Green Winslow*, pp. 13, 14.

[115]Brooke, *op. cit.*, p. 9.

[116]*The Juvenile Biographer*, pp. 82, 83.

[117]Brooke, *op. cit.*, pp. 12-14.

[118]*Ibid.*, p. 15.

[119]*Ibid.*, pp. 16-18. The new fashions for boys are an example of the child leading the mode; for long trousers had been worn by little boys nearly forty years before they became fashionable for their fathers, though this doubtless was to save the wear and tear on knees and stockings.

[120]*Ibid.*, pp. 30-32.

[121]*Ibid.*, pp. 34-38.

[122]Eliza Ware Farrar, *The Young Lady's Friend*, pp. 95, 96.

[123]Oliver Wendell Holmes, "My Aunt," *Complete Poetical Works*, p. 8.

[124]Elisha S. Horace, *Men and Manners in America One Hundred Years Ago*, pp. 233-36.

[125]James Schouler, *Americans of 1776*, p. 91; Lucy Larcom, *A New England Girlhood*, pp. 120-21.

[126]Elisha S. Horace, *op. cit.*, p. 241.

[127]*The New School of Good Manners*, by the Preceptor of the Ladies Academy in New-London, p. 12.

[128]*A Present to Children*, p. 11.

[129]Martin G. Brumbaugh, *op. cit.*, p. 109.

[130]Hersey, *op. cit.*, p. 92; Mrs. Louisa Hoare, *Hints for the Improvement of Early Education and Nursery Discipline*.

[131]Hoare, *op. cit.*, p. 93.

[132]*Ibid.*, p. 94; Maria Edgeworth, *Idleness and Industry, Exemplified in the History of James Preston and Lazy Lawrence*, pp. 1-72.

[133]Eleazer Moodey, *op. cit.*, pp. 78, 79.

[134]*Original Poems for Infant Minds. By several young persons*, p. 28.

[135]Benjamin Franklin, *The Way to Wealth; or Poor Richard Improved*, p. 8.

[136]George Tuttle, *My Mother's Story of Her Own Home and Girlhood (about 1800)*.

[137]Quoted by Kate Dickinson Sweetzer, "The American Girl 1719-1919," *D. A. R. Magazine*, No. 9.

[138]Quoted by Alice M. Earle, *Child Life in Colonial Days*, pp. 307, 308.

[139]Sarah R. Fackenthal, "Child Life During the American Revolution," *A Collection of Papers read before the Bucks County Historical Society*, IV (1932), 203, 294.

[140]Society for the Establishment of Charity Schools, *Manual of the System of Teaching Reading, Writing, Arithmetic, and Needle-Work in the Elementary Schools of the British and Foreign Society*. Pages unnumbered.

[141]Sarah R. Fackenthal, *op. cit.*, p. 522.

[142]Lydia M. Child, *The Mother's Book*, p. 113.

[143]*Ibid.*, p. 114.

[144]*Cares About the Nurserie*, p. 11.

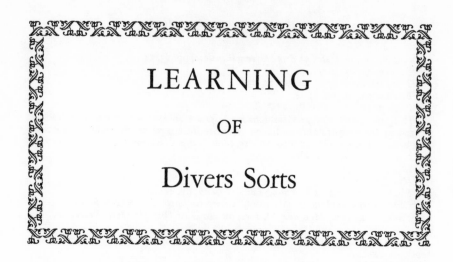

LEARNING

OF

Divers Sorts

The establishment of a school system in Colonial America, with the possible exception of that in New England, was a haphazard undertaking. During the troubled decades of the seventeenth and eighteenth centuries, the energies of the American colonists were absorbed in planting and defending their settlements. Education or the revered "learning of divers sorts" owed little therefore to formal instruction, for both schools and teachers were few and usually of poor quality, and the time allotted children for their studies was brief. Although the requisites for a well-rounded educational program were thus limited, there was little actual disparagement of educational opportunities for the young— especially for boys.

Elementary education was indeed valued as the process by which the child could acquire the definite habits, skills, and attitudes, and that fund of knowledge which civilization had prepared for him. Since American civilization along the Atlantic seaboard stemmed mainly from the English, the educational system of the colonies was but a modification of that used in the mother country; and the chief goal was to transmit this cultural heritage unchanged to succeeding generations. Besides religion, its most prominent characteristic, this "learning of divers sorts" included a medley of folklore, superstition, and scientific truth, adapted as far as possible to New World conditions.[1]

The Protestant Revolt had strengthened the position of the Church as the controlling power in education in order to assure the training of youth in a definite code of religious principles. This ecclesiastical dominance was also a part of the heritage transmitted by England to her colonies. Cotton Mather upheld the jurisdiction of the church over both secular and religious education when he deplored the decline of enthusiasm for the maintenance of common schools in New England. He saw in this apathy a direct blow at the very purpose of Colonial settlements:

The Colonies of New England were planted on the design of pursuing the Holy Reformation; and now the Devil cannot give a greater blow to the Reformation among us, than by causing Schools to languish under discouragements. If our General Courts decline to contrive and provide Laws for the Support of Schools; or if particular Towns Employ their Wits, for Cheats to elude the wholesome Laws; little do they consider how much they expose themselves to that rebuke of God, "Thou hast destroyed thy self, O New England."[2]

The success of society, according to Colonial thinking, depended on the fidelity with which the European cultural heritage was transmitted to the isolated American settlements, just as the success of the individual settler depended upon his acquiring this store of useful knowledge. There was always a haunting fear of losing this legacy of an old civilization and of reverting to barbarism. This apprehension has been indicated in the preceding chapter on manners, which traced the measures taken to safeguard time-honored customs in the primitive American environment. A similar attitude was carried over to education, and the important function of the school as an antidote to barbarism was persistently stressed. Again it was Cotton Mather who expressed his forebodings about this impending cultural doom in his *Prognostication upon the Future State of New England*—a document which might easily be taken as a norm of Colonial thought in any section of the country. Mather's warning read:

Where Schools are not Vigorously and Honourably Encouraged, whole *Colonies* will sink apace, into a Degenerate and Contemptible Condition, & at last become horribly Barbarous. If you have any love to God . . . you would not betray your Posterity into the very Circumstances of *Salvages*, let Schools have more Encouragement.[3]

The Colonial system of elementary education indeed lost few of its original features in the transfer from England to America. England had dame schools, and this type of school was transplanted successfully in the colonies, particularly in Massachusetts. England used the tutorial system of instruction, and so did the colonies, especially those in the middle and southern sections. England almost completely disregarded the education of women, and this same neglect prevailed in the colonies. Not only did English apprenticeship and poor-law traditions take root in this country, but so did the English charity school—an enterprise that definitely impeded the growth of a free, publicly controlled, non-sectarian school system.[4] Thus in almost every detail the British pattern of education served as a guide to the colonists; up to the time of the Revolution the traditions and practices of this model were reproduced with remarkable fidelity in American school life.

Besides the negative function of the church-controlled school system which was described by Mather, there were, as was gradually believed, two positive advantages to be gained from a well-ordered educational system. First, since most Protestant denominations at this time considered an educated clergy as a safeguard for their particular form of faith, provision had to be made for the training of aspirants to the ministry. Second, since the Bible was the chief source of divine truth for the laity, it was incumbent on all Christians to teach their children to read that they might investigate this source for themselves.

Utilitarian philosophy was another powerful factor in education during the eighteenth century. Everywhere it stimulated scientific inquiry, in order that man might master the forces of nature. Out of this intellectual curiosity, a threefold scheme for the education of youth developed. One phase was evident in the practical education given some middle-class boys, who were trained as apprentices in those crafts and trades that would enhance production and increase the physical comforts of life. The vast majority of children of this same social stratum lived in a rural environment and thus came into daily contact with plants, animals, tools, and the soil. These boys and girls in early childhood became acquainted with the processes of agricultural production—a useful, informal type of education which was particularly adapted to the needs of the new nation. Although life in rural America during the Colonial period offered many opportunities for ambitious youth to rise to success, this same isolated existence also tended to underrate culture and gentility. As a result, the children of the back country commonly failed to appreciate the potentialities of the fine and liberal arts, and often despised even the ordinary amenities of social life.[5]

In producing a group of ignorant but liberty-loving youth, the educational system of the Colonies further reflected the class distinctions of Europe, where higher learning was the badge of the upper classes. Besides its disciplinary training, higher education also provided the well-to-do with intellectual adornments which distinguished them from the poor. The correct use of language, a cultured accent, a knowledge of Latin and Greek, and eventually an acquaintance with the classics, combined to form a system which separated the child of wealth from his less fortunate fellow beings. On the assumption that their economic and intellectual superiority presupposed supremacy in other fields, the youth of the upper classes usually studied law, theology, and the military arts—those professions which formed the basis of social and political power.

Children of the lower classes, disciplined by poverty and hard work and almost completely deprived of leisure, were forced to confine themselves to useful studies, and only the more fortunate of this group received even these morsels of knowledge. Meager instruction in the rudiments of practical studies—reading, writing, and arithmetic—generally constituted the store of "book learning" for this submerged element. It was deemed a universal safeguard to society to have the poor acquire habits of honesty, obedience, and industry, as well as to develop their physical strength in certain skills.[6]

The middle-class colonists, in their attempt to emulate the educational achievements in the decorative studies attained by those of wealth and distinction, ultimately achieved a unique compromise by uniting in their curriculum many useful and some ornamental studies. Middle-class youths had to prepare themselves to make a living by some gainful art or skilled trade; so their interests were directed to business, law, medicine, or to scientific agriculture. Just as the upper classes set the intellectual pace for those immediately below them in the social scale, so did the middle class, in turn, exert a powerful influence in popularizing educational opportunities for the lower classes, at least on an elementary level.[7]

To understand the scope of Colonial education it is necessary to examine briefly the types of schools which supplied the young with what the Roxbury trustees called their "scholastic, theological, and moral discipline." The New England school system was in some respects superior to that of any other section by the middle of the eighteenth century. The people of that section were not of a superior character, but their compact villages and towns were more favorable for the establishment of schools and, with the exception of Rhode Island, the inhabitants of these towns belonged to the same religious denomination. This twofold unity made it easier for New Englanders to establish a common school system than it was for the scattered rural population of other colonies, or for communities of different religious denominations, to carry out a similar scheme.[8]

New England Puritans, like other Protestants, believed that the key to salvation lay in exact obedience to the teachings of the Bible; consequently a thorough knowledge of the Scriptures was both a religious and an educational requirement for their children. To fill this need a system of elementary parish schools of various degrees of efficiency was organized which at the same time buttressed the church and taught boys and girls the rudiments of secular learning. An "other-worldliness" colored the child's life; and, as already noted, many features of his educational system were directed to preparing him for that future existence.[9]

These parish schools, or the private schools of the same level, were usually taught by the local minister or by a lay teacher whose chief qualification was a knowledge of the faith rather than a solid foundation in the intellectual or cultural attainments of the times. Since these masters were not satisfied that the ability to read the Bible would of itself insure the preservation of their religious beliefs and practices, they prepared numerous catechisms containing interpretations of important biblical passages as well as points of dogma and rules of conduct. The catechism of their own denomination became an integral part of the school equipment of Colonial boys and girls. Still doubting the adequacy of this method, the educational leaders of New England and elsewhere made sure that the secular textbooks were fortified by a sufficient amount of moralization. Their goal could easily be reached, since in a majority of schools the only subjects taught were religion, reading, writing, and arithmetic; and few books were used in this course of study.[10]

Sometimes a mother held classes for her own children, and gave instruction of a still more elementary character than that imparted in the common schools; or a maiden lady was employed to drill the girls and small boys of a neighborhood in the elements of learning.[11] In these so-called dame schools, pupils as young as three or four years were taught the alphabet and a little reading and writing; but reading for the very small rarely extended beyond the crisscross row of the hornbook or the simple lessons of the *New England Primer*. Some towns in New England supported dame schools as their only source of primary education; in other colonies, private schools of this type, maintained on a tuition basis, held sway until well into the nineteenth century.[12] In his *True Relation of the Flourishing State of Philadelphia,* Judge Thomas Holme wrote in 1696 of the dame schools of that vicinity:

> Here are schools of divers sorts,
> To which our youth daily resorts,
> Good women, who do very well
> Bring little ones to read and spell,
> Which fits them for their writing; and then
> Here's men to bring them to their pen,
> And to instruct and make them quick
> In all sorts of arithmetic.[13]

Well-to-do parents in all the Colonies employed private tutors for their own families and for those close relatives who then lived under the

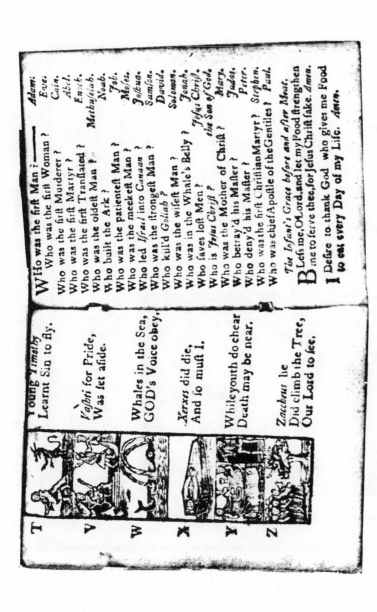

T   Young Timothy
    Learnt Sin to fly.

V   Vashti for Pride,
    Was set aside.

W   Whales in the Sea,
    GOD's Voice obey.

X   Xerxes did die,
    And so must I.

Y   While youth do chear
    Death may be near.

Z   Zaccheus he
    Did climb the Tree,
    Our Lord to see.

WHo was the first Man? —— Adam.
Who was the first Woman? — Eve.
Who was the first Murderer? — Cain.
Who was the first Martyr? — Abel.
Who was the first Translated? — Enoch.
Who was the oldest Man? — Methuselah.
Who built the Ark? — Noah.
Who was the patientest Man? — Job.
Who was the meekest Man? — Moses.
Who led Israel into Canaan? — Joshua.
Who was the strongest Man? — Samson.
Who kill'd Goliah? — David.
Who was the wisest Man? — Solomon.
Who was in the Whale's Belly? — Jonah.
Who saves lost Men? — Jesus Christ.
Who is Jesus Christ? — the Son of God.
Who was the Mother of Christ? — Mary.
Who betray'd his Master? — Judas.
Who deny'd his Master? — Peter.
Who was the first Christian Martyr? — Stephen.
Who was chief Apostle of the Gentiles? — Paul.

The Infant's Grace before and after Meat.

BLess me, O Lord, and let my Food strengthen me to serve thee, for Jesus Christ sake. *Amen.*

I Desire to thank God who gives me Food to eat every Day of my Life. *Amen.*

From the NEW ENGLAND PRIMER, 1775

THE

HISTORY

OF

AMERICA,

ABRIDGED FOR THE USE OF CHILDREN
OF ALL DENOMINATIONS.

Adorned with Cuts.

Unto children give suck, and to maturity ripe fruit.

PHILADELPHIA:
Printed by WRIGLEY & BERRIMAN, for
JOHN CURTIS.—1795.

*Columbus's first interview with the
Natives of America.*

From the first American history text published for children

same roof. Classes of this type were held in the home or in a special building on the grounds, and followed much the same curriculum as did the privately conducted or church-controlled elementary schools in various parts of the country. In the sparsely settled Southern Colonies, this tutorial system was generally adopted not only for its convenience, but because the sharp class distinctions made wealthy planters reluctant to send their boys and girls to the few common schools, which were also attended by the offspring of their less prosperous neighbors. The tutor might be an indentured servant with a slight store of knowledge, an Anglican minister, or in rare cases an English university graduate. Boys were generally prepared by such tutors or by their female relatives for the classical schools of this country or for the English universities.

Private schools—often of a secondary grade—were quite numerous in the larger towns. This type was supported by tuition fees and conducted by masters or mistresses who usually supplemented their meager income by the sale of books and school supplies. To give proper instruction for the boys who aspired to such careers as ships' officers, surveyors, clerks, or business men, or even to posts in the civil service of the government, a few "mathmetical" and English schools were established about the middle of the century in the larger towns. At the same time, night schools offering a wide choice of useful studies, such as mathematics, languages, surveying, bookkeeping, and navigation, were opened for the benefit of apprentices and other employed youth.[14]

Elementary charity schools, particularly those established by the Society for the Propagation of the Gospel in Foreign Parts, were found in New York, New Jersey, New England, Pennsylvania, and South Carolina, but they were not confined entirely to these colonies. The work of the S. P. G. among the German Quietist sects, such as the Moravians, Mennonites, and Dunkards, was especially important, since the aim of the Society was to promote the unity of the colony by teaching these people to read and speak the English language. Although the Quietists resisted all efforts at Anglicanization and clung tenaciously to their own language and religion, the project does indeed represent an early attempt to provide free elementary education in this country.[15]

The academy was also planned in the early eighteenth century to prepare boys more adequately for industrial and business pursuits. These institutions provided a liberal education of a new type and supplied vocational training. Thus, by offering a course of studies adapted to the intellectual and practical interests of the middle class, academies became immensely popular, and played their important role even through the next century. The academy was for decades the accepted pre-professional school for boys, and the finishing school for girls. Boys were there prepared for the study of law, medicine, or divinity; while girls, after what now seems a superficial program of studies, took up the serious business of life in the management of a home.[16]

Enough has already been said in previous sections of this study to demonstrate that at the beginning of the eighteenth century the theory and practice of child training was in every respect determined by adult standards and interests. Although no sudden or striking change can be detected in the Colonial system of education during the first three-quarters of the century, this was a period of transition, dominated by a growing trend towards secularization, and marked by sporadic efforts to find a more humane approach to child training. The old order was being repeatedly challenged from Europe by such writers as Comenius, Locke, Rousseau, Basedow, and Pestalozzi, who boldly proclaimed that the world did not understand the needs of childhood since it treated boys and girls like miniature adults.

John Amos Comenius, 1592-1671, a Moravian bishop, was one of the first of a series of European reformers whose influence extended to Colonial America and inspired the radical innovation in the school system of the nineteenth century. Comenius held that education should be a natural process in harmony with man's constitution and destiny, and should afford a well-rounded foundation for complete living. To this end he planned a regular system of graded schools and led in advocating instruction for very young children. He held that a knowledge of geography, history, and the elements of the arts and sciences was essential, but also stressed the need of physical education. Not only did he correlate the various subjects, but he subordinated Latin to the vernacular and taught it from the use of common objects known to the child. His educational system, which was more interesting and effective than any previously devised, was based on textbooks that were also far in advance of the times.

The first of his works, published in 1631, was the *Janua Linguarum Reserata* ("Gate of Languages Unlocked"). The English version of this book was used particularly by the children of the Middle Colonies where the Moravian sect was most numerous. The record shows, however, that by the middle of the seventeenth century a Boston town meeting selected a committee to introduce the Comenian texbooks and inductive methods into their Latin schools.[17]

In content the *Janua* consisted of sentences composed of several thousand Latin words for familiar objects and ideas. The Latin was printed in the column on the right, and the English translation on the left. By this arrangement the pupil was expected to acquire the rudiments of ordinary knowledge and to improve his Latin vocabulary.

As a supplement to the *Janua,* Comenius produced the *Orbis Sensualism, Pictus* ("The World of Sense Objects Pictured"), which, as the first illustrated reading book on record, was popular for two centuries. Its alphabet consisted of appropriate woodcuts the size of a postage stamp with such explanatory sentences as the following:

A a *Cornix cornicatur,*
The crow crieth.

B b *Agnus balat,*
The lamb blaiteth.

C c *Cicada stridet,*
The grasshopper chirpeth[18]

Comenius not only demanded that the "young must be educated in common . . . and all the young of both sexes should be sent to school," but he set down the principle that "what has to be learned, must be learned by doing." Reading, writing, singing, and foreign languages were to be learned by practise just as virtue and morality were to be acquired by prayer, good example, and sympathetic guidance. Since humanism was strongly entrenched, these realistic theories had only limited appeal, and their author was regarded as fanatic. Reformers of succeeding generations, however, were so strongly influenced by the principles of Comenius, that he may be considered a precursor of modern educators.[19]

Perhaps the most potent of all European influences on American educational standards was exerted by John Locke, 1632-1704, the English philosopher. His ideas and very words are found in the writings and speeches of the Founding Fathers, especially in those of Thomas Jefferson. Locke's outline for intellectual training was formulated in the famous *Essay concerning the Human Understanding* and to some extent in his *Thoughts concerning Education.* Like the French writer Montaigne, Locke held that book knowledge and intellectual training were less important than the development of character and good manners. Like Comenius, Locke leaned toward sense realism and recommended a wide utilitarian range of subjects for the education of a gentleman.[20] He also suggested that "contrivances might be made to teach children to read whilst they thought they were only playing." To this end he recommended pasting the letters of the alphabet upon the sides of dice—and "when by these gentle ways he begins to read, some easy pleasant Book, suited to his capacity, should be put into his Hands."[21]

As a corollary to these pleasant teaching devices, Locke declared in his *Thoughts* that "great Severity of Punishment does but very little good, nay, great Harm in Education." He preferred as effective means of intellectual discipline "Esteem or Disgrace," and reserved corporal punishment for moral offenses.

In his *Essay,* Locke proclaimed his famous *tabula rasa* doctrine—that all knowledge comes from experience, and the mind is like "white paper or wax, to be molded and fashioned as one pleases.'' On this "paper," ideas are painted by sensation and reflection. Locke not only advocated teaching the child mathematics and other subjects to cultivate "general power," but urged his "denial of desires" in moral education, and the "hardening process" in physical training.[22] His theory of "formal discipline" was to become the basic principle of early American education.

Few writers have had as great influence upon the organization, method, and content of education as Jean Jacques Rousseau, 1712-78, the French philosopher. By advocating naturalism and seeking to destroy traditionalism, his works caused men to rush to the defense of the old systems, and when they failed they undertook the construction of something better. He held that children should be taught the virtues of the primitive man, that they should be trained to contribute to their own support and to be sympathetic and benevolent to their fellow men. Through this doctrine, education became more closely related to human welfare.[23]

Rousseau advocated making the child and his needs the center of a new educational system which would allow the young to act and grow in harmony with the laws of nature. Not only did Rousseau dare to defy the age-old theory which held that since the child was naturally depraved it was the office of education to correct his evil tendencies, but he even maintained that the child was naturally good, and that he was only corrupted by human institutions and chiefly by a faulty educational system.[24]

In this country recognition of Rousseau's ideas came slowly, since he was opposed to the basic premise of the American educational philosophy —that education of the young was primarily a preparation for adult life. Rousseau contended that every age had its proper perfection and its own peculiar sort of maturity. Childhood, then, was not to be made miserable by preparation for some pretended advantage of the future which the child would probably never enjoy. Instead, the new aim of education was to teach the child what would be of use to him at the time rather than to impose upon him studies for an age he might never reach. In this era of formal discipline, the warning of the future emancipation of childhood came as a shock when Rousseau declared that "the age of mirth was not to be spent in the midst of tears, chastisements, threats, and slavery."[25]

In his *Emile*, Rousseau abandoned all compulsion for the growing child so that he might be free to develop a rich, moral personality. Emerson later seized from *Emile* the idea that man is inherently good, and carried it on to its logical conclusion, proclaiming man to be a child of God. The divinity of man was the great belief of all New England Transcendentalists. Man as the child of God, they said, possesses a divine nature. *Emile* may thus be said to have inaugurated a new era in the history of education.[26]

Such educators as Johann Bernhard Basedow, 1723-90, of Hamburg, were responsible for much of the emphasis given to nature study in the juvenile literature of the early nineteenth century. Basedow, who had been captivated by Rousseau's doctrine, developed a method of teaching through association of ideas in play and conversation. In an endowed school called the "Philanthropium," the reformer's principle of directing, not suppressing, the natural instincts of children was carried out by improved methods. Languages were taught by conversation, games, pictures, drawing, interesting reading, and plays. Grammar was not introduced until late in the course. Methods in other subjects were fully as progressive—arithmetic was taught by mental processes; geometry, by drawing neat, accurate figures; and geography, by learning about one's own country and then proceeding to the continents. Most notable was the plan for teaching the naturalistic religion of deism. To learn the existence of God, the child noted the various features and phenomena of nature and was asked their cause. Little ones were also kept in a darkened room for four or five days in order that they might be impressed more deeply with the wonders of nature when they were finally released and told of the God who had created these marvels.[27]

It remained for the reformer Johann Pestalozzi, 1746-1827, a native of Zurich and a disciple of Rousseau, to psychologize education. To explain his educational creed and practice, Pestalozzi in 1801 published a series of books—the *A B C of Observation*, the *Book for Mothers*, and *How Gertrude Teaches Her Children*. By these texts children were taught to observe correctly, to estimate proper relationships, and to express their ideas clearly. To this end syllabaries and tables of units and fractions were used in reading and arithmetic. Such subjects as drawing, writing, and geometry were taught through elements of form. Children arranged sticks in the desired designs and then drew lines representing these models on a board or slate. This was done until all elementary forms, straight and curved, were mastered. Nature study and geography were learned from actual observation; music, from its simplest tone elements; and religion and morality, from concrete examples.

Pestalozzi's method of control was mild and may be best described in his own words: "The relations between master and pupil, especially so far as discipline is concerned, must be established and regulated by love." In his teaching and works he maintained that the school should be modeled as closely as possible on the home; and that the main incentives to well-doing were not fear and compulsion, but kindness and love. Thus, in a happy homelike atmosphere where children were busy with interesting activities and where due regard was taken for their moral, intellectual, and physical needs, there was little necessity for severe punishments. Pestalozzi respectfully affirmed that he objected to the use of corporal punishment "when the teacher or the method is at fault and not the children."[28]

These liberal educational ideas from abroad were not the most disturbing elements in American academic circles, for there was also much in the native environment that created dissatisfaction with the kind of training given the young. In many aspects of life and in education particularly, America was breaking with the past and with Europe. All during the eighteenth century foreign ideals and experiences were not the great factors in American life, for the colonists were extremely provincial. Only a few were inclined to discover what lessons in social progress Europe had for America. On the one important social subject—politics— Americans regarded themselves as authorities. As a result, European reformers exerted but slight influence before the nineteenth century brought ambitions for real educational development. By 1700, the Colonies had reached adolescence; many of the older families were two or three generations removed from their European origins. The immigrants who came here from England or from the northern countries of Europe were quickly assimilated into the American pattern of life and soon developed a pride in their adopted land. A growing sense of security and a new realization of power marked this era. Along the Atlantic seaboard and inland to the eastern highland the fertile lands abundantly supplied the wants of the colonists; while the burdens of government, with few exceptions and in spite of protests to the contrary, bore lightly on the inhabitants. Ideas of the individual's independence and a sense of self-sufficiency developed apace and tended to produce those political repercussions which marked the last quarter of the century.[29]

Education, from the opening of the century to the outbreak of the Revolution, reflected the influence of the increasing self-sufficiency of the colonists as well as the disturbing potency of the Age of Enlightenment.

The period is characterized by a growing appreciation of the intellectual powers, and by repeated efforts to establish proper institutions to develop these faculties. American educators, who by mid-century, were dissatisfied with the narrow theological basis of the old school system, were seeking to broaden the scope of elementary and secondary education by including a wider range of human interests. This revolt against the theological basis of the old educational system, as well as the agitation for the more practical training of youth, received its impetus mainly in Pennsylvania from the writings and labors of such peerless exponents of the new Enlightenment as Benjamin Franklin, Anthony Benezet, and Benjamin Rush. Their principles, of course, were to be generally accepted by the close of the century. By that time education was no longer dedicated exclusively to religious training and dogma, because the layman with his interests in the practical pursuits of life was beginning to charge the school with a great variety of responsibilities. The prosperous merchants and traders along the Atlantic seaboard, eager to promote their business interests and to enhance their social prestige, demanded a type of education in line with their ambitions. Other incentives for secularizing the curriculum were furnished by those aspiring young men who saw possibilities of wealth and influence if they possessed some knowledge of the modern languages needed in commerce, or if they could obtain some skill in useful trades such as bookkeeping or surveying.[30]

The new conception of American education did not immediately discard religion or the classics, but aimed rather to have them better taught; and by introducing new subjects into a curriculum so long dominated by religious interests, to serve more adequately the needs of the growing nation. Benjamin Franklin, who was foremost among the advocates of the new trend, incorporated his ideas for the useful training of the young in his *Proposals for the Education of Youth in Pennsylvania*. This document, which reveals how heavily educational responsibilities weighed on the author, began with the words: "The good Education of Youth has been esteemed by wise Men in all Ages, as the surest Foundation of Happiness both of private Families and of Commonwealths."[31] For the next century, two aims—practical utility and formal culture—threatened the priority of religion in the child's intellectual world.

These influences, to be sure, touched the lives of only a small portion of Colonial children; the masses, in spite of aims, were to be poorly instructed as long as education remained largely an individual responsibility. Very few boys and girls of the rural districts or in the back country had access to schools of any kind. But from a consideration of the meager opportunities for formal schooling, one cannot conclude that youths who were less fortunately situated than their wealthier neighbors were for that reason wholly uneducated. The discipline of life and work of the isolated home, farm, or shop fostered a unique wisdom.[32]

Influenced by the pragmatism of the times, schools began to offer vocational or quasi-vocational training. French, music, and dancing were included in the school's curriculum for their social value, just as classics were taught for their alleged cultural values and for the dignity accruing to the young gentleman who could quote "elegant" sources with ease. Liberalism—in the sense of a broadening interest in youth—had become the outstanding feature of the Colonial educational system by the last quarter of the century; but this characteristic can be best examined in the new program of studies and in the English schools and academies established to develop that program.

The budding liberalism of the eighteenth century may be seen in Franklin's well-known plans of 1749 for the proposed Philadelphia Academy. Franklin, in mapping the course of studies, contemplated an English school, but after several patrons of the project demanded a system that would also give a classical training, he abandoned his first plan for another, making a threefold division of interests: mathematics, English, and the classics. This new type of school placed emphasis on the teaching of the English language, of literature, and of oratory; introduced scientific courses; and provided for the non-sectarian control of the institution by a self-perpetuating board of trustees.[33] The institution, in the scope and diversity of its curriculum, was simply the fruition of Franklin's hope, expressed when he proposed that in the Academy the boys should learn "those Things that are likely to be *most useful* and *most ornamental:* Regard being had for the several Professions for which they are intended."[34]

Richard Peters, in his address at the opening of the Academy, January 7, 1751, indicated the need of providing vocational guidance for youth as well as training in the useful pursuits. Peters deplored the common "misapplications of genius" as a major evil of the educational system in all the colonies:

My fellow Citizens, you ought to represent to yourselves the State of the Infant Geniuses of the Place; How many are totally lost thro' Idleness and Inactivity? How many are forced, as it were, in Opposition to their natural Temper and Genius, into wrong Trades, Offices, Professions and Employments; and by these Means become the Objects of Wants, Wretchedness, and Misery? What numbers are ever peevish and fretful, a Torment to themselves and all about them. . . . Their undiscerning Neighbors can assign no cause for it; or if they do, attribute it to a perverseness of Temper. Alas! . . . you will find the man is put to the wrong Business, he likes some other much better. . . .[35]

This speech of Richard Peters also furnishes some idea of the current standards of school discipline, as well as the new methods of rewarding diligence employed by such progressive educators as Franklin. After exhorting parents and teachers to be firm in holding youth to the line of duty, and to see that the young students "adhered to disagreeable studies," the orator outlined the method of disciplining a refractory youth:

Be sure to keep a strict Hand over him, reprove, Chastise, correct, use Severity, if necessary, but let this be seldom, and when the Fault is glaring; nor give over when you have begun, till you have quelled the tyrannical spirit.[36]

Franklin, on the other hand, would reward annually with much pomp those boys who distinguished themselves and excelled their companions in any branch of learning. To these he advised "fine gilt Books be given as Prizes" at special exercises in the "Hall" in the presence of the trustees and the citizens of the town. According to this plan, awards were to be given to the three boys ranking highest, and "Commendations, Encouragement, and Advice to the rest; keeping up their Hopes that by Industry they may excel another time."[37] Franklin insisted that the idea of true merit should always be presented to youth as consisting in "an Inclination join'd with an Ability to serve Mankind, one's Country, Friends, and Family; which Ability is to be greatly encreased by true learning."[38]

In setting the entrance requirements for his new Academy, Franklin also gave an interesting revelation of the meager scholastic standards for what would constitute a high school course in modern times. He wrote in his *Proposals:* "It is to be expected that every Scholar to be admitted into this school, be at least able to pronounce and divide the syllables in Reading, and to write in a legible hand."[39] It is important in this connection to examine briefly the books that were used in the homes and schools to establish this seemingly weak foundation for a secondary education.

Very small Colonial children learned the elements of reading from the hornbook, a small thin piece of wood that closely resembled a paddle, upon which a sheet of paper was placed containing the alphabet in both large and small letters, some simple syllables such as "ba, be, bi, bo, bu, etc.," and the Lord's Prayer. This single page was covered by a sheet of yellowish horn; and both paper and horn were secured to the wood by narrow strips of metal fastened by tiny hand-wrought nails. At the two upper corners of the page were crosses; hence a recitation from the hornbook was commonly called "reading the crisscross row." Since the wooden back usually had a perforated handle at the bottom, the hornbook could be conveniently carried in the hand by a string, hung by the child's side, or worn around the neck. The teacher in the dame schools or the mother at home pointed to the letters with a quill or knitting needle while their smallest pupils read them aloud; or the teacher heard the older ones in chorus lustily shout their "a-b ab's," spell out their prayer, and read the crisscross row. And since this simple textbook so closely resembled a paddle, the record shows it was also used in that capacity as the need arose.[40] The battledore was an offshoot of the hornbook, and was printed on a double fold of stiff cardboard. In school it was used as a text for the study of the alphabet and crudely illustrated short sentences; but outdoors it served as a bat in the game of shuttlecock and battledore.

American "infant scholars" for more than a hundred years usually turned from the hornbook or its cousin the battledore to the *New England Primer*. This book was so religious in content that it has been aptly called the "Little Bible of New England," although it was used universally in the Colonies—even by the Quaker children of Pennsylvania. The 1749 edition of the *Primer* contained, among other items, the alphabet in hornbook form and in illustrated couplets, a syllabary, rules for decent behavior, selections from Watts' *Divine Hymns,* and the Shorter Catechism.[41] An idea of its tone and content may be indicated by two extracts from the "Alphabet of Lessons for Youth":

> F   Foolishness is bound up in the Heart of a Child,
>   but the Rod of Correction shall drive it from him.
>
> G   Grieve not the Holy Spirit.[42]

With the growth of the secular spirit in education, the *Primer* by 1800 had lost some of its pietistic tone. The alphabet of that year read in part:

> A   was an Angler, and fished with a hook.
> B   was a Blockhead, and ne'er learn'd his book.
> C   The Cat doth play and after slay.[43]

In the same blithe spirit, the illustration for the last line represented a cat playing a fiddle to a group of mice dancing on their hind legs. This was probably in reference to the nonsense rhyme "Hey diddle, diddle, the cat and the fiddle," found in the *Mother Goose's Melodies* which were then gaining popularity.

When the Colonial child had completed the hornbook and primer, he was considered ready for grammar; but through the decades almost to the Revolution this meant not English, but Latin grammar. One of the earliest Latin texts used in this country was Leonard Culman's *Sententiae Pueriles Anglo-Latinae*. It was intended for beginners, so the selections were graduated from two-Latin-word examples—*Amicis utere*. "Make use of thy friends"[44]—to sentences five or six lines in length. Among the "Holy Sentences to be taught Scholars upon Holydays," are found such remarkable bits as:

Patrem mores non sunt arguendi, sed ferendi.
Our fathers manners are not to be found fault withal, but endured.

Varia & mutabilis semper faemina.
A woman is always wavering and inconstant.[45]

Another book of Latin syntax, published in Philadelphia in 1761, has the same title as Culman's work, but was not the same text; it was advertised as a "short and easy method to exercise children in parsing." From a host of similar sentences, the following may indicate how faithfully this tiny volume reflected the current utilitarian trend of educational philosophy:

Cessator consequitor nec honorem, nec opes.
A Loiterer gets neither Honor nor Riches.[46]

Cole literas, quae fecundas res ornant.
Pursue Learning which adorns prosperity.[47]

The most popular Latin text used by Colonial boys was that prepared by the New England schoolmaster Nathan Bailey, and published under the explanatory title: *English and Latine Exercises for School-Boys, Comprising all the Rules of Syntaxes with Explanations and other necessary Observations on each Rule*. In his preface the author explained that the larger exercises contained "such precepts of religion and morality as ought to be inculcated into the heads of all learners"; and that the whole book was so contrived that besides "Latine, the children may suck in such Principles, as will be of use to them afterwards, in the manly Conduct and Ordering of their Lives.[48]

The quaint sentences found in this work illustrate rules of Latin syntax more or less accurately, and also give the modern reader intimate revelations of the current academic procedure. For example, to show the use of the nominative case before and after the verb "sum" a sentence reads: "Joanna sum spurcus," with its translation, "Jane is a nasty girl."

Disclosures of the following type exemplified other rules: "I slept sound under a form in the school. The Master is angry; you will be sure to smart. School-boys love the chimney corner when their limbs are cold. New and sudden things please Boys; but they soon weary of everything but Play. A rod is prepared for the fool's back."[49] The master counseled his students: "If thou knowest thy Schoolfellow guilty of a Crime, admonish him privately, and tell me not of him, For I delight not in punishing . . . but if he hearken not, make me acquainted. . . . Yet I would by no means have Thee a Telltale or common Accuser."[50]

The schoolmaster, Edward Whittenhall, in 1762 prepared his *Short Introduction to Grammar for the Use of the College and Academy in Philadelphia.* He published his work with some hestitation, for he said in his preface: "It may be thought improper to trouble the World with any new Attempts to improve the Latin Grammar, after such a Variety of Books on this subject." Whittenhall explained the existence of his book by announcing that his experience as a teacher had shown him that some grammars were too short, others too long, but that his book "sought to remove these difficulties." Since it was only after taking second thought that the founders of the Philadelphia Academy had included the classics in their course of studies, Whittenhall evidently sought to justify the compromise, for he wrote of the merits of Latin grammar:

Grammar is the Sacrist that bears the Key of Knowledge by whome alone admittance can be had into the Temple of the Muses, and Treasures of Arts; even whatever can enrich the Mind, and raise it from the Level of a Barbarian and Ideot, to the Dignity of an Intelligence. But this Sacrist is a severe Mistress, who being once contemned, will certainly revenge the Injury. . . .[51]

Even from this brief consideration of the importance attached to the study of Latin grammar by most educators of this time, the modern reader can appreciate Franklin's demand for more advanced training in English—the language spoken by the masses of Colonial children. Distressed by the general indifference to the teaching of the mother tongue, Franklin gave expression to his dissatisfaction when he wrote:

But where is English taught at present? Who thinks it of use to study correctly that Language which he is to use every Day of his Life. . . . ? Every one is suffered to form his own Stile by Chance; to imitate the first wretched model which falls in his Way. . . . Few think their Children qualified for a Trade till they have been whipt at a Latin school for five or six years, to learn a little of that which they are obliged to forget; when in those years right Education would have improv'd their Minds, and taught them to acquire Habits of writting their own Language easily under right direction.[52]

Although Franklin recommended the use of the Brightland and Greenwood *English Grammar,* a British work, the first text of this type to be used extensively in Colonial schools was *A New Guide to the English Tongue,* written by Thomas Dilworth in London in 1740, and reprinted by the Franklin press in 1747. Besides alphabets, syllabaries, and illustrated fables, the grammar also contained for the first time word lists for spelling, which ranged in the order of their difficulty from those of "two letters—one vowel and one consonant, such as go and ox," to those of six syllables, like Me-so-po-ta-mi-a.[53] Previous to the appearance of this book, most American children had learned spelling incidentally with their reading, and generally from selections in the Bible. The reader may get an idea of the pronunciations of the time from selections found in Dilworth's table of words, "the same in sound, but different in spelling and significance," two groups of which follow:

> Air, one of the Elements
> Are, they are
> Heir, to an Estate
>
> Barbara, a woman's name
> Barbary, a Country
> Barberry, a Fruit[54]

Almost from the beginning of the century, boys and girls in the Quaker schools of Pennsylvania used George Fox's *Instructions for Right Spelling and Plain Directions for Reading and Writing True English.* This work also contained a surprising section on homonyms similar to that found in Dilworth's *Guide:*

> He has 3 *Sutes* of Apparel, and 3 *Suits* in Law.
> Ask the Carpenter for his *Ax.*
> He *cool'd* his milk because he *could* not eat it so hot.
> A *Parson* or Priest, a third *Person.*
> The highest *Room* in the House, the City of *Rome*
> If he *were* wise, he would *wear* warmer clothes.
> For want of *Victuals,* his *Vitals* were faint.
> A *Tomb* or Sepulchre; the first *tome* of a Book.
> It is *neither* thee nor I can lift the *nether* millstone.[55]

Among the interesting items included in this book is a long section devoted to the "signification of the Proper Names in Scripture," and another on the "weights, measures, and coyns" mentioned in the Bible.[56] The spelling words of this work were not given in lists, but underscored in selections which frequently contained vital points of conduct or an exposition of Quaker belief:

Sarah was a good Woman. Jezebel was a bad Woman who killed the Just, and turned against the Lord's Prophets with her attired Head and painted Face peeping out of the Window.

Christ I must feel within me who is my Life and my Light, and Truth; and that is God that Shewth me my Thoughts and Imaginations of my Heart.[57]

It was probably to improve the methods of such "instruction in spelling and pronunciation" as the foregoing that Franklin advocated his *Proposals:* "To form their Pronunciation, they may be put on making Declamations, repeating Speeches, and delivering Orations; the Tutor assisting at the Rehearsals, teaching, and correcting their accent."[58]

Anthony Benezet, the great Quaker reformer, taught in the Philadelphia schools about the middle of the century, and shared Franklin's enthusiasm for improving the civil as well as the religious education of American children. Although Benezet's text, *The Pennsylvania Spelling Book, or Youth's Friendly Instructor and Monitor,* did not differ greatly from other spellers then in use, it did contain some "necessary remarks on the education of the Youth in the country parts of this and neighboring Governments." Benezet deplored the crude methods of instruction employed in almost all the elementary schools in the land, and also denounced the apathy of his neighbors in regard to the training of youth:

When we cast our eyes over the country and consider the little attention and pains employed therein, we must allow that people either do not speak what they think, or that what they mean by education is something else than to qualify their children to be useful and serviceable in life; and to fit them for eternal happiness.[59]

In Benezet's work the reader finds evidences of the double aim expressed by the author and other reformers of this first transitional period for the American educational system: namely, to teach children to be useful in life and to fit them for happiness in eternity. In his advice to overseers and tutors in the common schools of the colony, Benezet set down four rules for their direction in teaching the English language:

1st. That in teaching English, particular care should be taken to make children spell correctly, by exercising them frequently in that necessary branch of their learning.

2nd. That endeavours be used to make the scholars read with proper emphasis and punctuation, to which purpose it will be also necessary, besides the Bible to make use of Historical and Religious Authors, of which the School ought to be furnished with proper setts.

3d. That such parts of grammar as are applicable to the English tongue be taught those Boys who are fit for it, in order to make them write properly.

4th. That the Master as often as is convenient make a practice of dictating to such Scholars some sentence out of some good Author which they are to write after him; then the Master carefully correct it.[60]

Benjamin Franklin made one of the most practical contributions to the store of Colonial textbooks when he revised and reprinted a compendium written by an Englishman, George Fisher. Franklin renamed the book to suit its new environment, and it appeared under the lengthy title: *The American Instructor: or, Young Man's Best Companion; Containing Spelling, Reading, Writing, and Arithmetic, in an Easier Way than any yet published. . . . And also Prudent advice to young Tradesmen and Dealers. The Whole Being better adapted to these American Colonies, than any other Book of the like Kind.* Nothing shows better the progress that had been made in the secularization both of the curricula of the schools and of juvenile reading than does this compendium of useful knowledge. Except for a few oblique references to God, it completely ignores religious topics and concentrates on such interests as bookkeeping, the gauging of various kinds of vessels, precedents of legal writings—such as bonds, bills, indentures, wills, etc.—medical advice, and even "instructions to young women how to pickle and preserve all kinds of fruits and flowers."[61]

Ancient history was required in the study of the classics in the Colonial Latin schools, but it was not until the second half of the eighteenth century that history was treated as a separate subject. Franklin believed that almost all useful knowledge could "be introduced to advantage and with pleasure to the student by his reading the translations of the Greek and Roman historians, and by the modern histories of ancient Greece and Rome." Hence it is not surprising that he devoted more than half the space in his *Proposals* to an exposition of the merits and importance of this comprehensive study.

Franklin, dissatisfied with the old rote method of teaching boys "chronology," laid down several basic rules for a new approach to history by reducing the subject to order and method, and by observing what related to "usuage and custom." Both instructor and student were counseled:

1. To enquire particularly and above all things after the Truth.
2. To endeavour to find out the causes of the Rise and Fall of States.
3. To study the character of the Nations and great Men mentioned in history.
4. To be attentive to such instructions as concern Moral Excellence and the Conduct of Life.
5. Carefully to note every Thing that relates to Religion.[62]

Franklin affirmed that history had a moral value in private economy, since it not only mirrored "all the passions of the human heart" and the snares and vicissitudes of human life, but also explained the reason for the "rules of Prudence, Decency, Justice, and Integrity." To the boys of the 1750's, Franklin's last appeal for the study of history must have been especially alluring, for he showed that historical knowledge furnished youth with the basis of sound politics by revealing the "Advantages of Liberty, the Mischief of Licentiousness, the Benefits arising from good Laws, and a due Execution of Justice."[63] He pointed out the special appreciation for the advantages of liberty and justice which youth might acquire from a careful study of the past, and recommended the *Universal History* in the following paragraph of his *Proposals:*

If the new Universal History were also read, it would give a connected Idea of Human Affairs, which should be followed by the best modern Histories, particularly of our Mother Country; then of these Colonies; which should be accompanied with Observations on their Rise, Encrease, Use to Great Britain, Encouragements, and Discouragements, and the Means to make them flourish and secure their Liberties.[64]

Franklin's plan for teaching American history was delayed for almost half a century, for not only was the idea novel but there were no textbooks available for giving the desired instruction; then too, the war with England turned the attention of potential historians from scholastic pursuits to military or political enterprises. The first American history written especially for children was not produced until the close of the century.[65] Within the next decade, Noah Webster compiled a "Chronological Table of Remarkable Events from the Creation of the World and Adam and Eve, B. C. 4004, to the Death of Lord Nelson, October, 1805." These works gave nothing but the barest outline of events. For example, Webster made no entries in his table between the year 1773, when he noted: "The society of Jesuits suppressed by the pope August 25th"; and the year 1782, when he recorded: "Balloons discovered by S. and J. Montgolfier in France."[66]

As a result of this dearth of historical works, children for the first three-quarters of the century had to be satisfied with general histories, which undoubtedly filled to some extent their need for a more comprehensive understanding of ancient and medieval peoples and customs. Among the texts for universal history, used about the middle of the century, was a work in two small volumes entitled: *A Compendious History of the World from the Creation to the Dissolution of the Roman Republic.* The opening lines of Volume Two give the general tone of the texts in common use, and reveal as well the amount of human interest provided American boys and girls in the books used as supplementary readers or in connection with the study of geography:

The death of Alexander was succeeded by such horrid crimes as generally arise from wild ambition, and inordinate thirst for dominion. The generals who at first governed the provinces . . . thought only of engrossing what power they could into their own hands. For this purpose, the mother, wives, children, brother, and sisters of Alexander, were all in a little while inhumanely murdered; so that not one of this Prince's family was permitted to enjoy a foot of the land he had conquered.[67]

Perhaps a more accurate appraisal of historical thinking and teaching can be gained from some of the sermons, poems, or speeches addressed to Colonial children in the troubled years immediately preceding the War for Independence. Two boys, Philip Freneau and Hugh Brackenridge, in 1771 jointly composed a long poem for their commencement exercises at the College of New Jersey. In this work, entitled *The Rising Glory of America,* the young authors showed that the blessings of agriculture had planted the Colonies from north to south; they recalled the wealth and comforts that science and the "golden stream of commerce" had brought to the land:

> New-York emerging rears her lofty domes,
> And hails from far her num'rous ships of trade,
> Homeward returning annually they bring
> The richest produce of the various climes.
> And Philadelphia mistress of our world,
> The seat of arts, of science, and of fame
> Derives her grandeur from the pow'r of trade.
> Hail happy city where the muses stray,
> Where deep philosophy convenes her sons
> And opens all her secrets to their view!
> Bids them ascend with Newton to the skies,
> And trace the orbits of the rolling spheres,
> Survey the glories of the universe,
> Its suns and moons and ever blazing stars!
> Hail city blest with liberty's fair beams,
> And with the rays of mild religion blest![68]

Assuming the role of prophets, these boys sketched their vision of the rising glory of America:

> And here fair freedom shall forever reign.
> I see a train, a glorious train appear,
> Of Patriots plac'd in equal fame with those
> Who nobly fell for Athens or for Rome.

> The sons of Boston resolute and brave
> The firm supporters of our injur'd rights,
> Shall lose their splendours in the brighter beams
> Of patriots fam'd and heroes yet unborn.[69]

That the young authors just quoted reflected the same optimism which inspired their elders at the opening of the Revolutionary War, is shown in an address made by Timothy Dwight, a tutor at Yale College in 1776. Dwight not only pointed out the advantages accruing to the thirteen colonies from their unique sameness in manners, interests, language, religion, and essential principles of civil government; he also reminded his young audience that their ancestors, with the same attachment to science as to freedom, had instituted schools, and had diffused knowledge in every part of their settlements.[70] He also predicted, with extraordinary foresight, the important place the future held for the United States in global affairs; and sought accordingly to raise his pupils from their provincial interpretation of life to his own clear, broad view of America as a world power:

The period in which your lot is cast, is possibly the happiest in the roll of time. It is true, you will scarcely live to enjoy the summit of American glory; but you now see the foundations of that glory laid. . . . You should by no means consider yourselves as members of a small neighborhood, town or colony only, but as beings concerned in laying the foundations of American greatness. Your wishes, your designs, your labours are not confined by the narrow bounds of the present age, but are to comprehend succeeding generations, and to be pointed to immortality. You are to act not like inhabitants of a village, nor like beings of an hour, but like citizens of a world, and like candidates for a name that shall survive the conflagration.[71]

Mathematics in the most progressive Colonial schools included arithmetic, accounts, and some of the first principles of geometry and astronomy. In the ordinary seats of learning, the fundamentals of arithmetic were taught without textbooks.[72] The masters of the common schools were usually equipped with a painfully prepared manuscript "sumbook" which they had made in their own school days. Although this subject was not obligatory, even in those sections where the Colonial governments controlled education, the knowledge of arithmetic, because it was practical, was a decided asset to any teacher in obtaining a new school or private pupils. Those persons were considered learned who had a reputation for being "good at figures." The ability "to do any sum in arithmetic" invariably raised a teacher above his less talented colleagues in the estimation of his pupils and patrons.[73] Besides a section given to mathematics in such works as the *American Preceptor,* or in Bradford's *Young Man's Companion,* the first purely arithmetical text published in the colonies was Hodder's *Arithmetick; or, that Necessary Art Made Most Easy.*[74] This English work was most popular with the apprentices who desired to improve their "cyphering" in the short periods the masters allowed such boys for self-advancement.

The ordinary method of teaching arithmetic was quite easy; it simply meant assigning a pupil who could read and write a page from the master's homemade sum-book or from a printed text. Any student who could read a problem was expected to be able to solve it without special explanation from his master; hence it is not surprising to find recorded of the American artist, Jonathan Trumbull, that he spent three weeks before his lone efforts "over a single sum in long division" were crowned with success.[75]

Anthony Benezet, renowned in the Quaker schools of Philadelphia, tried to remedy this haphazard method of instruction by recommending that teachers and overseers give first place to the most practical rules of arithmetic, "leaving those that are abstruse and not generally necessary, to boys of the brightest genius or leisure." Benezet also suggested his own method of providing each boy with "a small but very plain set of Merchant Account Books, viz., a Day Book, or Journal and Ledger," just sufficient to acquaint the students with the simplest entries of debtor and creditor. Boys were to copy these "in a neat and correct manner," and the master was to see that they understood what they were doing.[76]

Most adults took a firm stand in demanding that boys and girls should write a "fair hand and swift,"[77] since the ability to write well was not only a useful accomplishment, but also the unfailing mark of good breeding. To promote the strong freehand desired by the upper and middle classes as a badge of their social status, children's books cautioned the masters to be particularly careful to make the pupils sit in the proper position at their writing desks, and to insist that they hold their quill pens at the prescribed angle; for on these points, it was affirmed, "their perfection in writing very much depended."[78]

The teacher generally made model copies of extracts from the Bible or from the *School of Good Manners* for his pupils' imitation, but there were also samples of various styles of script in the "compendiums of knowledge" used in many schools. One of these books, *The American Instructor,* gave the children directions for making quill pens and indicated in verse other equipment needed by the young penman for his writing lesson:

A Pen-knife, Razor Metal, Quills good store
Gum Sandrick Powder, to pounce paper o'er;
Ink, shining black; Paper more white than Snow,
Round and flat Rulers on yourself bestow,
With willing Mind, these, and industrious Hand
Will make this Art your Servant at Command.[79]

Colonial girls, commonly discriminated against in the matter of educational opportunities, were generally denied the advantages which enlightened educators sought for boys. Benjamin Franklin, the ardent reformer of the old school system, directed not one sentence of his *Proposals for the Education of the Youth of Pensilvania* to the girls of that colony. Anthony Benezet, on the other hand, defied the prevailing traditions, and in 1755 established a school of his own for the "instruction of females." In this regard, it is perhaps significant that Benezet also interested himself in the status of the Negro slaves of America, and founded an evening school in Philadelphia for people of that race.[80]

A brief examination of the educational philosophy of James Nelson is interesting, because the training usually given Colonial girls mirrored so faithfully his ideas. In his *Essay on the Government of Children* Nelson cautioned parents to make their offspring "pleasing and useful." From his infancy the boy was to be taught to consider himself as continually seen by someone for the first time; and thus to conduct himself in such a manner as to deserve esteem. Since the other aim of education was to make the lad useful, he was to be trained in those studies that would insure his success and happiness, as well as best develop his natural talents. Because the law gave men superior power, the father was advised to be careful to foster in his son a "tender regard for the opposite sex." The boy was not to become a slave, or to degenerate into effeminacy, or to be the "dupe of those who study to allure," but he was to have a just sense of the merits of girls, and to resolve never to insult or oppress them.[81]

Nelson pointed out that the education of the girl should consist of a rudimentary knowledge of her own tongue, a little French, music, arithmetic, drawing, and geography. She should not aim at deeper or more learned studies, because they would make her affected or pedantic; for the educated female, in this author's opinion, was "a pain to herself and disgustful to all who converse with her, particularly her own sex." Since a degree of subjection was the allotted status of the girl, the fruits of her education were to appear in her actions. Besides her knowledge of books, the "exercise of her needle and her pen," and an ability to cast simple accounts, she was to understand the management of a house, to be acquainted with the various times for storing provisions, with market prices, skill in carving, demeanor at table—in a word, the whole economy of a family. Above all, the girl was to know that her province was to please and that every deviation from this objective was thwarting nature; but that a cheerful fulfillment of her duties would secure her own happiness and the esteem of others.[82]

James Burgh, an English contemporary of Nelson, did not fully agree with him in this pinched view of female training; for he argued that "a foolish head was always contemptible, whether it was covered with a girl's cap or a boy's wig." Burgh pointed out that "without some acquaintance of history and the sciences in addition to the accomplishments just described, a woman's conversation must be confined within a very narrow compass, and that she would give and receive little pleasure in the company of her husband and his friends, if she could discuss no topics "except fashions and scandals."[83] The view that a woman should receive something more than an elementary and domestic training in order to be pleasing to her male associates was later to prove an entering wedge in opening for her the door to secondary education.

Educational trends in the life of the Colonial child for the first seventy-five years of the eighteenth century indicate that potent social forces were at work altering imperceptibly the basis of the old system of juvenile instruction. Although most schools were still church-controlled and continued to emphasize the traditional classical curriculum, there were also increasing numbers of private institutions of learning offering a quasi-vocational training. Most Colonial scholars viewed with suspicion and alarm the secularization of the course of studies by the introduction of useful subjects. But taken together, church and private schools were not sufficiently numerous or available to educate all children, and thus the system in that respect did not meet the needs of the decades when the masses were chanting, "All men are created equal."

One of the chief aims of American Colonial education was to fit boys and girls for their probable vocation in life, so that they might go forth from the training received in the church, in the school, and in the home equipped to perform properly the duties of a useful and responsible career. This triple system of education, in spite of its patent shortcomings, may have answered the needs of the disturbed decades at the close of the century better than is usually supposed. Colonial boys were trained to be good farmers, merchants, mechanics, or professional men—each coached in the mysteries of his own calling. From their deep religious instruction and from the emphasis placed on "decent behaviour," which formed the very foundation of their training, the boys apparently acquired definite ideas of their responsibilities as founders and heads of families, as well as a salutary self-respect and exalted ideas of their civic duties. Although the girl's schooling was usually confined to a most elemental course of study, her scope of knowledge was extended by the training she received in the management of a home as an almost self-sufficient economic unit. In addition to her traditional round of household duties, the girl's powers were further exercised by child care and by the spinning and weaving of garments. When the acid test of wartime demands was applied to this educational system at the close of the century, the men who had been trained by its tenets went forth to win and establish a new free government; while the women whose morale had roots in the same source provided food, clothing, and blankets for the patriot army, and seemed to have been able to manage their households during that long, trying crisis. If the aim of child-training was to fit boys and girls for life, and to develop in them a proper sense of values—both temporal and eternal—these first groping attempts of Colonial educators seem to have attained a fair measure of success.

The enthusiasm of the Founding Fathers of the United States for more perfect government manifested itself in a crusade for educational reforms as well as in the establishment of a new nation. The realm of education was to be made more perfect by the extension of human knowledge through the instruction of the masses, and by making the curriculum of the common schools more useful. Although the new federal Constitution provided for the separation of church and state and thus gave a free hand to patriotic statesmen who dreamed of training all children for the duties of citizenship, a free public school system was not immediately forthcoming. The legislators were indeed willing to prepare the children of all social and economic levels for an intelligent participation in government; but the resolution of the first national politicians wavered when confronted with the necessity of levying taxes for school support. The question of taxes had been a dangerous, vital issue from Colonial days; and consequently it was avoided for several decades.[84]

The political leaders, in spite of this initial hesitation to embark on a more comprehensive program of instruction, did effect some significant achievements. The chief of these was the forthright statement of their educational aims in the Northwest Ordinance of 1787, in which they affirmed: "Religion, morality, and knowledge, being necessary to good government and the happiness of mankind, schools and the means of education shall forever be encouraged."[85] In these words the Founding

Fathers clearly envisioned a simultaneous development of the country and its school system. Washington, in his message to Congress in January 1790, supported the proposals for popular education: "Knowledge is in every country the surest basis of public happiness. In one, in which the measures of government receive their impression so immediately from the sense of the community, as in ours, it is proportionably essential."[86]

Although liberal national leaders aspired to democracy in education, the plans for such a system were slow in forming and still slower in being realized, because much of the energy and attention of this group was directed to buttressing the foundation of the new government. As a temporary measure to fill immediate needs while the government was in its formative stage, numerous philanthropic citizens formed themselves into school societies or propaganda agencies. This propaganda finally fructified after the middle of the century in the present system of public instruction. In the meantime incorporated schools—either under the direction of these organizations or under the control of local communities—implemented such long-established institutions as the academy or church school by supplying elementary knowledge to those American children whose parents did not meet this need in the home.[87]

The monitorial system of instruction borrowed from England did much from 1806 to 1840 to popularize the common elementary school not only by substituting group training for individual instruction, but by reducing the cost of schooling. Joseph Lancaster, the promoter of these schools, spent much time in this country between 1818 and 1838, in interesting philanthropic societies in the project and in establishing and directing institutions for teaching the three R's to underprivileged children. Although the system was short-lived, its branches spread throughout New York, Pennsylvania, and Connecticut, where the governors endorsed the plan, and also in the new western cities such as Detroit, Cincinnati, and Louisville, and in New Orleans.[88]

Under the highly organized Lancasterian system as many as a thousand pupils could be assembled in one room under the direction of one teacher; for the children were assorted according to their age and ability, and were seated in rows of ten under the immediate care of monitors. These monitors were first taught reading, writing, spelling, simple arithmetic, and in some cases catechism, which they in turn taught the thirty or more pupils assigned to them. To guide the monitors a *Manual of Instruction* was prepared which covered such problems as classification, the use of the library, and the approved method for group recitation as well as discipline. The following sections, for example, illustrate some of the disciplinary devices employed and also the function of the library:

Badges of merit and disgrace marks are made of little pieces of wood 6 inches long, 3 broad, and ¼ of an inch thick. They have two holes in them, to admit a piece of packthread by which they are suspended around the neck of the children. On one side of the badge are written the words, "First Boy" "Playing Mark" "Idle Mark" "Dirty Mark" etc.

The school should have a collection of amusing and instructive books, to be chosen by the committee, which may be lent to the best pupils in the school as a reward for their good conduct. The library is placed upon a platform either at the side or behind the master's desk.[89]

The regular cost of instructing a pupil by this system was estimated to be about four or five dollars for a year; but the record shows that in some cases even smaller allowances were made to suffice. In Philadelphia during the winter of 1799, thirty "indigent boys" were taught the ordinary branches of an English school at night classes with a total revenue of $16.37.[90] This unusual management evoked a classic remark from one of the sponsors to the effect that "the teachers evinced an extraordinary exercise of economy, and close devotion of their time and talents to the object of their association."[91] Even though this remarkable economy had a strong appeal to most Americans, other features of the Lancasterian system were obnoxious, and eventually spelled the doom of an institution still regarded by some as "the branch of that wonderful providence which is destined to usher in the millennial day." Advocates of this type of charity school pointed out the democratic aims of the system:

All the children of a village or a neighborhood may meet together on the same footing, be disciplined by the same rules, inspired by the same emulation, influenced by the same motives, taught the same lessons, impressed with the same moral sentiments, and fitted for life on an equality that no other system can afford.[92]

The Lancasterian charity school, from the first decade of its existence, had convinced many observers that it was to be permanent in the United States. Most Americans cherished deeply ingrained ideals of independence, and were reluctant to accept any English educational theory that branded its pupils with the stigma of poverty and inferiority. Some evidence of this independent spirit, even among America's destitute, may be found in a rather plaintive report of a philanthropic group:

In the United States the benevolence of the inhabitants has led to the establishment of Charity Schools which though affording individual advantages, are not likely to be followed by the political benefits kindly contemplated by their founders. *There is a disposition in the people averse to dependence. In the country, a parent will raise children in ignorance sooner than place them in Charity Schools. It is only in the larger cities that Charity Schools succeed to any extent.*[93]

Different types of schools were not only brought under examination and criticism, but the methods and books of instruction, and the government of the child were also much-debated subjects. Public opinion proclaimed the need of useful knowledge among Americans and was reflected in a tiny juvenile book, *Wisdom in Miniature:* "Useful knowledge can have no enemies, except the ignorant: It cherishes youth, delights the aged, is an ornament in prosperity, and yields comfort in adversity."[94] Although the goal of perfection in the education of boys and girls was maintained in the middle thirties by leaders of American thought, most laymen did not yet consider a public school system to be the medium of that perfection. The small numbers of public schools that existed were poorly subsidized—in some states by local taxes, and in others by meager returns from the land grants—hence free public instruction was without prestige except in a few isolated communities. Public schools were usually disdained by the rich and the poor, as a result of the injudicious economy of state legislatures in their appropriations for education.[95] Noah Webster, in his *Elements of Useful Knowledge,* reviewed the status of education at the turn of the century:

Notwithstanding the numerous improvements in the means of education within the last twenty or thirty years, much remains to be done towards facilitating the acquisition of general knowledge and useful science. . . . The elementary works on geography, biography, natural history, and other subjects proper for the use of schools seem to be imperfect.

Our whole system of instruction is still more defective in the number of sciences taught in ordinary schools and academies. Many of the most useful sciences and arts are not taught at all, or very imperfectly—nor have we books well calculated for the purpose.

Most of the books now used in schools for reading are composed of solemn didactic discourses, general lessons of morality, or detached pages of history. These are indeed useful; but may not children read for common lessons the known and established principles in philosophy, natural history, botany, rhetoric, mechanics, and other sciences?[96]

The dissatisfaction with the school system and with the books employed in the teaching approximated a humanitarian crusade, and in zeal almost rivaled the antislavery agitation or the temperance movement.[97] Among the feminine reformers was Lydia Huntley Sigourney, who in 1810 at the age of nineteen had established a school for girls at Norwich, Connecticut, and subsequently devoted herself to teaching and writing in behalf of the young. To raise the standards of the common schools, Mrs. Sigourney suggested that they be made more select, since they were often so crowded, and the groups "exhibited such disparity of age," that individual improvement was necessarily impeded. Hence the Prussian plan was repeatedly advocated, whereby fifteen students were considered an "ample number for a single mind to rule and operate upon to advantage."[98]

Some idea of the existing faults of the schools can be gained from the reforms suggested. For instance, it was proposed that those institutions that sought improvement should establish habits of order and punctuality; that the school hours should be divided into a schedule for the different studies and adapted to the needs of each class; that rules embracing the duties and deportment of the students should be drawn up, explained, daily read, and, if necessary, the signatures of the pupils taken as a pledge of their assistance in improving classroom discipline.[99] For many years the question of enforcing proper school discipline had disturbed American educators. The first vestige of that freedom and self-expression which now characterize American youth appeared simultaneously with the change in adult methods from repressing the young to entertaining them.

Caleb Bingham, "an experienced instructor" of New England, and the author of the *American Preceptor,* discussed at length in 1821 the growing difficulties confronting the members of his profession as a result of children's complaints about school. Familiar echoes of Bingham's sentiments might be heard today at educational conventions. He asked that parents consider the variety of circumstances that exaggerated the "evil reports of children respecting their teachers." Citing the natural defects and weaknesses of their age, he showed that children usually judged hastily and too often misrepresented things. He remarked that the young not only hated those who restrained them, but resented any correction in exact proportion to their love of "change, idleness, and the indulgencies of their home." Like all human beings, they did not know when they were well off, and were wont to complain. Parents were warned to be slow in abusing the character and disturbing the happiness of teachers who "probably deserved thanks rather than ill usage; whose office at best was full of care and anxiety; and when it was interrupted by the interference of parents became intolerably burdensome." Speaking from his long experience, Bingham declared that the "whole business of managing a large school, and training pupils in learning and virtue was nothing in comparison to the trouble made by whimsical, ignorant, and discontented parents."[100] In pursuing his "hints to parents" and his comments on the current trends of child training, Bingham wrote:

The time was when modesty was considered an accomplishment in children, and deference to their superiors a duty. But now, almost as soon as they can walk, children are sent to the dancing academy to get rid of their modesty, and to learn disregard for their elders and superiors. . . . It is no wonder that so many of our young people decorate their persons instead of adorning their minds, and parade at the corners of our streets, instead of attending to their business or studies.[101]

The low salaries paid the teachers were another cause for grievance with the school system. These were generally not sufficient to induce well-educated men to choose the work of instruction as a life profession. The point was often made that schools would acquire prestige and enjoy a more permanent policy if the communities could be convinced that parsimony was ill-placed where the mental and moral culture of youth was concerned. Most teachers who engaged in teaching for a transient period, using their schools as stepping-stones to more lucrative positions, were often occupied at the same time with the study of the profession on which their future living was to depend. Hence the charge was made that many brought "but wandering thoughts and divided affections to a service which demanded a concentration of both." To remedy this defect, there were insistent demands by the 1830's for the establishment of normal schools. It was thought these training centers would be "a great blessing" to the country, since in the primary and in the ungraded district schools, where reformation was needed, the education of the teachers was most defective.[102]

The need for a well-chosen library in connection with the remote village school was clearly apparent by the 'thirties. Writers often proposed that a regular system of drawing out and returning books be established, and the right of reading books be used as a reward for good scholarship and correct conduct. In the few schools equipped with a library, a common rule prevailed that those who were "favored with the perusal of a volume, should render some account of its contents to the teacher in the presence of the school, that all may share the benefit."

The new interest in the personality of the child deepened the conviction that some specialized knowledge was requisite for the teacher in order to guide even the youngest pupils to improvement. Yet it was noted that in obscure villages, "if there was any decayed old woman, who was too feeble to earn a living by the spinning wheel or needle, it was thought that she would do to keep a school for the little ones—

at that most plastic period of life when the impressions received were to last forever."[103] Since most male teachers were woefully underpaid, the teaching career, on the primary level, was no longer attractive to men. The only alternative then in replacing the "decayed old women" of the dame schools was to convince "young ladies of affluence" that the work of instruction was not beneath them. Those interested in school reform were not slow to organize their propaganda around this theme, or to direct it at prospective "schoolmarms." It was pointed out that teaching was one of the best modes for young ladies to complete their own education, to consolidate their knowledge, or even to prepare themselves for marriage, since teaching induced habits of order, industry, and self-control, and gave besides "that knowledge of human nature so valuable in the management of a household."

Reasons peculiar to the United States were advanced to show why women should qualify themselves to conduct the whole education of their sex. In this country, the roads to wealth and distinction were thrown open to all classes. Men were constantly induced by tempting possibilities to forsake teaching for greater gain. Individuals of every rank of American society were stimulated by some form of competition and were restless to acquire a fortune. Most energetic men, motivated by incentives to wealth and power, would not stoop to the drudgery of teaching ignorant children. These men, attuned to the idea of living eventually in easy circumstances, were not usually contented with the petty salary of a teacher.[104]

Although a few learned or benevolent men devoted themselves permanently to the work of education, their number was small in proportion to the wants of the country, in which the population was rapidly increasing and constantly migrating. The pioneers of the unplanted wilds or the settlers on the western prairies could scarcely be expected to gather around them the children of an infant settlement to teach them the rudiments of science or to direct the development of morals and character. Much less would men of enterprise turn from their schemes of railroads, canals, or land speculation to submit to the tedious process of teaching, or to study the nameless refinements of "female culture." The wealthy secured men of talents to educate their sons and daughters, but these were exceptions. Here then was a sphere into which the "patience and quietness" of the early American woman could enter and win a permanent niche in the economic and social life of the nation that had offered her so few places of honor.[105]

Much of the discontent with the system of instructing the young had its roots in the scarcity of good textbooks for the few subjects taught in the elementary schools. When the major political crises had passed after 1787, and men could again turn their thoughts to perfecting the educational system, numerous regrets were voiced about the lack of proper juvenile books. In the preface of *Miscellanies, Moral and Instructive,* the author stated this common grievance: "Very few attempts have been made to supply this deficiency by introducing something on such a plan as might, besides improving the understanding and morals, instructively amuse the vacant hours of young people, and have a tendency to render the task a more agreeable employment."[106]

This little book also defined for its young readers the aim of education: "The use of learning is not to procure popular applause or to excite vain admiration, but to make the possessor more virtuous and useful to society, and his virtue a more conspicuous example to those that are illiterate."[107] To achieve the ends of education—to make boys and girls more virtuous and more useful to society—the new texts stressed the importance of reading. In the decades from the opening of the Revolutionary War to 1835, a host of little readers had supplanted the *New England Primer.* The majority of these books were published in the middle states, particularly in the cities of Philadelphia and New York. Most of the primers attempted to simplify and improve the instructional procedure, but much confidence was still placed in the old rote method. One author observed:

The minds of little children are extremely liable to be confused, and in giving them instruction, too much care cannot be taken to have but a few objects before them at one time. The most expeditious method of teaching the alphabet is by dividing it into lessons of from three to six letters, and by making the scholar perfect master of the first, before he proceeds to the second, and so on through every lesson.[108]

Among the first of the new primers was the *A B C with the Church of England Catechism* which was published in Philadelphia in 1785 for the Episcopal Academy of that city. Besides the usual introduction to reading, this little book contained the Christmas hymn, "While Shepherds Watch'd Their Flocks by Night," and an Easter hymn which began with the words: "So count yourselves as dead to sin. . . ."[109] An American adaptation of two primers by the English writer Mrs. Barbauld was prepared in Philadelphia by "A Mother" for her own children. In the first of these books, *Lessons for Children from Two to Four Years Old,* the editor explained that the "climate and familiar objects suggested alterations of the English texts." The form and content of the old texts were coming under scrutiny, for the American editor remarked that "amid the multitude of books written professedly for children," there was not one for the very small. A modern reader would be astounded by the comment that "a grave remark or a connected story is above the capacity of a two-year-old, and nonsense is always below it; for Folly is worse than Ignorance." Other defects of the old primers—the want of good paper, a clear, large type, and adequate spaces between letters and words—were supposedly remedied in the new baby books. Since these works were among the first attempts at this reform, the American editor explained that only those who had actually taught young children could appreciate "how necessary these assistances were," for she affirmed that the eye of a child could "not catch a small, obscure, ill-formed word, amidst a number of others all equally unknown to him." The tiny folk of that generation apparently owed much gratitude to that progressive but anonymous mother for sparing their eyesight—a reform which she described as "laying the first stone of a noble building."[110]

To illustrate how far even these first departures from the *New England Primer* had gone in laying aside the religious tone of that work and in using the tools of realistic writers, the following reading lesson may be noted:

Bring the tea things. Bring the little boy's milk. Where is the bread and butter? Where is the toast and the muffin? Little boys do not eat butter. Sop the bread in your tea. The tea is too hot, you must not drink it yet. Pour it into your saucer. The sugar is not melted.[111]

Volume II of this work continued in the same secular tone to tell "pretty stories" to children of four. When Charles, the hero, was asked why he was better than Puss, the answer made no reference to his immortal soul, as earlier books most certainly would have done:

Puss can play as well as you; and Puss can drink milk, and lie upon the carpet; and she can run as fast as you, and climb trees better; and she can catch mice which you can not do. But can Puss talk? No. Can Puss read? No. Then that is the reason why you are better than Puss—because you can talk and read.[112]

The Fortune Teller; or an Alphabet without Tears, which was a reprint of an English work by the same title, was published in Philadelphia in 1793. This little primer not only shows the trend towards the secularization of textbooks which was going apace, but also the first stirrings of the reform movements, particularly that of temperance:

> B   Blockhead, throw by the book and run to play,
>   Nor take the killing pains to learn great A.
>   But soon thou shalt thy wretched fate deplore,
>   And poor and ragged beg from door to door.

D Drunkard, go fill thy glass and banish care,
    And in the sparkling bowl drown every fear,
    But wealth consum'd and health forever lost,
    Shall end thy mirth and be the fatal cost.[113]

Easy Lessons for Children by an anonymous author was published in Philadelphia in 1794, and held between its fancy flowered covers some of the happiest lessons for beginners so far offered the American child. Its little stories must have made a strong appeal to both boys and girls. The first lesson, for instance, was written for the child who loved her dolls:

Miss Jane Smith had a new doll bought for her, and her good Aunt gave her some cloth to make her a shift, and a coat, and a pair of stays, and a yard of twist with a tag to it for a lace; she gave her a pair of red shoes, and a piece of blue silk to make her a slip, and some gauze for a frock, and a broad white sash. Now these were nice things, you know, but Miss Jane had no thread, so she could not make Doll's cloaths when she had cut them out; but her dear good Aunt, gave her some thread too, and then she went hard to work, and made Doll quite smart in a short time.[114]

Little boys were taken to see the sights of Philadelphia:

I shall take you to Philadelphia, William, said Mr. Chandler to his son, on purpose to shew you some sights. . . . First they went to see the city library, then the museum . . . then the Market Street Meeting House, which is a very fine place indeed; afterwards they went to the congress-hall and saw the President deliver an address to both houses of congress amidst many fine gentlemen. . . .[115]

Another attempt to revive interest in the old primer resulted in a small book entitled *Beauties of the New England Primer*. Its editor stated that as the old work had become almost useless "on account of its catechism," he had compiled the new version. This edition he hoped would be acceptable to the children of his own day, and "to those which may follow, and afford an opportunity to gather some good hints from a work that for generations had been a first book for their forefathers." Appearing as it did with other primers whose contents were more attractive to the young than the selections "As runs the glass, our life doth pass," or "Youth should delight in doing right,"[116] this work retarded slightly, but did not prevent, the passing of the old primer.

The Wonderful History of an Enchanted Castle Kept by the Giant Grumbo was quite pietistic in tone, but not oppressively so, for its element of mystery offered a perpetual appeal to children. The young reader was told that the Enchanted Castle occupied by the Giant Grumbo could be visited by good children. Although Grumbo was described as "the most

humane and tenderhearted giant in the known world," he did not pre-
side as host in the castle. When children sounded the knocker, the porter
would ask them whether they had been good and had said their prayers;
if they could answer in the affirmative, he would bid them look at the
opposite wall where the little ones could find a number of verses written
in golden letters:

> B is a beauty all cheerful and gay,
> But her beauty soon fades like a flower in May.
>
> Y is a youth who loved reading and writing,
> Which he found was far better than swearing and fighting.[117]

The American Primer, printed and sold by Mathew Carey of Philadelphia in 1813, was probably one of the worst offenders of aesthetic
taste among the juvenile books published in this country. Besides syllabaries and lists of spelling words, this primer also contained an alphabet,
illustrated by birds and beasts and by certain depraved types of human
beings, beginning with "A stands for Ape," to "Z for Zany"—a weeping
boy wearing a dunce cap. Short selections for reading accompanied some
of the letters. "Zany," for instance, was followed by the comments: "If
you do not take pains to spell, you will not know how to read, but will
be a great dunce. I would not have my dear child a dunce for all the
world; it is a shame."[118] In preparing his woodcuts, the engraver apparently gave little thought to proportion in his illustrations of birds and
beasts. The mouse is at least half as large as the "nag," the rat is larger
than the bear or the elephant, while the pig and the hare are of equal size.

Traces of the Federalist influence may be detected in the denunciation
of the radical trends of the French Revolution as they were recorded
for young readers in the stories written by French émigrés in England
and later copied in this country. One of these juvenile works, *The Remarkable History of Augi: or a Picture of True Happiness,* shows the
prevailing sentiment in its closing sentence:

Augi, who had the solid advantages of a rationalistic education, was married to
an amiable wife, and found himself the happiest of mortals. This happy
family by the effort of skillful labour, and without oppression or injustice
to the poor, became extremely rich. . . . The great Revolution in the year 1789
arrived . . . the eager multitude surrounded his house, his property was pillaged,
his life destroyed. . . . His aged parents perished in the flames that consumed his
mansion. His distracted wife, unable to support the dreadful shock, left him
six female orphans, who were at first conducted to the receptacle for foundlings,
and afterwards turned adrift to seek their fortunes through the unfeeling world.
O Liberty! how dearly do thy blessings cost a nation who purchases thee by
crimes![119]

Anti-war propaganda found in the little books for boys and girls published between the years 1812 and 1815 was particularly vehement. *The Seven Wonders of the World,* printed by Samuel Wood of New York in 1814, makes nice distinctions between natural and artificial evils, and declares that the miseries of the poor are chiefly occasioned "by the oppression, cruelty, or sordid and unjust stewardship of those who have power." This train of thought leads directly to the sufferings of war:

A wise man observed: 'The very trimmings of the vain world would clothe the naked one.' More lamentable is the immense destruction of time and property to say nothing of depravity of morals, loss of lives, or the soul, occasioned by war. When the noble hero who has ransacked cities, villages, and laid waste countries is obliged to view the past without any false coloring, to stand the test of an awful tribunal, and his conscience is suffered to do its duty, what must be his sensations?[120]

Among the best examples of temperance and antislavery propaganda for youthful consumption was the *Instructive Alphabet,* a New York publication of 1814. Under the picture of a jug, the young reader found the warning:

Jugs are often filled with ardent spirits, which when used with care, is a useful medicine; but, unhappily for mortals, the too free use of this article has destroyed its thousands and ten of thousands: yea it slays even more than the sword.[121]

The antislavery sentiment expressed in "The Negroe's Complaint" is more bitter:

> Deem our nation brutes no longer,
> Till some reason you shall find
> Worthier of regard, and stronger
> Than the colour of our kind.
> Slaves to gold, whose sordid dealings
> Tarnish all your boasted pow'rs,
> Prove that you have human feelings
> Ere you proudly question ours.[122]

The Humorous Alphabet published at Newbury about 1814 was unique in its Celtic gayety. This Irish primer began with the words: "Come here you little O'Shaughnessy, bring your primmer in your hand, and your copper in your fist . . . hold up your head like a man. . . . Don't be hunting the flies across the ceiling, but cock your eye and look straight at your book." An explanation of the alphabet followed, similar in style to the above: "You see that letter which looks for all the world like the gable of your father's cabin, with a beam across it—now that is called

A . . . and the next door neighbor is namesake to the little gentleman that sucks the flowers; fills the honey pots; and carries a long sting in his tail; that is master bee—B."[123] At the end of the last lesson was a woodcut of the hero showing his sisters how well he could read; the cut was headed with an invitation to O'Shaughnessy's friends: "Come Read and Learn from the Battledore."[124]

Primers improved with the years, and by 1835 a few delightful toy books such as *The Little Sketch Book, Tom Thumb's Picture Alphabet in Rhyme,* and the *Book of the Sea for the Instruction of Little Sailors* could easily suggest some of the modern juvenile works in their appreciation of the child's tastes. In the *Little Sketch Book,* such selections as "The Log Cabin" must have piqued the curiosity of boys and girls in older sections of the country who were not compelled to live in such crude homes: "Huts like the one shown above are very common in the wild woods of the western parts of our country. But when the country gets settled, and they have mills for sawing logs into timber and boards, they can build better homes."[125]

Tom Thumb's Picture Alphabet was also far removed in the sentiment of its selections from its pietistic ancestors of the previous century:

> A   is an angler, young but expert,
> B   is a butcher who wears a red shirt.
>
> I   is an iceboat propelled by steam,
> J   is a jockey who drives a gay team.
>
> O   is the farmer's ox that is fattened for beef,
> P   is the parson whose sermons are brief.[126]

Boys must have thrilled especially to the pictures, the sprightly rhymes and descriptions found in *The Book of the Sea for the Instruction of Little Sailors.* Its very title opened for them the door to a world of make-believe, into which none of the dangers of the real sea could enter:

> Like prisoned eagles sailors pine
> On the dull and quiet shore;
> They long for the flashing brine,
> The spray and the tempest roar.
>
> To shoot through the sparkling foam,
> Like an ocean bird set free—
> Like the ocean bird their home
> They find on the raging sea.[127]

Noah Webster's *American Spelling Book* was a minor result of two great forces—the intense patriotism of Revolutionary days and the improvement in scholarship. This work was especially designed to supplant such British texts as Dilworth's *New Guide to the English Tongue.* Webster gave his aim in the preface of this famous "Blue Back Speller": "To diffuse a uniformity and purity of language in America . . . to destroy the provincial prejudices that originate in the trifling differences of dialect and produce reciprocal ridicule . . . to promote the interests of literature and the harmony of the United States."[128]

Webster expressed his contempt of both Dilworth and Fenning, the English authors of standard spellers, on the question of homonyms. He objected to their classing together such words as *consort* and *concert,* and said he had omitted several of their words from his lists: "I choose to admit no words but such as sound exactly alike." In spite of his protestations, Webster classed together: *Bow,* to bend, *Bough,* a branch, *Bow,* to shoot with, and *Beau,* a gay fellow. Dilworth placed these words in two groups as in the modern pronunciation.[129] Webster's sentences of advice were apt and terse, but whether they were inspiring to children is doubtful. He warned schoolboys, for example: "Play no tricks on them that sit next to you; for if you do, good boys will shun you as they would a dog that they knew would bite them."[130] Webster's little speller with its sound moral precepts was used for decades to dictate the "orthography" of American youth; just as, during the same period, the portrait of the author with his immense piercing eyes and his hair standing on end was said to have terrified children when they first opened a copy of the "Old Blue Back."

Benjamin Johnson, who published the *New Philadelphia Speller* in 1809, gave attention to its aesthetic value. Although the book never attained the popularity of Webster's, it did offer a new approach to the subject; for besides spelling lists, it contained selections in prose and verse from the works of various children's authors, including the story, "The Whistler," by Benjamin Franklin. Among the attractive illustrations were those of the cataract of Niagara and the falls of Passaic. The compiler explained that the chief distinctions of his work were "the fairness of the paper, the size of the type, and the beauty of the ornaments"— points to which he had given much care—"since the children as well as their tutors were often disgusted with the appearance of books badly printed and on dark paper." All were pleased with good printing, he pointed out, and the attention of even dull children was sometimes excited by well-engraved cuts representing objects familiar to them. Frequently boys and girls of small mental capacity were "induced to take the first steps over the threshold of literature by this pleasant route, when otherwise, perhaps the rod or the dunce cap would be employed to urge them forward." An interesting feature of this work was the list of proper names, which included the following for males: Aaron, Caleb, Cyrus, Ephraim, Isaac, Nathan, Jonathan, Joshua, Ezekiel, Nathaniel, and Theophilus. Feminine names also indicated their biblical or mythological origins: Esther, Phebe, Sarah, Martha, Abigail, Deborah, Margaret, and Penelope.[131]

Reference to the scarcity of English grammars for colonial children has been made previously in this study. To help fill this need, Henry Osborne of Charleston, South Carolina, compiled in 1785 *An English Grammar Adapted to the Capacities of Children.* Among the subscribers to this little book were General Pinckney, Colonel Laurens, Peter Freneau, and Mrs. Pierce Butler. In the preface, the author declared that "English grammar was now considered by liberal educators as one of those essential parts of education, which every one has now decided upon. . . . The many barbarisms which, from a variety of sources, have mixed with the language of these States, make a book of this kind particularly desirable."[132] His attempt to supply the great variety of rules "which were applicable to every case that could occur," robbed Osborne's work of much of the human interest found in other texts of this type, and reduced his book to a bewildering collection of dry and rather pointless forms.

The Philadelphia Vocabulary, compiled by the English grammarian, James Greenwood, in 1787, made another contribution to the widening curriculum of the American schools. Considering the date and the strained relations with England, the modern reader might be surprised at the woodcut on the title page, which represented the cities of Philadelphia and London with the Atlantic between them, and Britannia greeting the "Cradle of Liberty." Greenwood assured his young readers of the gentleness of his methods by stating that the "burthening of the memory with more than is necessary at the entrance upon any study is certainly a great discouragement to the Learner." He attempted to avoid everything in this Latin-English vocabulary that was not of immediate use; but one of the first words offered to the young student was "vibex" defined as "a wale on the flesh after whipping." On point of variety, the contents of this small book were unique, for they covered such widely ranging subjects as plants, insects, diseases, meats and drinks, apparel, household goods, country affairs, judicial matters, and naval affairs, besides the parts of speech.[133]

One of the best opportunities for observing the change in the status of the child is offered by a comparison of the grammars prepared for children in the decade after 1825 with those published in the late eighteenth century. The new technique of amusing the child and arousing his interest by making forms and principles come to life had quite supplanted the dry formal rules imposed on earlier generations. *The Infant's Grammar,* published in Baltimore in 1825, affords an interesting insight into this happy new approach to language study. Lightly spiced with nonsense, the introduction in verse begins:

> One day, I am told, and, as it was cold,
> I suppose it occur'd in cold weather,
> The Nine Parts of Speech, having no one to teach,
> Resolv'd on a Pic-nic together.

Gaily colored illustrations helped to introduce the child to such guests as the nouns and the verbs found in the verse:

> Some actors of eminence made their appearance,
> And the servants, nouns common, with speed made a clearance
> Of tables, chairs, stools, and such movable things,
> As wherever it goes, the Noun always brings.
> These actors, the Verbs, when they'd room to display,
> Both wrestl'd and tumbl'd; and gambol'd away;
> They play'd and they ran, they jump'd and they danc'd,
> Frisk'd ambl'd, and kick'd, laugh'd, chatter'd and pranc'd.[134]

From his own experiences on such occasions, the ordinary child could readily picture to himself the disorder that greeted the little servant Interjection after the Parts of Speech had enjoyed their feast and fun:

> Having finish'd their Pic-nic without much apology,
> The party all quitted the Hall Etymology;
> But such a litter was scattered about in the room,
> That, when Interjection came up with her broom,
> Her surprise was so great that she nothing could say,
> But, Oh! Ah! Good Lack! Well-a-Day![135]

Punctuation Personified, a little book that might have been used as a supplement to this sprightly grammar, was published a few years later in Steubenville, Ohio. Since there were apparently many young scholars like the hero, Robert, who "could read but he gabbled so fast that he lost all the meaning of his lesson," this work proposed to prove that

> When the stops were plac'd aright,
> The real sense was brought to light.

During Robert's interview with Mr. Stops, one of the most important punctuation marks was introduced:

This fullfaced gentelman here shown,
To all my friends, no doubt, is known:
In him the period we behold,
Who stands his ground whilst four are told;
And always ends a perfect sentence,
As "Crime is followed by repentence."[136]

These attempts to call to life the dry bones of grammatical rules, and also to make the mysteries of arithmetic more appealing to the young, reveal the new interest in childhood. Daniel Fenning in 1795 made an effort to replace the British texts in mathematics, which had been used in those limited cases when books were employed, by publishing his *American Youth's Instructor; or a New and Easy Guide to Practical Arithmetic.* In keeping with the new educational trends, this small volume was written in "a natural and familiar dialogue, in order to render the work more easy and diverting as well as useful to learners." Fenning plainly recognized the meager educational advantages offered most children, for in his preface he noted that his work was intended for those who "had much neglected" the study of arithmetic, and for "others who had neither time nor opportunity to apply to a proper master." For the sake of those living in the country he gave some instruction in measuring a regular piece of timber or a plot of land and for calculating "tyling" and brick work, as well as gauging a cistern or a cask of malt. In spite of his interest in its "practical points," a reader today would find the dialogue tiresome and distracting and would miss the scientific precision of modern texts. But more than a century ago its obscure rules assisted the underprivileged youth "of himself, in a short time to become acquainted with every thing necessary to the knowledge of business."[137]

The arts of penmanship and letter writing had been traditionally developed in the young as the badge of good breeding. In the surge of patriotic ardor that followed the Revolution, numerous guides for these branches were produced by Americans. One of the first works, *The American Letter-Writer,* published in Philadelphia in 1793, set the pace for many others, was subsequently praised by some educators for encouraging children to write naturally, and was blamed by others because, according to its principles, "every idle, thoughtless, superficial scribbler fancies that natural ease consists in dashing upon paper all his insipid trifles, his silly conceits, and his tiresome repetitions."[138]

The question had been settled in Congress, and so the *American Letter-Writer* proceeded to denounce the use of such terms as "Majesty, Royal Highness, Excellency, Worshipful, and the like down to the humble

Esquire," because they were not suitable in a country where all men were declared to be equal.[139] Strangely enough, although royal titles were tabooed, class distinctions were clearly recognized as compatible even where "all men were declared to be equal." This fine distinction of quality is evident in the introductory chapter covering the general rules of letter writing:

When you write to your friend, your letter should be a true picture of your heart, the stile loose and irregular, the thoughts themselves should appear naked, and not dressed in the borrowed robes of rhetoric, for a friend will be more pleased with that part of a letter which flows from the heart, than with that which is the product of the mind.... Above all learn to write correct ... a blot in writing is by no means so bad as a blunder in the sense.... Always subscribe your name in a larger hand than the body part of your letter.... *Letters should be wrote on fine gilt post paper to persons of distinction; but if to your equals or inferiors, you are at your own option to use what sort and size you please; but take care never to seal your letter with a wafer unless to the latter.*

On the subject of letter writing, educators had charged that telling the child his "letters should be easy and natural, had given a sort of sanction to the most careless, slovenly, and incoherent effusions." But the student letters edited by the Boston teacher Caleb Bingham were models of literary propriety. Today they form a valuable contribution to social history by presenting unexpected flashes of early American life. Sophronia Bellmont, who has been quoted before, wrote from Hanover, New Hampshire, to a friend in Boston:

Travellers are well entertained at the public houses here. Notwithstanding which, there are some to be found, who call themselves *gentlefolks,* who, to show their *good breeding,* affect too much delicacy to relish *country* cooking; and carry their disgust so far, as to throw their tea and toast out at the window! I hope such ladies do not come from Boston....

We ventured into the untried wilderness, and have safely reached this place, about sixty miles from Dartmouth College.... We saw many log huts, and out of curiosity called at a number of them. Some were miserable dwellings, having no floors and being poorly covered with bark. I pitied some of the poor children for they were extremely ragged. I hope they do not suffer for food as they do for clothing. The inhabitants are very obliging. It is but ten or twelve years since the first settlers established themselves in this town; and already we see a handsome building for an academy nearly completed. It is pleasing to see such early attention paid to the education of youth.[141]

Laura Lyttleton, in her letters from Northampton to her friend Matilda Maitland, reveals the popular educational objectives for girls:

I have the pleasure to inform you that I have lately been learning to spin. . . . I knit and sew as well as girls in general of my age. My mamma you know is an industrious woman; and though she is anxious to give her children a good education, she is determined that they will all learn how to work. That she says, is an essential part of a good education. To encourage us girls, however, in our labors, she has adopted the following plan. After we have finished our day's work at wheel, we all take our knitting, and seat ourselves around the fire; where each one takes her turn in reading some useful lesson to the rest. We generally gain an hour to spend in this way, before bed time. The story read last evening is found in Park's Travels into the interior parts of Africa.[142]

"Illegible penmanship" was the chief defect in letter writing in the 'thirties, if the numerous complaints on this score are to be taken as an index. One of the most tolerant treatments of this subject is found in *The Daughter's Own Book,* which was first published in Boston in 1833, but later went through numerous editions. The author, a father, informed his daughter that he did not regard it so important that she should attain high excellence in penmanship; yet he desired that her attainments "in this department should be at least respectable." He recommended an easy graceful hand, but above all he would have it possess "the attribute of being legible." Present-day remonstrances on the illegibility of much juvenile handwriting are probably the echoes of this parental ultimatum:

A more odd conceit never entered the human head than seems to have got possession of some at the present day—that a hand which put ones inventions to the torture, is a sure mark of genius. If that be the test, I will only say that I choose to have you run the hazard of being considered a dunce, rather than torment me and your friends with illegible communications. . . . Take up no practice on this subject that will prevent you from being a neat, plain, and if you will, elegant writer.[143]

Patriotic writers sought to pay tribute to their Revolutionary heroes, and particularly to George Washington, even before a history of the new republic had been prepared. A small work was published in 1794 at Philadelphia with the explanatory title: *The Life of General Washington, Commander in Chief of the American Army during the Late War, and present President of the United States. Also of the Grave General Montgomery.* This little book did not recount Washington's achievements "in the late war," but gave intimate glimpses of his home life and of his reactions to the publicity which his services had brought. Of his Philadelphia days this anonymous biographer wrote: "The conspicuous character he has acted on the theatre of human affairs made many official and literary persons, on both sides of the ocean, ambitious of a correspondence with him. These correspondencies unavoidably engross a great portion of his time, and . . . render him the *focus of political intelligence for the new world*."[144] In 1810 John Corry gave a thumb-nail sketch of Washington which he dedicated to the youth of America. This work emphasized the "tall majestic person" of the hero, his manly countenance and strong, well-governed mind, and remarked that although his perceptions were not quick, when once he had taken a position "it was generally well-chosen." Corry thus concluded his summation of Washington's personality:

Neither wit nor vivacity brightened his features; it was a face of care, of doubt, of caution, all was calmness and deliberation—Washington's greatest forte was prudence or discretion; it covered him like a shield in the days of prosperity; by this single talent he acquired all his wealth, and obtained all his celebrity. . . .[145]

The History of America published in Philadelphia in 1795 was the earliest work of its kind written for the children of the United States. The author informed his young readers that a spirit of patriotism had "excited" him to the production of this work, because it was generally acknowledged that the mind "takes a turn in future life suitable to the tincture it hath received." Since the history of the new republic furnished an instructive account of human actions, it was judged important for children to examine the record—"for what the nature of a nation has been, so it is now, and its operations are the same, making due allowance for diversity of circumstances." To make the book more attractive, woodcuts of discoverers, heroes, and the governors of the various states were included, but the greatest economy was practised in this respect. Six woodcuts were designed, all of a striking similarity, but falling roughly into two classes; in one, a tricorn hat with or without a cockade was the distinctive mark, while the other was characterized by a braided periwig. This series of pictures was used over and over, regardless of the time or nationality of the hero. As a result, Christopher Columbus, dressed in the ruffles and frock coat of an eighteenth-century gentleman, and wearing a tricorn hat, is identical with General Montgomery; while Americus Vespucius and John Sullivan, the Governor of New Hampshire, bear a strong family likeness. No special account of Washington is given in the book, although his picture precedes the record for the state of Pennsylvania. The modern reader might question the effect of this interpretation of the Revolutionary period on the patriots of the middle and southern states:

The New England Colonists inherited a love of liberty from their forefathers who had suffered much for their principles in Old England, and sought in a wilderness that freedom which was denied them in the mother country. As they grew in power, they carefully watched over and guarded against the encroachments of the British government. They paved the way for the rest of the colonies to come forward and join them in a united struggle against the unlawful claims of a country whose chains had galled them for many years; till finally the grand and astonishing stroke was struck, which demolished the power of Great Britain over the colonies and left them in possession of an envied sovereignty; as independent states, likely one day to become respectable and dreaded by all Europe for their opulence and power.[146]

Social history was not neglected in this little work; the inhabitants of New York were described as "healthy and robust, breathing a free and serene air, sprightly in their tempers, and instances of suicide rarely seen among them."[147] The child also learned that on the first planting of Maryland there were several nations of Indians there; but "now it is rare to see one in the state: It is, however, well stocked with negroes, which some people think a poor exchange."[148]

The Pilgrim, one of the few juvenile histories of a special section, was published in Philadelphia in 1825. This little work, written in verse, was amply illustrated by woodcuts, and covered the entire history of Massachusetts from the scene of the Pilgrims' leaving England to the details of the annual celebration of their landing in this country. A section of special interest described the Indian warfare:

> But soon the savage bent his bow,
> In wild inhuman strife;
> And oft the Pilgrims' blood did flow,
> Beneath the Indians' knife.[149]

In the illustrations depicting these savage attacks, the Pilgrims can be distinguished even during bloodiest battles by the very high hats which they always wear at the proper angle, for the fury of the fight did not displace one! The terrors spread through the colony by drunken Indians were also given consideration:

> Though fierce by nature, fiercer yet
> The savage would became
> When bought or stolen, he could get
> The poisonous draught of rum.[150]

Lydia Huntley Sigourney gave an account of the bicentenary celebration of the landing of the Pilgrims in her little work *Tales and Essays*

for Children. In describing the recurrence of famine and plague among
the settlers in 1623, she recalled for the edification of later generations
the sufferings of these voluntary exiles:

Scarcely any corn could be obtained. At one time the quantity distributed was
only five kernels to each person. These were parched and eaten. . . . On
December 22nd, 1820 was the second centennial celebration. Great pains were
taken by pious and eloquent men to impress upon the minds of a happy and
prosperous people what their ancestors had suffered in their first planting of
this land. At the public dinner, when the table was loaded with rich viands
of a plentiful country, by each plate, was placed five kernels of corn, as a
memorial of the firm endurance of their fathers.[151]

The place of history in the school curriculum was disputed by the
authors of children's books in the early 'thirties. Some held that the study
of history "was an important means of becoming acquainted with the
operations of the human heart." This group advised children to make
themselves "acquainted with some judicious outline," and as far as possible fill up every part of it by their supplementary reading and always
to give special attention to the story of their own country.[152] Others
denounced the usual method of writing history, and recommended that
it be composed on moral and philosophical principles instead of political.
These had little approbation for history as the "science that warns by
contraries," since it presented to the contemplative mind "a disgusting
detail of follies and crimes; and insolence of power, and the degradation
and misery of our kind." The subject was also blamed for throwing
a false gloss over names that deserved "nothing but execration"; and it
was consequently accused of poisoning the minds of unreflecting youth.
The destroyer of thousands was given a distinguished niche in the temple
of historic fame, while one who had spent his life humanizing and
illuminating mankind, or in diffusing the blessings of peace and civilization, was seldom honored with a line to preserve his name. Until a new
method of historical writing brought the actions "of the principal actors
on the stage of life to the test of reason, nature, religion, and truth,"
children were advised to read history with extreme caution, and to be
guarded by previous instruction "from bestowing applause where they
ought only to detest and despise."[153]

The new geographies appearing after the Revolution reflected the
national pride of American writers and their faith in the future of their
country. Among the first texts on this subject was *Geography Epitomized;
or a Tour Round the World,* which was "attempted in verse" by Robert
Davidson, a Philadelphia educator, in 1784. After touring Europe and
the Orient in spirit, the young reader was brought to the western shores

of what is now the United States, where he could join with the author
in the praise of his native land:

> Having cross'd the Pacific, we'll now take our stand,
> On this happy, prolific, and wide-spreading land,
> Where nature has wrought with a far nobler hand.
> No more let the Old World be proud of her mountains,
> Her rivers, her mines, her lakes, and her fountains,—
> Tho' great in themselves—they no longer appear
> To be great—when compar'd to the great that are here.[154]

A curious geographical reader was published in 1788 at Reading, Pennsylvania. It gave a general description of the government of the thirteen states of the Union, but failed to mention such important items
as the Federal Constitution or the Northwest Ordinance of 1787. It did
refer to the Articles of Confederation, and noted that the supreme power
of the United States was lodged in a congress of delegates, but that each
state retained its sovereignty and independence. Information about old
as well as new states was meager; for example, in regard to Connecticut,
the child read: "This state retains its ancient form of government. They
have a very respectable Seminary of Learning called Yale College."[155]
Concerning Georgia, he learned: "The soil is excellent and the timber
is good for ship building. The government of this state has recently
been new modelled, but we have not been able to obtain a copy."[156] No
reference was made to industry or manufacturing in any section of the
country.

The Short but Comprehensive Geography of the World prepared in
1795 by Nathaniel Dwight was most popular, if judged by its numerous
editions. Dwight informed his readers that during "an employment of
several years in school-keeping" in New England, he had observed the
little enthusiasm for geography—an indifference which he attributed to
the great expense of procuring books, or to the fact that most texts were
above the understanding of children. After this introduction, he gave
an interesting survey of social conditions in this country, as he interpreted them. There was probably no danger of any reader mistaking the
location of the writer's birthplace, for the comparison of accounts for
New England, Pennsylvania, and Virginia gave a highly sectional interpretation of the national scene. One might question the ultimate effects
of such works on national unity, or on that "promotion of social intercourse and mutual happiness" which the author declared to be the aim
of geographical knowledge. Witness the decline of virtue in the population as the author proceeded south from New England:

New Englanders. They are usually industrious and orderly people economical in their livings and frugal in their expenses, but very liberal when called on for valuable purposes, or by brethren in distress. They are well-informed in general; fond of reading; punctual in their observances of the laws, sociable and hospitable to each other, and to strangers; jealous and watchful over their liberties; almost every individual pursuing some gainful and useful calling. . . . Science is greatly cultivated, and more generally diffused among the inhabitants than in any other part of the world. . . .[157]

Pennsylvanians. They are of very different characters. They, however, generally agree in being temperate, plain, industrious, and frugal. Many of the yeomanry in some parts of this state . . . are impatient of good government, order and regularity.[158]

Virginians. They are sociable and hospitable, attached strongly to pleasure and dissipation and highly jealous of personal independence. The holders of slaves have the same character in all countries.[159]

In contrast to this book was *The Elements of Geography Made Easy,* published in Philadelphia in 1825 by an anonymous author. It treated chiefly of physical geography and laid special emphasis on the land and water divisions. It was not only beautifully illustrated, but had the novel advantage of being "embellished with nine neat coloured maps." Few books of this period had maps, for the "study of the globes" was a thing apart from history or geography.

Nature study was closely allied to the child's religious training and frequently formed a part of it in the early nineteenth century. Dozens of little books on the subject were written for youth or for adults who sought to guide the young "from the open book of nature to duty and to God." Most of these works proposed a novel laboratory technique, which at first must have intrigued young naturalists, although this continued sugar-coating of moral lessons probably dulled the interest of normal children. The mother, for example, was told to take the child's favorite kitten in her arms and, after pointing out its graceful proportions, to teach the little owner a lesson of kindness; or while the dog slept at the boy's feet to remind the child of its fidelity and enduring gratitude. The mother, instructing her children, was to "teach their little feet to turn aside from the worm, and to spare trampling the nest of the toiling ant." She could also point out the bird "laying the beams of its chambers" among the green leaves or in the thick grass, and make little ones shudder at childish cruelty which robbed such feathered friends of their treasures. She could explain the properties of the flower that the child held in his hand, and speak of Him whose "touch perfumes it, and whose pencil paints." The voice of the brook, the waving gestures of corn, the icicle sharpened by frost, the sleeted pane with its fantastic tracery, the nodding trees of the awful forest, and the fixed star "on its burning throne," were used to teach children the wonderful works of God.[160]

In the textbooks provided for the children of the early national period, one may detect the first strivings after that perfection in education which had been envisioned by the Founding Fathers. The later intellectual awakening associated with the actual founding of public school systems lies beyond the scope of this study. The fifty years following the Revolution were a period of liberalization and transition, during which time the growing interest in the personality of the child manifested itself in a broadened, secularized curriculum, and in sporadic attempts to find the proper system in which this curriculum could develop. But until education was regarded as a public, and not an individual, responsibility, collective action was inhibited, with the result that private schools and academies, or common schools and charity schools, had to serve as temporary agencies.

To reach the goal of mass education as a function of the government in seeking to educate citizens for a democracy, early education had to surmount many obstacles. Class distinctions were a barrier for both rich and poor—the one scorned contact with inferiors; the other despised the stamp of pauperism. Sectarian interests jealously guarded their rights to teach and preserve in private schools the dogmas of a particular faith. Many regarded state control of education as an invasion of family rights, while a few felt that the education of the masses would produce dangerous radicals in society. Since an enthusiasm for universal education could not develop properly while slavery existed, nation-wide plans for free schools, supported and controlled by the state, were not realized until after the Civil War.

[1]Frederick Eby and Charles F. Arrowood, *The Development of Modern Education in Theory, Organization, and Practice,* p. 467; see also Curtis P. Nettels, *The Roots of American Civilization,* pp. 484-514; Edgar W. Knight, *Twenty Centuries of Education,* pp. 230-51.

[2]Cotton Mather, *A Family Well-Ordered,* Appendix 2.

[3]*Ibid.,* pp. 4, 5.

[4]Knight, *op. cit.,* p. 231.

[5]Eby and Arrowood, *op. cit.,* p. 532.

[6]Nettels, *op. cit.,* pp. 486-487; see also Merle Curti, *The Social Ideals of American Educators,* Chapter I.

[7]Nettels, *op. cit.,* p. 487.

[8]Oliver P. Chitwood, *A History of Colonial America,* p. 551.

[9]Joseph Butterweck and J. Conrad Seegers, *An Orientation Course in Education,* pp. 64-67.

[10]Alice M. Earle, *Child Life in Colonial Days,* pp. 64-67.
[11]Eby and Arrowood, *op. cit.,* p. 532.
[12]*Ibid.,* p. 533.
[13]As quoted in Lillian Rhodes, *The Story of Philadelphia,* p. 69.
[14]Eby and Arrowood, *op. cit.,* p. 533; see also Chitwood, *op. cit.,* p. 559.
[15]*Ibid.,* p. 534; see also Chitwood, *op. cit.,* p. 562.
[16]Knight, *op. cit.,* pp. 162-63; see also Stuart G. Noble, *A History of American Education,* pp. 72, 73.
[17]Paul Monroe, *Founding of the American Public School System,* p. 159.
[18]John Comenius, *Orbis Pictus* (London, 1777), p. 3.
[19]Frank P. Graves, *Great Educators of Three Centuries,* pp. 37-47.
[20]Graves, *op. cit.,* p. 53.
[21]*Ibid.,* pp. 56, 57.
[22]*Ibid.,* p. 63.
[23]*Ibid.,* p. 107.
[24]Eby and Arrowood, *op. cit.,* pp. 465-70.
[25]*Ibid.,* p. 474.
[26]Harry Kelso Eversell, *Education and the Democratic Tradition,* p. 13. See also R. L. Archer, *Rousseau on Education,* p. 89.
[27]Graves, *op. cit.,* pp. 118, 119.
[28]Graves, *op. cit.,* p. 149.
[29]Noble, *op. cit.,* p. 59. See also Monroe, *op. cit.,* p. 204.
[30]*Ibid.,* p. 79.
[31]Benjamin Franklin, *Proposals Relating to the Education of Youth in Pensilvania* [*sic*] (Philadelphia, 1749), p. 5.
[32]Noble, *op. cit.,* p. 77; see also Knight, *op. cit.,* pp. 284, 285.
[33]Eby and Arrowood, *op. cit.,* p. 536; A similar non-sectarian control ot nospitals, libraries, etc., was developing in the English-speaking world of the Enlightenment, indicating a secular trend and the breakdown of denominational lines in Protestant lands. Evidences of the growth of such secular institutions can best be studied in the early history of Philadelphia.
[34]Franklin, *op. cit.,* p. 11.
[35]Richard Peters, *A Sermon on Education. Wherein some account is given of the Academy, Established in the City of Philadelphia, Preached at the Opening thereof,* p. 11.
[36]*Ibid.,* p. 13.
[37]*Ibid.,* Appendix, p. 8.
[38]Franklin, *op. cit.,* p. 30.
[39]Peters, *op. cit.,* Appendix 1.
[40]Alice M. Earle, *Child Life in Colonial Days,* p. 118; See also Andrew W. Tuer, *The History of the Hornbook,* 2 vols. (1898); There is a rare collection of hornbooks in gilt, ivory, and wood in the Yale University Library.
[41]*The New England Primer,* pages unnumbered.
[42]*Ibid.*
[43]*The New England Primer* (Hartford, 1800), p. 5.
[44]Leonard Culman, *Sententiae Pueriles Anglo-Latinae. Collected out of sundry Authors long since . . . for the first Entrers* [*sic*] *into Latin,* p. 1.
[45]*Ibid.,* pp. 24-28.
[46]*Sententiae Pueriles; or Sentences for Children, fitted to the fundamental Rules of Latin Syntax,* p. 32.
[47]*Ibid.,* p. 36.
[48]Nathan Bailey, *English and Latine Exercises for School-Boys Comprising all the Rules of Syntax,* Preface.
[49]*Ibid.,* p. 14.

[50]*Ibid.*, pp. 29-33.

[51]Edward Whittenhall, *A Short Introduction to Grammar for the Use of the College and Academy in Philadelphia,* Preface, ii, iii.

[52]Benjamin Franklin, *op. cit.,* p. 18. Judging from the mass of material on the liberalizing education that was published in Philadelphia, the reader is forced to the conclusion that as compared to other sections, the Enlightenment found its great center in Pennsylvania.

[53]Thomas Dilworth, *A New Guide to the English Tongue,* pp. 5-78.

[54]*Ibid.*, p. 79.

[55]George Fox, *Instructions for Right-Spelling and Plain Directions for Reading and Writing True English,* pp. 71-82.

[56]*Ibid.*, pp. 15-32.

[57]*Ibid.*, p. 11.

[58]Benjamin Franklin, *op. cit.,* p. 19.

[59]Anthony Benezet, *The Pennsylvania Spelling-Book; or Youth's Friendly Instructor and Monitor,* pp. 161, 162.

[60]*Ibid.*, p. 156.

[61]George Fisher, *The American Instructor: or, The Young Man's Best Companion,* Preface, pp. iii-v.

[62]Franklin, *op. cit.,* p. 19.

[63]*Ibid.*

[64]*Ibid.*, p. 25.

[65]*The History of America, abridged for the use of children of all denomnations.*

[66]Noah Webster, *A Dictionary of the English Language; Compiled for the use of Common Schools in the United States.*

[67]*A Compendious History of the World from the Creation to the Dissolution of the Roman Republic,* 2 vols. (1774), 3, 4; An edition of this work was published by John Newberry in 1763, in England; See A. S. W. Rosenbach, *Early American Children's Books,* p. 35.

[68]Philip Freneau and Hugh Brackenridge, *A Poem on the Rising Glory of America; being an Exercise Delivered at the Public Commencement at Nassau-Hall, September 25, 1771,* pp. 16, 17.

[69]*Ibid.*, p. 23.

[70]Timothy Dwight, *A Valedictory Address to the Young Gentlemen who commended Bachelors of Arts, at Yale-College,* July 25, 1776, pp. 10-12.

[71]Timothy Dwight, *op. cit.,* pp. 15, 16.

[72]Benjamin Franklin, *op. cit.,* p. 12.

[73]Clifton Johnson, *Old-Time Schools and School Books,* p. 301.

[74]James Hodder, *Hodder's Arithmetick: or that Necessary Art Made Most Easy. Being Explained in a way Familiar to the Capacity of any that desire to learn it in a Little Time. The Five and Twentieth Edition, Revised and Augmented, and above a Thousand Faults Amended by Henry Mose.*

[75]Alice M. Earle, *Child Life in Colonial Days,* p. 138.

[76]Benezet, *op. cit.,* p. 166.

[77]*Ibid.*, p. 168. See also Franklin, *op. cit.,* p. 12.

[78]Benezet, *op. cit.,* p. 165.

[79]George Fisher, *The American Instructor,* p. 28.

[80]A. S. W. Rosenbach, *op. cit.,* p. 40.

[81]James Nelson, *An Essay on the Government of Children,* p. 367.

[82]*Ibid.*, p. 368.

[83]James Burgh, *Rules of the Conduct of Life,* pp. 126, 127. This work was so popular in America that as late as 1846 it was reprinted in Philadelphia.

[84]Stuart G. Noble, *op. cit.,* pp. 96-131; See also Frederick Eby and Charles Arrowood, *op. cit.,* pp. 540-52.

[85]As quoted in James Truslow Adams, *Dictionary of American History*, IV (1940), 181.

[86]As quoted in Noble, *op. cit.*, pp. 104-5.

[87]Edgar Knight, *Twenty Centuries of Education*, pp. 236-46. See also Joseph Butterweck and J. Conrad Seegers, *An Orientation Course in Education*, p. 83.

[88]Stuart G. Noble, *op. cit.*, p. 123.

[89]Philadelphia Society for the Establishment of Charity Schools, *Manual of the System of teaching Reading, Writing, Arithmetic, and Needle-Work in the Elementary Schools of the British and Foreign Society*, pp. 9, 10.

[90]*Ibid.*, Preface, v.

[91]*Ibid.*

[92]*Ibid.*, x.

[93]*Ibid.*, xi (Italics mine).

[94]*Wisdom in Miniature: or the Young Gentleman and Lady's Magazine*, p. 5.

[95]Noble, *op. cit.*, p. 149.

[96]Noah Webster, *Elements of Useful Knowledge*, Preface.

[97]Educational reform was, of course, ultimately a product of the same general humanitarianism which also produced the other reform movements noted.

[98]Lydia Huntley Sigourney, *Letters to Mothers*, p. 140.

[99]*Ibid.*

[100]Caleb Bingham, *The American Preceptor; Being a Selection of Lessons for Reading and Speaking*, p. 12; see also John Hall, *On the Education of Children While under the Care of Parents or Guardians*, pp. 118, 119.

[101]John Hall, *op. cit.*, p. 116.

[102]Sigourney, *op. cit.*, pp. 141, 142. See also Theodore Dwight, *The Father's Book or Suggestions for the Government and Instruction of Young Children in Principles Appropriate to a Christian Country*, p. 201.

[103]Sigourney, *op. cit.*, pp. 143-45.

[104]*Ibid.*, pp. 147, 148.

[105]*Ibid.*, p. 149.

[106]*Miscellanies, Moral and Instructive in Prose and Verse Collected from Various Authors for the Use of Schools and Improvement of Young of Both Sexes*. Preface, iii.

[107]*Ibid.*, p. 21.

[108]*The Child's Spelling Book*, p. 25.

[109]*The A B C with the Church of England Catechism*, pp. 11, 12.

[110]*Lessons for Children from Two to Four Years Old*, Part One, pp. 77-79.

[111]*Ibid.*

[112]*Lessons for Children of Four Years Old*, Part Two, pp. 4-6.

[113]*The Fortune Teller*, pp. 26-28.

[114]*Easy Lessons for Children*, pp. 6, 7.

[115]*Ibid.*, pp. 58-61.

[116]*The Beauties of the New England Primer.*

[117]*The Wonderful History of an Enchanted Castle Kept by Giant Grumbo*, pp. 16-20.

[118]*The American Primers; or an Easy Introduction to Spelling and Reading*, p. 28.

[119]*The Remarkable Story of Augi: or a Picture of True Happiness*, First American edition. Translated and reprinted by Isaiah Thomas, pp. 15-25.

[120]*The Seven Wonders of the World; and Other Magnificent Buildings*, p. 41.

[121]*The Instructive Alphabet*, pages unnumbered.

[122]*Ibid.* Two other books of a similar mild religious tone were the *Progressive Primer Adapted to Infant School Instruction* and *The Washington Primer; or First Book for Children.*

[123]*The Humorous Alphabet*, pp. 4, 5.

[124]*Ibid.*, p. 15.

[125]*The Little Sketch Book*, p. 7.

[126]*Tom Thumb's Picture Alphabet in Rhyme*, pp. 2-7.

[127]*The Book of the Sea for the Instruction of Little Sailors*, p. 2.

[128]Noah Webster, *The American Spelling Book*, Fifth Edition, Preface.

[129]*Ibid.*, p. 116.

[130]*Ibid.*, p. 65.

[131]*Ibid.*, p. 63.

[132]Henry Osborne, *An English Grammar adapted to the Capacities of Children*, Preface.

[133]James Greenwood, *The Philadelphia Vocabulary; English and Latin*, pp. 1-132.

[134]*The Infant's Grammar*, p. 7.

[135]*Ibid.*, p. 12.

[136]*Punctuation Personified: or Pointing Made Easy*. Pages unnumbered.

[137]Daniel Fenning, *The American Youth's Instructor; or, a New and Easy Guide TO Practical Arithmetic*, Preface.

[138]William Milns, *The Well-Bred Scholar*, p. 18.

[139]*The American Letter-Writer*, p. 7.

[140]*Ibid.*, p. 3 (italics mine).

[141]Caleb Bingham, *Juvenile Letters; Being a Correspondence between Children from eight to fifteen years of age*, p. 87.

[142]*Ibid.*, p. 87.

[143]*A Father to His Daughter: The Daughter's Own Book, or Practical Hints*, p. 43.

[144]*The Life of General Washington, Commander in Chief of the Army during the late War, and present President of the United States. Also of the Brave General Montgomery*, p. 17.

[145]John Corry, *Biographical Memoirs of the Illustrious General George Washington*, p. 144.

[146]*History of America, abridged for the use of children of all denominations*, Adorned with cuts, pp. 23, 24.

[147]*Ibid.*, p. 37.

[148]*Ibid.*, p. 58.

[149]*The Pilgrims, or the First Settlers of New England*, p. 8.

[150]*Ibid.*, p. 9.

[151]Lydia Huntley Sigourney, *Tales and Essays for Children*, p. 74.

[152]*The Daughter's Own Book*, pp. 51, 52.

[153]*The Boy's Manual: Comprising a Summary of the Studies, Accomplishments, and Principles of Conduct Best Studied for Promoting Respectibility*, pp. 158-160.

[154]Robert Davidson, *Geography Epitomized; or, A Tour Round the World; attempted in verse for the sake of the memory; and principally designed for the use of schools*, p. 60.

[155]*A General Description of the Thirteen United States*, p. 10.

[156]*Ibid.*, p. 23.

[157]Nathaniel Dwight, *A Short but Comprehensive System of Geography of the World; by way of question and answer. Principally designed for Children and the Common Schools*, p. 141.

[158]*Ibid.*, p. 164.

[159]*Ibid.*, p. 174.

[160]Lydia Huntley Sigourney, *Letter to Mothers*, p. 95; see also Johannes F. Martinet, *The Catechism of Nature for the Use of Children*, translated from the Dutch by John Hall; *Natural History of Four-Footed Beasts; The Youth's Cabinet of Nature;* William Mavor, *Catechism of Animated Nature*, reprinted from the English edition; *The History of Animals.*

Young Victims

OF

KITCHEN PHYSICK

Pediatrics in its modern connotation was an unknown science in Colonial days, for child care, even in its primitive state, lay beneath the dignity and recognition of the regular medical profession. Although medical works gave some attention to childhood diseases, the care and treatment of children were based largely on conjecture and superstition. Child health and healing were casually consigned to "old grandmothers" who were commonly credited with understanding best the needs of the very young. These "wise women," utterly devoid of scientific training, developed the most absurd procedures and loathsome dosings in the execution of their folk practice. In view of the appallingly high child mortality, it is evident that these ignorant practitioners of "kitchen physick" offered slight protection against the ills of youth, and even lessened chances of survival by imposing hideous ordeals on the young victims of disease.

No actual statistics for disease and death were kept in the colonies, but they may be deduced from those of the mother country, where morbidity and mortality rates for children in such British cities as London had reached alarming peaks by the decade after 1750. During some of these years mortality records reveal that 74 per cent of all children born in that city died under two years of age, and that this loss comprised about half the total death rate.[1] Although the American story of child health was different, it could have been no better than that of Europe; for living conditions in the colonies were primitive and health hazards universal.

The new clearings abounded in malaria and dysentery. The rigors of the climate, with its extremes of heat and cold, endangered the lives of children in the winter by exposure in the cold, drafty houses, and in the summer by the lack of protection against insects. Rough frontier life increased the ills of childhood and brought innumerable casualties from accidents. The drinking water obtained from surface wells was always liable to pollution and caused frequent epidemics of typhoid. Scourges like smallpox came from Europe, just as hookworm followed in the wake of the African slaves. On rare occasions sperm or lard oil lamps were used, but the usual source of illumination was candles, whose light doubtless did much to ruin juvenile eyesight. Even the largest towns did not provide sanitary services, so that ashes and garbage were piled about in offensive heaps, and hogs roaming through the streets served as scavengers by eating up the scraps of meat and vegetables thrown out by housewives. The senior members of the large families were so deeply engrossed in making a living that children were often neglected or denied the simplest hygienic care, and were frequently obliged to share the rough, hard work. Although the argument has been made that the fresh air, sunshine, and plain, wholesome food enjoyed by the young in the rural districts provided compensating advantages, these gains were offset by the natural hardships and by the clouds of ignorance and superstition that surrounded childlife.[2]

England displayed little concern in safeguarding public health in the Colonies by failing to eliminate the frightful epidemics that regularly depleted the population. When the old methods of prevention—quarantines, isolation, and the destruction of contaminated goods—had proved unsatisfactory in arresting the progress of epidemics, public attention shifted to sanitary reform on the supposition that certain plagues could be traced to noxious airs and waters. But this shift was retarded by a bitter controversy on the part of physicians as to the contagious or non-contagious nature of various diseases. Colonial legislatures, on their part, made only the feeblest efforts to provide social control by enacting such health codes as those of Massachusetts and Connecticut. This legislation, more formidable on paper than in its application, called for isolating cases of contagious diseases, the impressment of nurses in emergencies, the killing of dangerous dogs, the destruction or fumigation of materials, and the flying of white notification signals.[3]

The apathy that relegated child care to the level of "kitchen physick" was but one phase of the general Colonial indifference to scientific progress. An example of this unconcern may be found in the fact that although William Harvey had discovered the circulation of the blood as early as 1616, his ideas found few supporters among the physicians who came to the Colonies. And even if the barbers, bloodletters, and bonesetters who practised the roughest sort of physic and surgery in the pioneer settlements had heard of Harvey's ideas, they were probably un-impressed by such novelties. Much less was the confidence and mystery of folk medicine disturbed by any scientific discovery. The practice of midwives and old women was not based on science but on ancient traditions, and it employed remedies as old as Hippocrates himself. The institutions of higher learning were also tradition-bound, for in 1699, seventy-one years after Harvey had written his famous treatise, the circu-lation of the blood was still a debated question at Harvard.[4]

A brief examination of the popular notions of child care at the begin-ning of the eighteenth century is required to understand the apparent insensibility to such vital points as hygiene and preventive medicine. The colonists had inherited from Galen the belief in humoral pathology, which held that the body consisted of four elements—earth, air, fire, and water—and that it also contained four humors or liquids to correspond neatly with the elements. In the mystical lore of this era these humors, catalogued as bile or choler, blood, melancholy or black bile, and phlegm, were supposed to have some mysterious relation to the elements of the body. Since disease was attributed to an excess of a certain humor, or to its being too hot or cold, too moist or dry, an early writer had listed the possible unhappy variations of the humors at about eighty thousand—a system of diagnois that might well have impressed an ordinary patient.[5]

To restore health by removing morbid humors, or by invigorating the liver, which was commonly considered the center of life, Colonial physicians made use of a prodigious variety of simples and nostrums handed down from antiquity. The only plausible justification in the popular mind for these drastic dosings probably lay in the assumed necessity of eliminating those restive humors that sent poisonous vapors to the brain. For almost every pathological disturbance of man, woman, or child, the favorite panacea was bloodletting. Infants a few days old and aged persons on the brink of the grave alike had their "peccant" humors expelled by the poorly trained "chirurgeon," or by clergymen, barbers, and other medical dabblers who practised this depletion. Having ascertained the age of their victims, these impostors usually consulted an old almanac to discover the proper time of the moon for letting blood.[6] Americans were thus only indirectly affected by the great medical dis-coveries that stirred Europe; for in their isolation and sufferings most of them eagerly utilized any quackery or ignorant folk physic that promised relief.

Colonial Americans also attached great importance to the doctrine of signatures, which was originally based on the primitive medical theory of savages, and later, in the sixteenth century, was supported by the Swiss chemist Paracelsus as part of the prevalent philosophy of correspondences. The fundamental thesis of this practice was the belief that God had put a signature on each substance to show the disease it was intended to cure, so that even the uneducated, with their native genius, could read the signs correctly and achieve success. Influenced by the belief that like is cured by like, or contraries by contraries, the spotted leaves of St. John's wort were applied to abrasions; the warts of the toad were taken because of their value against skin eruptions; while milk, being white, was supposed to clear black humors. The much-desired gold of the alchemists was still being sought, for it was argued that since gold was the most precious metal it would also be a most potent remedy if it could be reduced to liquid form. John Winthrop and his son Wait compounded the heaviest liquid mercury with gold, and thus produced a "tincture of the sun." As the tincture was thought capable of "destroying the Root and Seminaries of all malignant and poisonous diseases," many New England children were dosed with this mystical concoction.[7]

Another expression of the long-sought universal medicament was theriac, or what was known in England as Venice treacle, a preparation of viper's flesh containing some sixty ingredients. All poisons, as well as a variety of diseases, were supposed to be controlled by this complex mixture. In the more simple American practice, the flesh of the rattlesnake was used in broths for the sick; its oil was endorsed for gout, and was believed to be "very sovraign for frozen limbs"—a common calamity in the icy winters of New England. The bezoar stone, "the queen of poisons," claimed to be taken from the intestines of wild goats found in the Orient, was used in its pulverized form by the colonists as a valuable antidote for snake bites. Remarkable virtues were also accorded the use of dittany, or American pennyroyal, which was thought to be particularly effective in driving away and "astonishing" serpents, mad dogs, and venomous beasts. Other favorite herbs were brought from England to America, and Colonial mothers were careful to cultivate in their kitchen gardens the wild plants of medicinal value that they had been accustomed to gather from the British hedgerows.[8]

The medical notions of the British colonists coincided nicely with those of the Indians since both affirmed that all things were made with reference to man. The common use of American plants and animals had accordingly little relation to scientific research. The woods were full of creatures reputed to possess potent curative powers; their efficacy simply depended on the ability of the gatherer to interpret accurately the label fixed on the flora and fauna by a beneficent Creator. Thus the very appearance of the familiar kidney bean grown in Indian gardens plainly revealed that it was "good to strengthen the kidneys." The brains of the screech owl were indicated for headache, just as a necklace of caterpillars was believed to cure ague by the shuddering it induced in a sensitive patient. Obviously, remedies used in this early medical practice had nothing to recommend them but the popular illusion that disgust was potently curative.[9]

Among those who best appreciated the widespread ignorance, bad judgment, and superstition behind the stupendous problems of child welfare was Dr. William Dewees, Professor of Midwifery at the University of Pennsylvania, who wrote as follows:

It is our firm conviction, that the mortality among children is unnecessarily great; and that this excess originates, in very many instances, in the mal-administration of the means of life, rather than to the operation of natural and inevitable causes. Some are nursed to death, while many others die because they are not nursed at all; some are fed to death, while many others die from inanition; some are physicked to death, while others die from the want of a single dose of it—all of which goes to prove how much experience and judgment are required to administer with success, to the wants and infirmities of children.[10]

Limited reforms were made in therapeutics as the eighteenth century came to its close, and children were relieved of some of the horrors incidental to the dosings with revolting herb and animal concoctions prescribed by the Colonial "kitchen physick." A revolution in health and sanitation banished dirt and much disease from the ordinary home early in the new century. In the large cities drains were installed in most houses, the streets were paved and cleaned, and drinking water became safer after sanitary systems had been installed at public expense. Children were either given a cold morning bath or were scrubbed with soap and warm water in a vigorously weekly ritual on Saturday night. Beer and heavy improper foods were withheld from them, and the diet of tiny folk was reduced to such simple items as cocoa, milk, porridge, eggs, and bread or toast thinly spread with butter and jam. The training given nurses was still elemental and unsatisfactory, but when children fell ill, regular doctors were summoned with greater confidence than formerly. To trace this gradual improvement in the attitudes and techniques of child care, as it is revealed in juvenile books and in the manuals for parents' guidance, is to record an important if inconspicuous phase of the first revolution in the history of American child life.

This literature discloses the fact that in Colonial days most aspects of the hygienic care of youth were highlighted against a backdrop of religious beliefs and practises. In the drama of child life the watchful care of parents and the medical skill of physicians were alike considered the inconsequential instruments employed by Providence for the interpretation of the Divine Will. Pains and ills, in this setting, were regarded as the first means of instructing the child, since it was believed that suffering not only taught him to avoid certain dangers, but made him provident, compassionate, humane, and courageous. For instance, to complete the disillusionment of carefree youth on the prospects of health and happiness, as well as to banish any hopes of longevity, such lines as "Disappointment" were addressed to the young American:

> Oh think not my child as you grow in life,
> That pleasures unceasing will flow;
> Disappointment, and trouble, and sorrow, and strife,
> Will follow wherever you go.
>
> Tho' now the bright prospect seems opening fair,
> And hope paints a scene of delight,
> Too soon you will see it all vanished in air,
> And leave you to darkness and night.[11]

Several juvenile books on the novel subjects of health and safety were published in Philadelphia. Among these works were three volumes of William Darton's *Chapter of Accidents and Remarkable Events: Containing Caution and Instruction for Children,* which had been pirated and printed from the English edition by Jacob Johnson. The printer localized some of the stories in his own city, and included such delightful bits as "Cautions to Walkers in Streets of Philadelphia." Young pedestrians on Market Street were warned never to "turn hastily round the corner of the street, by this some have been greatly hurt. One young woman in so doing, ran against a porter's load, and nearly lost one of her eyes by the blow she received; but this was partly owing to the porter not being in his proper place for he was close to the wall, when he should have been the farthest from it."[12] The child was told to avoid any crowds that assembled in the streets "as much as may be"; yet when accidents occurred, he should assist the afflicted if possible. Only the natives were entirely dependable for honesty and courtesy, for strangers were warned to inquire at "houses or of shop-keepers for any place they may want to find, and not of persons in the street, lest they be deliberately misdirected."[13]

Another book relating to juvenile safety, *The Post Boy,* was thoroughly American in its content, and contained some rather harrowing lessons. In passages headed "The Post Boy's Bag Opened," were discovered the following terse "Packets":

Packet 1. James had cut his hand, so he cannot write; his knife was falling from off the desk, and he strove to stop it by catching at it: His hand bled freely, but now being bound up in the warm blood, with a clean linen rag, it is in a fair way to do well.—Never catch a knife!

Packet 3. Two little boys lost their lives in a pond! They went in to bathe, and did not know how deep the water was. They asked to take a walk into the field, and as it was a hot day, they went into the water. They were both put into one grave.[14]

That children, especially those living within the shadow of Independence Hall and within the sight and sound of the Liberty Hall, should celebrate their national holiday on July fourth with enthusiasm is not at all surprising; but the grown-ups of the early nineteenth century prudently placed restraining hands on the young patriots who commemorated the day with firecrackers. Adults, to the detriment of juvenile jollity it is feared, were commonly of the opinion that "playing with gunpowder" was the most dangerous of all sports, hence another little safety guide gave the following pronouncement:

Boys are very fond of letting off squibs and crackers, but many have severely repented the consequence of this amusement. . . . How many accidents have happened on rejoicing days, particularly on the 4th of July! As we commemorate the escape from the dreadful effects of gunpowder, it is rather absurd that it should on that day be made the principal agent for amusement.[15]

Influenced by the spiritual values placed on sickness and suffering, Colonial parents, who knew very little of the causes of disease, were less interested in preventing sickness than they were in seeking cures for the ills that already afflicted their offspring. The adult attitude discounted medical skill and accepted with apparent resignation the shocking record of juvenile morbidity and mortality as a part of the Divine plan for child life. This stand in matters of child welfare, reflecting as it did the spiritual standards of early American life, found clear expression in children's books. For example, an old textbook, published in 1720, aptly taught the children a commonly accepted lesson of life—that of hesitating to place too much confidence in material aids:

If it please God, Physick shall do a Man good; but if God withhold his Blessing, all Endeavors are vain: For God makes use of Physicians as his Instruments, and therefore it best agreeth with Religion to join Prayer with Physick. God is always at leisure to do good to those that ask him.[16]

Thus it was that health, like many other problems of child life, was left largely in the hands of God to be resolved as He saw fit.

The very scarcity of children's books on the subject of child care before 1800 is further evidence of adult indifference to juvenile health habits, and another proof of the common acceptance of health, sickness, and death as acts of God. Juvenile works on a variety of other topics unintentionally give a fair idea of prevailing attitudes on child care. One of the little gilt books published by Isaiah Thomas in 1787, a rare type of work in its day, contained some valuable suggestions to parents on the management of their progeny:

Would you have your *Child Strong* . . . give him what Meat and Drink is necessary, and such only as affords good Nutrition, not salt Meat, rich Tarts, Sauces, Wines, etc. A Practice too common amongst some indulgent People. Also Let the Child have due Exercise; for this it is What gives Life and Spirits, circulates the Blood, strengthens the Sinews, and keeps the whole Machinery in order.

Would you have a *Hardy Child*, give him common Diet only, clothe him thin, let him have good exercise, and be as much exposed to Hardships as his natural Constitution will admit.

Would you have a *Healthy Son*, observe the directions already laid down with regard to Diet and Exercise, and keep him as much as possible from Physick; For Physick is to the Body, as Arms to the State; both are necessary, but neither *to be used but in cases of Emergency and Danger.*[17]

One finds, in various sources, numerous references to the untimely deaths of little ones. This is particularly true in funeral elegies for children, which were often printed and distributed for the edification of surviving companions. Benjamin Coleman, for example, exclaimed in dismay at the high rate of child mortality. "What multitudes die in infancy! In Childhood the blooming flower falls too. If through a million Dangers mortal to others, we get up to Youth, yet how suddenly and how often does Death cut the verdant budding plant! . . . Those that are really pious and godly in their childhood, do die young."[18]

Noah Webster, writing in 1800 about "Diseases and Remarkable Events" experienced by early Americans, is more specific as to the causes of child mortality; for he points out that these little ones had to contend with hardships, scarcity of provisions, an uncomfortable degree of heat and cold, as well as with the diseases of this country such as influenza, malaria, scarlet fever, and diphtheria or "malignant sore throat." This last-named was the scourge of childhood, and he shows that from the year 1735 to 1800 it was epidemic six times in the northern states.[19]

The prevalence of these diseases fatal to children, as well as the general ignorance and superstition attending medical treatments, led Benjamin

Franklin to make the following comment in his revision of a textbook: "In the British Edition of the Book, there were many Things of little or no Use in these Parts of the World: In this Edition those Things are omitted, and in their Room many other Matters inserted, more immediately useful to us Americans."[20] Among the "useful things" was a treatise entitled "Every Man His own Doctor: or the Poor Planter's Physician: Wrote by a Gentleman in Virginia." The object of this work, frankly stated, was "to lead the poorer Sort into the pleasant Paths of Health; and when they have the Misfortune to be sick, to shew them the cheapest and easiest Ways of getting well again."[21]

Expressing much commiseration for his suffering neighbors, the author complained that his countrymen were subject to "several sharp distempers" because the marshes, swamps, and great rivers sent forth so many "fogs and exhalations" that the air was continually damp. He showed that fevers, coughs, quinseys, pleurisies, and consumptions, along with a dismal train of other diseases, made as "fatal Havock" here as did the plague in the eastern parts of the world. This bad health was deplored as a "cruel check" to the growth of the colony, which otherwise, by the "fruitfulness of its women" and the great number of settlers sent by the mother country, would have grown very populous in a few years.[22]

While bewailing the "melancholy truth" that many poor people perished for want of a timely remedy, the author revealed the general distrust of medical aid: "One Mischief is, most of our Inhabitants have such an unreasonable aversion to *Physick* (even when they have it from their charitable Neighbors for nothing), that they neglect to take any; till their case grows desperate, and Death begins to glare them in the Face." Although today one has more sympathy than blame for these distrustful souls, whose wariness perhaps resulted from bitter experience in dosing, nevertheless this book stressed with great firmness the importance of professional assistance. It was promised that "a moderate skill may recover a Patient while he has the Strength to go thro' all the necessary Operations." That these "necessary Operations" were a formidable test of Christian fortitude may be gathered from such suggestive phrases as blistering, purging, bleeding in the jugular vein, and "whipping with smart little rods," descriptive of the current medical technique. Timorous sufferers were warned that the "whole College" would not be able to save them after their spirits had sunk and the "principles of life were nearly extinguished."

It was this "unhappy temper" on the part of fearful adults, and not the ignorance and crudities that marked the professional treatment of diseases, which was blamed for the great mortality that "fell the heaviest

on the Younger Sort who were most susceptible to hurrying distempers."
But the author of this work admits extenuating circumstances for certain
cautious parents, some of whom would have been glad of professional
medical assistance for their families if they had not believed that the
"Remedy was almost as bad as the Disease." Since doctors' fees were
commonly so exorbitant "whether they killed or cured," many parents
in ordinary circumstances preferred to trust rather to the sick child's
constitution than "to run the risk of beggaring their whole family."[23]

Medical authorities repeatedly disapproved of the injudicious dosing
of children by ignorant adults and warned that to those who were in
health medicines were worse than useless, and that even to the sick
they often did more harm than good. One finds, however, that the practice of "kitchen physick" went on with obdurate eagerness during this
entire period.[24] The desperation that filled parental hearts at the sight
of so many of their children carried off by death while the medical world
looked helplessly on, undoubtedly prompted mothers or nurses to make
use of household remedies or, at times, of dangerous drugs. At any rate,
when the first symptoms of illness appeared, these misguided souls forthwith administered some concoction to the ailing child. After repeating
the dose, parents would often become alarmed and feel compelled, in
conscience, to send for a medical adviser. For example, in one such case
the physician was gravely informed that the child had become slightly
ill, and in spite of the fact that "full and repeated doses of calomel, mag-
nesia, rhubarb, and laudanum had been given, it had continued getting
worse and worse."[25]

It was almost an article of faith that Providence had wisely furnished
every country with the medicines proper for the "distempers" incident
to its climate; and that such domestic remedies were always sufficient
for the poor who lived upon "homely fare," or for the temperate who
made right use of God's blessings. Hence several manuals and catechisms
of health were published, explaining to parents the use of numerous
nostrums and cures that could be concocted and administered in the
home.

In this respect, the "Virginia Gentleman" modestly claimed that he
did not "cram his patients with much physick," neither did he ransack
the universe for outlandish drugs which would waste and decay on a
long voyage; but he was contented to "do all his execution with the
weapons of our own country." Among the ingredients used in the preparation of his nostrums he listed such simples as "bears-oyl," cresses, garlic,
parsley, tobacco, honey, linseed, wormwood, and whey. To explain the
absence on his list of mercury, opium, and "Peruvian Bark," which were

widely used at that time and no doubt were frequently injurious to the patient, this gentleman asserted that such drugs ought to be administered with the greatest discernment. As he was writing for the poor, who had to judge for themselves, he feared "putting such dangerous weapons in their hands." In this respect at least, the poor probably fared better than did their more opulent neighbors who were dosed with mercury until they were properly "salivated."[26]

For simple ailments such as a cough, the child was told to drink "brandy treacle and sallad oil" when he went to bed; or to take a mixture of butter and brown sugar. When a child "fell into" a more serious "distemper," a sort of slow torture seemed to be the traditional procedure. In the case of quinsy, a common complaint of childhood, the procedure was to "bleed immediately ten ounces, rather in the jugular vein than in the arm"; to apply a blister to the neck and, if the inflamation continued, to bleed again the next day. The following morning the child was to take a purge of the "decoction of mallows" and syrup of peach blossoms; while from the beginning he was to gargle with Dr. Papa's Liquor, and to drink half a pint "of the same night and morning." To prevent these throat complaints and their torturous treatments, the child was told to wash his neck and behind his ears every morning in cold water, and not to "muffle himself up too warm either night or day."[27]

So few precautions were taken against infection that tuberculosis was a common disease among early American children, and one frequently reads of boys and girls falling into a "decline" or a "consumption." If few preventive measures were taken against this plague, the scope of attempted cures fully compensated for this lack. Regarding the painful and disgusting treatment given those in a decline, parents were told that the only course of cure they could give in this "melancholy distemper must be done when the consumption is apprehended and not actually begun."[28] At that stage "blisters and issues might revulse the humour, and prevent the mischief." In comparison to the modern rest cure, the little consumptives of that day were subjected to the following strenuous regimen:

I would recommend Bleeding 2 or 3 Ounces every third Day, with a constant Riding on Horseback, and Change of Air. This will help Nature throw off the Evil that threatens her, by calming the Blood, opening the Pores, and promoting insensible Perspiration. It may also enable her to make a vigorous Effort, by Means of a seasonable Boil . . . under the arms apply Poultices in order to draw the Mischief if possible that Way. And for inward Medicines, let him only chew Sassafras Root every Morning fasting. I would likewise entreat him before he goes to Bed, to take three Pills, made of Turpentine and

Deer's Dung, in equal Quantities: and besides these let him take once a Week a Purge of Mallows and Syrup of Peach-Blossoms. Let his Diet be without Meat, and mixt with Abundance of Turnips, roasted Apples, Raisins, and Liquorice; and let his Drink be, Bear brew'd with Ground-ivy; avoiding strong liquors of every sort, as he would poison.

The way to prevent this wasting Disease, is never to suffer a Cough to dwell upon you; but bleed in time, and purge gently once a week, in the meantime eat not one morsel of Meat, nor drink anything stronger than a little sound Cyder; and to make the Game sure, ride every fair Day, and breathe as much as possible in the Open Air.[30]

Since mid-eighteenth century girls were often subject to fainting fits and to "vapours" or hysterics, there were also directions for treating these "miserable conditions." It was declared that the young girl experienced a great heaviness and dejection of spirits, during which "a cloud seemed to hang over her senses." In this debilitated condition she had no "relish for anything," and was continually out of humor. In all probability, such children were suffering either from the ordinary depression of the adolescent period or from a vitamin deficiency induced by unbalanced meals of "hog and hominy," and from the cruel slimming methods which the fashionably laced wasp-waist demanded of young females. Whatever the cause, the parents of that day were advised to give the hysterical one a cure for vapours according to these rules:

Endeavour to preserve a chearful Spirit putting the best Construction upon every Body's Words and Behaviour; Plunge, 3 mornings every Week, into Cold Water, over Head and Ears; . . . it will have the same effect if you suffer yourself to be whipp'd with smart little rods. It can't be imagined how this will brace the Nerves and rouse the sluggish Spirits. Observe a strict Regularity and Temperance in your Diet; and ride every fair Day, small Journeys on Horseback. Stir nimbly about your Affairs, quick Motion being as necessary for Health of Body as for Dispatch of Business.

Her food must be fresh, and easy of Digestion; nor may she eat one Morsel of Beef, which affords a gross nourishment, and inclines People too much to hang themselves. And for her Drink she must forbear Beer, and stick to bawn Tea intirely.[31]

Walter Harris, in his *Treatise on the Acute Diseases of Infants* published in 1742, thus described his treatment of a "beautiful girl of eleven years of age" who was suffering from epileptic fits, which he cured by powders prepared according to the following formula:

Earth worms prepared one Ounce, human Skull prepared two Drams, lesser Cardamoms two scruples. Reduce them all to a fine powder, and divide it into twelve Papers.

The physician told his reader that because the little girl "loathed such a great quantity of nauseous powder," she followed each dose with a few drops of oil of nutmeg! After the fits had discontinued, he advised the child to continue for some time to take the powders "three days before every New and Full Moon, and to have issues opened in each leg." From that time on she had no return of epileptic fits.[31]

After noting such distressing physical and mental symptoms among young girls, Dr. Faust, a German authority, in his *Catechism of Health* published in 1795, declared that the most pernicious consequences to the youth of that generation came from separating "female children" at the earliest period of their existence from males, from dressing them like adults, from preventing their taking the proper kind of exercise, and from compelling them to lead a sedentary life.[32] A few years later a German medical authority, Christian Augustus Struve, whose work, *A Familiar View of the Domestic Education of Children during the Early Period of Their Lives,* was widely read in this country, insisted that girls should not be excluded from active exercise, and that it was an error in physical education "to make that ill-founded distinction between the two sexes." Young females were thus condemned almost from their cradles to a sedentary existence by keeping them at their needles, and by giving them "dolls and tinsel work or trinkets," while sprightly boys amused themselves with their noisy drums and active games. Struve warned the priggish parents of his day that such female "modesty" was purchased at the expense of health and a cheerful mind.[33]

Dr. G. Akerley, an English physician, lamented that girls were not encouraged to partake more fully of active exercises. Boys, he noted, found gratification in their lively sports, but little girls were required to pass a great part of their time at needlework or in idleness, frequently from a feeling on the part of their parents that "active play was improper for them."[34] To this same end, Lydia H. Sigourney wrote in her *Letters to Mothers:*

I plead for the little girl, that she may have air and exercise as well as her brother, and that she may not be too much blamed, if in her earnest play she happen to tear, or soil her apparel. I plead that she be not punished as a romp, if she keenly enjoys those active sports which city gentility proscribes.[35]

William Mavor, an English reform writer, in the preface to his *Catechism of Health* published in 1819, deplored the fact that in every country, and particularly in the United States, the "economy of health," especially in the matter of children's food, was frightfully neglected. Even among enlightened persons the most absurd customs continued in the management of the young, and in all classes of society, in every section of the land, dangerous practices persisted in defiance of reason and science. Parents had not yet been sufficiently impressed with the old maxim— "Prevention is better than cure."[36]

The few progressive parents could not hope to preserve the health of their children unimpaired without subjecting them to a strict regimen in regard to the quality and quantity of their food and the mode of taking it, hence the current ideas on this subject were reduced to a few simple precepts. Boys and girls were to be confined to plain food with pies, pastries, gravies, hotbreads, and all sorts of rich and highly seasoned foods omitted. Ordinarily they were to take but one dish at the same meal; for instance, if they dined on "baked meat," they could take it with potatoes and bread, and accompany this by a drink of water, milk, or "small beer." This plan was to accustom the young to expect but one kind of food besides bread at dinner; and for the other two meals to be contented with bread and milk.[37]

Although a change of diet from meal to meal might have pleased most children, the practice was discouraged on the grounds that the stomach "digests a single kind of food with more ease than a compound of various kinds." Moreover, children would eat far less if there was but one kind of food before them than they would if there were many, because it was declared that a variety of dishes was one of the strongest temptations to gluttony.[38] Indeed, in this moral age, the little reader could find frequent reference to the sin of gluttony; for instance, there is the story in verse of a "Notorious Glutton"—

> A Duck who had got such a habit of stuffing,
> That all the day long she was panting and puffing.

Children read that when she showed signs of "choaking after a plentiful dinner," Dr. Drake was summoned to attend her:

> The Doctor was just to his business proceeding,
> By gentle emetics, a blister, and bleeding,
> When all on a sudden she roll'd on her side,
> Gave a horrible quackle, a struggle, and died!

> Her remains were inter'd in a neighboring swamp
> By her friends, with a great deal of funeral pomp.
> But I've heard this inscription her tomb was put on,
> "Here lies Mrs. Duck, the Notorious Glutton;"
> And all the young ducklings are brought by their friends,
> To learn the disgrace in which gluttony ends.[40]

Despite such literature, Americans had not universally established proper eating habits by 1835, as an interesting description of the mode of living in a large city reveals.[40] City children were customarily seated at the breakfast table with their parents, and allowed an indigestible meal of salted dried fish or sausages, with coffee and hot bread or buckwheat cakes.[41] Although the powers of digestion of healthy children are exceedingly vigorous and could for a time withstand such irritating diet, yet by the constant repetition of such meals, the little creatures were made peevish and fretful, and were frequently corrected for bad temper. After a breakfast of this sort the children's digestive organs were in no condition to dispose of a substantial luncheon; consequently, their natural craving for food during the afternoon was satisfied by unlimited quantities of bread and butter. At the evening meal the little ones were further deprived of sufficient nourishment by having set before them generous supplies of "sweetmeats" and rich cakes.[42]

Members of the medical profession, to underscore the lesson of correct diet, gave directions for avoiding the disagreeable skin diseases so common among youth at that time. They stressed the need for exercise in the open air to stimulate poor appetites, and pointed out the comforting fact that by a balanced diet children's teeth "would not be set to ache by every slight exposure to change of temperature the climate is so peculiarly subject to."[43]

The types of food usually approved for children point a striking contrast to modern principles of child-feeding. Bread was the staple food of childhood in the eighteenth century. Parents who had a child who was really fond of bread felt that they could guard him against many of the dangers that beset other children who ate improper foods. In order to develop an appetite for this simple food, adults were told that when a child was hungry between meals he was to be promised a piece of dry bread; and that after he had become accustomed to this snack, he would eat it "as eagerly as a great dainty." To see children walking about the house with tarts or bread and butter in their hands, "daubing everything and everybody they touched," was certainly a sad reflection on their parents' good sense. Since this indulgence was judged to be detrimental not only to the health of the young, but to their manners as well, it was denounced as "inexpressibly vulgar."[44]

Although butter was believed to be nourishing, it was not thought the best food for the young, because by obstructing some of the glands it caused a "breaking out" on children.[45] That the little ones had no greater relish then for plain dry bread than they do today may be inferred from instructions directing the mother to tempt her hungry child by promising him a piece of "nice white bread, made of fine flour from the wheat which God makes to grow on purpose for us in the fields." If the idea of dry bread was then not promptly seized by the child, the mother was to praise the taste of bread beforehand, to take a bite herself, and to ask the child if it were not good. On the other hand, eating crusts of bread had from the earliest times been thought by parents to be a proof of good training, and was recommended to children as a duty. Writers of the 'thirties denounced the "foolish doctrine, that eating crusts will make the hair curl," not only because it encouraged vanity and showed that parents trifled with the truth for the sake of expediency, but for the more practical reason that the crusts commonly offered to children were too large for their little mouths and teeth.[46]

There is an interesting account of the early methods of supplying the quantities of milk consumed by city youth. *The Cries of New York* informed the young reader that milk in that city was carried around from door to door twice a day in summer and once in winter. A man carrying the large twelve-gallon kettles from a yoke on his shoulders trudged through the streets and called out to his customers: "Here's Milk, Ho!" Farmers who kept cows on the outskirts of the city drove around with milk carts, "which were mostly covered," and sold their beverage at from six to ten cents a quart.[47]

Only infrequent references were made to vegetables, even when they might accompany the "vehicle" of meat and bread in the principal meal. Most works insisted that little ones eat "a great deal of bread." A few directed them to "blend their meat and bread with greens, turnips, or other garden stuff," but warned that pickles and all "high sauce" should not be touched by children.[48] It may have been understood by the readers of those days that children in an agricultural country would naturally be supplied with an abundance of fresh vegetables, at least in season; but whatever the cause for the omission in works of this type, the modern reader is led to believe that little importance was attached to vegetables, as such, in the child's "economy of health."

Fruits at best were given only a half-hearted approval. One reads: "Children should not be debarred from fruit; but the use of it requires some attention." This "attention" demanded that the fruit be ripe, limited in quantity, and of a kind that would agree with the child. It was a disputed point whether children should eat fruit in the morning, since to reach the pulp and juice which refreshed them they had to eat the surrounding skin. This "tough kind of coat in which nature had wrapped the fruit" was considered unfit to take into the stomach.[49] As late as 1835, Dr. William Dewees of Philadelphia wrote on this head:

It is an error to suppose, that any fruit is positively useful, as a nourishment or as a medicine, to young children. . . . We have known them to be useful, but we have very often known them to be injurious. . . . Fruit of almost every kind is less digestible than any of the farinaceous substances in common use.[51]

Fish was among the foods held extremely improper for children, and the prudent parent was warned never to let the child so much as taste it for his first seven years, at least, if for no other reason than for the danger of bones sticking in his throat. Since fish of all kinds was regarded as naturally "flabby, cold, and watery," it was of itself deemed unfit for young stomachs, and was usually made more so by rich sauces. Nuts also fell into the category of forbidden foods that "should never be meddled with because they were apt to create a thirst, or even produce coughs by cording up the whole chest." It was also believed that nuts loosened children's teeth—a process which foolish youth assisted by their repeated attempts to crack the hard shells.[51]

William Cobbett further observed on the question of foods outlawed for children:

This love of what is called "good eating and drinking," if very unamiable in grown up persons, is perfectly hateful in youth; and if he indulges in the propensity he is already half ruined. Let me beseech you to free yourselves from the slavery of tea and coffee, and other slop kettle. . . . Experience has taught me that those slops are injurious to health.[53]

The practice of giving children wine, cider, beer, and brandy aroused even more vehement protests. This custom, rather common in some sections, was condemned as a gross error because it "clouded the understanding," rendered young people unfit for study, and laid "the foundation of a sot for life."[53] Such authorities as Benjamin Rush, on the other hand, recommended the use of "sound old wine, from a teaspoonful to one half a glassful according to the age of the child" to be taken as a prophylactic medicine in the summertime. He also sanctioned the custom of upper-class children sipping a glass of wine after dinner now and then with their parents.[54] William Buchan, an English doctor, listed milk, water, buttermilk, or whey as the most proper beverages for children.[55] In recommending pure cold water as the best drink for healthy youth, a Philadelphia physician described the excessive intemperance of his day:

In the western parts of our state, where ardent spirits has become almost the substitute for water, whiskey is given daily in large quantities, from the youngest to the oldest child; and, so quickly do they become accustomed to this pernicious liquor, that we have seen a child of six or seven years old, drink a wine-glass full at a draught. . . . [57]

In contrast to the advice given the young in the previous century "To eat as fast as possible," health authorities of the early 1800's recognized in this habit the besetting table fault of American children. Parents were told to allow their offspring at least twenty minutes for each meal, and for adults to set the young the proper example by eating slowly.[57] Another change in juvenile eating habits may be noted in the contrasting instructions given on this point. In Colonial days the child was told to eat everything that was put on his trencher without asking questions or making remarks; nor was he to "look sour or to murmur" at what was given him.[58] Parents of the new day were thus advised to regard the child's personality:

As the child grows up its own palate should in some degree be consulted, in selecting its food; and if not *positively improper,* it should be indulged in its little likings to a certain extent. Children, if observed will be found to show a fondness for particular things, and an aversion to others. It is an innate feeling, and is as various and as natural as in the adult; and although it has not been viewed generally in this light, it ought not to be disregarded.[60]

The evil of allowing children "spiritous liquors" did not evoke nearly so much denunciation from writers on child health as did the simple matter of "confectionary." Numerous sources indicate how children "on their morning walks" too commonly visited confectioners' shops, there to jeopardize their health by eating a variety of "sweetmeats and pastry." Those tempted to such indiscretions were advised to let their luncheon of sweets serve them instead of a dinner, and to eat no more that day "till their stomachs were entirely emptied of those contents that were so difficult to digestion."[60] Other writers pointed out that although sweetmeats and toys of confectionery had a peculiar charm for children, these same devices were usually covered with poisonous paint and hence were positively injurious as articles of food.[61]

This question of confectionery also had a moral side that transcended even the important issue of health. According to the moralists, these forbidden sweetmeats not only tended to undermine the health of children, but such delicacies destroyed the "tone of their minds" and laid foundations of ingratitude and discontent in the young. When parents failed to supply the sweets as often as the pampered appetites of youth demanded, children then forgot all former kindnesses and either loudly complained of their parents' parsimony or in sullen discontent murmured because they were so cruelly treated.[62]

While it was regarded as an ill omen to find the young very fond of confectionery, some allowance was made for a fondness for fruits, since they were supposed to be of a "cooling nature" and came at a season when refreshing foods were especially needed. Sweets taken between meals had a "heating tendency" which interfered with digestion, and, if they were taken with the child's meals, would weaken his stomach. From any such simple indulgence, the child's "several animal appetites" became vitiated—not instantly, indeed, but such was the tendency. When the child thus departed from the strict rules of temperance in any given article of food or drink, his progress was downward, with the result that either the quantity of food or drink was gradually increased or the quality more concentrated.[63]

For these reasons, reformers of the 1830's trembled to find the young so fond of exciting foods, condiments, and confectionery. In the case of children whose appetites were already vitiated, there was no assurance that they would not become worse and worse until they finally arrived at the lowest point on the scale of intemperance, gluttony, and debauchery. Although the matter seems of little moment today, it was a real issue in the early 1800's. Moralists pointed to the thousands of young people who "went down to ruin" by this alluring trail; and reformers sought to influence public opinion in favor of closing confectionery shops outright. To some degree prohibition of confections preceded prohibition of liquors as an American social reform movement.

In order to impress on the youthful minds the imminent perils to body and soul that lurked in a bag of candy or a box of cookies, reformers traced a gradation of evils. It was first pointed out that those unfortunates who felt the necessity of using confectionery merely for the sake of the pleasure and excitement it afforded uniformly lost their health. Then, dissatisfied with these feebler excitements, they proceeded to gratify the lower appetites with strong tea, coffee, fermented liquors, snuff, opium, or tobacco, and perhaps with several of them combined. Moralists also hinted that many descended by this broad road to indulgence "more disreputable, as well as more destructive."[64] After reading the horrible example of degenerates, the ordinary child must have required but little imagination to picture himself inexorably driven by a peppermint stick along the path to perdition.

It is easy for the modern reader to imagine the child's reaction to these reform measures of what now seems a really innocuous gratification. One of the most vehement writers, to point his moral on this subject, held up the female seminaries as impressive examples of delinquency in this regard. Although these institutions were respected by the reformer as the "hope of our country and of our race," nevertheless they still afforded abundant cause for gloomy forebodings. In almost every institution the preceptors found an "insurmountable fondness for confectionary." The record shows that they forthwith framed laws to check the evil and imposed severe penalties for existing abuses. Like other attempts at prohibition, these reform measures finally failed, and succeeding generations of American youth have led the world in the annual consumption of sweets.[65]

Fortunately the social historian has statistics to show the "alarming proportions" of these childish aberrations. In one city (presumably Boston) there was a large school about twenty rods from a fruit and confectionery shop. The owner of the shop frankly confessed that her daily profits on the "single article of molasses candy," most of which was sold to the school children, were seventy-five cents, and that her sales on this article sometimes amounted to ten dollars a week. After some rapid calculations, the writer reported that since the initial cost of molasses candy was very little, he could safely conclude that the pupils of the school purchased about one dollar's worth a day! As he contemplated the "uselessness" of such sweets, and sighed over the "alarming extent" to which they were used, he could offer only the most dismal prospects for the health and morality of American children.[66]

The question of sleep was another phase of child health that called forth much discussion. The English philosopher Locke, whose advice on many points was closely followed by American parents, declared that "of all which looks soft and effeminate," nothing is to be indulged children more than sleep. On the other hand, nothing was deemed more "injudicious and unnatural" than the custom many parents had of keeping their children up late; for the first law in making boys and girls healthy, temperate, and wise was to create in them habits of early rising and retiring.[67]

In regard to the place and manner of putting the child to bed, nearly all writers agreed that the room in which he slept should be "quiet, obscure, and large enough to allow a free circulation of air," that the windows of his apartment should always be kept open except at night; but at this point harmony of opinion ended. Some thought the child should be given only cold food for supper some hours before going to bed; others advocated warm bread and milk as the best evening meal. Although little ones for decades had worn nightcaps on the supposition that they were particularly good for the hair, eyes, and teeth, parents were advised by the middle of the eighteenth century to keep the child's head cool, and—even though the head was shaved—to dispense with the warm nightcap. Children, however, for another century continued, perhaps advisedly, to wear nightcaps in their cold, drafty homes. Tradition also drew the curtains closely around the bed of the child on the theory that night air had some noxious quality; and thus the child was confined almost entirely to the air within the small compass of the bed frame. There were those who considered this practice highly erroneous, and urged that parents would do well to let their children lie with the curtains undrawn or, at most, arranged to protect their heads.[68]

Charles Darwin, by 1835, was teaching that the "beds for young children could not be too soft," but he denounced the error of having "so deep a feather bed for a child that he sinks down into the middle of it," and remarked, "Perhaps beds made of soft leather, properly prepared and inflated with air, might be preferable, on this account to feather beds."[69] Locke, on the contrary, had said: "Let the child's bed be hard, and rather quilts than feathers." He affirmed that "hard lodgings" strengthened the body; but being "buried every night in feathers" melted and dissolved it, and that this practise was often the cause of weakness and the forerunner of early death. Since his conclusion was that "a tender weakly constitution was very much owing to down beds," he advised that children should sleep on a "mattrass" and use only a bolster with no pillow, for it was not good for them to have their heads high. Alcott, at variance with this opinion, had no objections to soft beds for any part of the community; in fact, he preferred them for obvious reasons. He was of the opinion that the person who slept on a hard board, though he might rest quite well, could not be as comfortable as if his bed were softer, since the weight of his body pressed on a few small spots.[70]

Although the form of the bed itself was much discussed by medical authorities, most children in the crowded homes of that day were tucked into cradles, cribs, trundles, or folding beds, without much theorizing on the part of their busy parents. There seems to have been little hesitancy either in shifting little ones from one place to another, or in crowding several children into one bed; and there was no fear that a change would affect them, since it was believed that children slept soundly wherever laid.[71] It was probably in reference to conditions in the crowded frontier cabins where a traveler found "six fine but dirty children" sleeping in an adjoining bed[72] that a doctor wrote, "In order to secure the advantage of undisturbed repose, it is important that too many children be not crowded together."[73] In any event, writers firmly insisted that all "the cares and burdens of the day were to be laid aside with the children's clothing." Even in the case of older boys and girls, no practice was judged more destructive than that of studying in bed, or of reading until sleep came.[74]

Though children of the eighteenth century were dressed in imitation of their parents, and were expected to conform as closely as possible to adult standards of living, even in the Colonial period there were occasional protests against the pernicious effects of costume on child health. The hazards involved in the dress of the young sprang from a fatal combination of ignorance and oversolicitude on the part of grown-ups, rather than from any deliberate intention to torture or annoy children—albeit the results were the same.

Mothers or nurses observed that a newborn child had not support of itself—that its head leaned on one side or the other, and the little body sank into a heap. To remedy this condition and to prop up the helpless babe, they put a stay to its neck, and rolled a long strip of flannel many times around its body. At the end of a month the infant was usually "coated"; that is, it was still bound by the roller when undressed for the night, but in the daytime when dressed, it wore a "stay" about the waist. Since popular opinion argued that children were helpless and could not sit upright or be tossed about as custom demanded without a support, the same kind of device was applied to both boys and girls. Only gradually was the child relieved of these cruel contrivances; after several months the neck stay was left off, and the roller was abandoned in about a year. Although the first three stays were rather soft and pliable, those used after the age of two were stiffer, and this was the type worn by boys until they were put into trousers at the age of six, and by girls throughout their lives.[75]

Fashion thus interfered with the comfort and even the health of children. Some adults always doubted whether a graceful form in children compensated for the tortures of these contraptions. Most mothers, however, for decades insisted on retaining this method of molding the youthful figure. The solicitude of parents for a good form related chiefly to the girls. Boys "twisted themselves like eels into a thousand forms," and eventually succeeded in holding their bodies erect without a framework of whalebone; but girls, with less freedom and more anxiety, seldom developed so well, although God had originally made both sexes equally upright.[76]

This peculiar type of torture in the form of juvenile clothing lasted until the close of the century. Since fashions came to America from France, the political revolution in France was also accompanied by a radical change in children's dress. This revolution in juvenile clothing was almost as significant as the overthrow of the Bourbon dynasty, for it banished for little ones on this side of the Atlantic wigs and buckles, powder and pomatum, stiff stays and full petticoats, long waists and high-heeled shoes.

During the Empire period, one extreme led to another. Little girls, who previously had been encased in whalebone and buckram and layers of quilted skirts, stepped forth as free as nymphs, without stays, petticoats, fullness to their garments, or even heels to their shoes. White muslin dresses of the scantiest dimensions, fitting closely around the figure, with the shortest possible waist and not an extra fold in the skirt, were the garments commonly worn by American girls of the early 1800's. Mothers, viewing the change and remembering their own hooped skirts and flowing drapery, groaned over their daughters, and declared that the scanty dresses made the girls look as though they had been "stuffed into bolster-cases."[77]

This apparent improvement in the hygiene of clothing was involuntary and only a capricious foreign influence in fashion. Within a decade the dress of the young gradually reverted to its former voluminous dimensions; even some additional atrocities were then introduced in the shape of stiff collars, high tight breeches and short waistcoats for boys, and cumbersome skirts and dangling pantalettes for girls. Reformers gave the matter of dress their serious attention and advocated definite measures for correcting the evils of the time:

The dress of children ought to be light and easy; their linen ought to be frequently changed, and all motions of the body should be unrestrained by ligatures of any kind . . . it ought to be comfortable, not fine: and it ought to differ in fashion from that worn by those in advanced life.[78]

Mavor argued that a simple costume would allow little ones to live with less restraint and greater happiness in the society of one another; and by contrast with that of adults, a distinctive dress for children would be an indication of their dependent status. He also believed that special juvenile styles would check the early temptations to "pride which led children to ape the customs and actions of grown-up persons"—a practice not only unbecoming to their age, but dangerous to their health and morals.[79] To achieve the desired simplicity in children's clothing and to protect their health and morals, Mavor advocated a uniform costume for boys and girls, to be worn from the age of three to eight. According to this plan, the head and neck of the child were to be free and bare; the body was to be clothed with a wide linen shirt and short-sleeved frock, while the feet were to be equipped with a pair of short socks

and low-heeled, well-fitting shoes.[80] Another authority with more advanced ideas believed that it would be better for children not to wear
stockings, because their "tender legs, though uncovered, were not easily
affected by the cold." It was asserted that if stockings were altogether
abandoned, children would be less subject to coughs and colds.[81]

The homemade shoes of Colonial days—designed to cover rather than
to fit—were generally too narrow and ill fitting to allow sufficient room
for motion, or they were so long and loose as to be easily trodden down
at the heels. In either case, the young wearer was likely to acquire a
deformity that resulted in an awkward and unsafe gait. To enable the
child to walk more steadily, low-heeled, waterproof half-boots that supported his ankles and fitted his legs were introduced late in the eighteenth
century.[82] This new design of shoes for both boys and girls, shaped as
they were to the form of the foot by separate lasts, and fastened with
strings instead of buckles, resulted in a more upright posture, and at the
same time enabled children to run and jump with freedom and comfort.[83]

It was fashionable by 1835 for children to be "more thinly clad" than
their parents, and some observers claimed that nothing was more common than to see little ones "with their arms, neck, and upper portions
of the chest bare." Many critics were slow in endorsing this process of
"hardening" the race at the risk of killing off its weaker members.[84]
Indeed, most parents were inclined to follow the more comfortable advice,
"Give children plenty of milk, plenty of sleep, and plenty of flannel."[85]
Flannel was considered the best material for underclothing "at all times
and at all seasons." Many adults believed that disease and death were
conveyed by every blast of air, hence a "due quantity of covering should
be employed." Some held that health was best protected even in the
hottest climates by the use of fine flannel next to the skin.[86] There was,
however, a diversity of opinion on the advisability of keeping children
in flannels during hot weather. This was evidenced in the bewildered
discomfort of an eleven-year-old boy who wrote from Georgia in mid-
summer:

tell dear mother that cousin Bet will not let me pull off my flannen that she
would if she was me take off everything but the flannen, I look so red and
harty that you would not know me, but Uncle says that I will never get harty
in the world untill I take off my flannen. . . . [88]

Long-needed reforms were inaugurated by the middle 'thirties, as a
result of the pleas made at the turn of the century for a distinct dress
for children. Although these reforms did not mature until much later,
most children were no longer pinioned by stiff stays. Moreover, linen

or cotton underclothing that could be changed more frequently was gradually replacing the cherished flannels of former days. Boys and girls also
found, in the short socks and sturdy new half-boots made to the shape
of their feet, more comfort and freedom of motion than Colonial children
had ever known in their crudely fashioned cloth or kid shoes. Although
children were still too much muffled up and overdressed in cold weather,
there was more insistence on outdoor exercise; and the sports garments
worn then were more simply and loosely designed. Nightcaps were still
in vogue in cold homes, but children were freshly dressed for bed in
a new type of warm nightclothing.[88] Umbrellas to shelter the head from
the sun and rain were also in common use, and rubbers protected the
feet of the well-to-do youth.[89] On the other hand, there were thousands
of frontier children of both sexes whose parents, following a policy of
salutary neglect, clad them day and night in single, scanty shifts. Evidence
of this custom may be found in the following report of a traveler: "In
some of the interior hovels, are seen little once-white boys sitting at the
table in their long shirts; and running half the summer with nothing
else on; which renders them hardy."[90]

That bathing was one of the most neglected aspects of child care in
Colonial America might be inferred from the infrequent references to
the subject in children's books. Indeed, the primitive mode of life characteristic of many communities inhibited the frequent bathing of children,
for it was not easy to wash at the pump in the yard or in a metal pan
on the back porch. In cold weather people naturally dispensed with all
but the briefest ablutions before the kitchen fire. To understand the
apparent unconcern in such matters one must keep in mind the lack
of the simplest facilities for cleanliness. In Revolutionary times only a
few wealthy families owned tubs and basins, and the traditional bowl
and pitcher were used by the middle classes; but even these simple devices
were denied the isolated people of rural districts.[91]

Besides the scarcity of tubs and warm water, other hardships made
the bath a trial of endurance for the young. Bathing on pleasant summer
days, in the manner described in an old story book, was indeed a sport
that might well be classified with baseball and leapfrog:

> When the Sun's Beams have warmed the Air,
> Our Youth to some cool Brook repair;
> In whose refreshing streams they play,
> To the last Remnant of the Day.[93]

But bathing on a frosty winter day in the drafty homes of that period
could scarcely have been mistaken for a sport by a shivering child. Even

from the vantage point before the open hearth there was small comfort, for in the frigid rooms water frequently froze in a pan before the fire, while the sudden blasts from the chimney chilled any zest for cleanliness even in the hardiest youth. Added misery was found in the coarse home-made lye soap which, even when used sparingly as advised, chapped and irritated the child's tender skin.[93] Although a mild castile soap and an innovation called a "bathing machine" were introduced early in the nineteenth century, bathing remained a rare experience for most children. On the grounds that the bathing machine helped the child to enjoy his bath, these large shallow vessels made of wood, tin, or canvas were widely advertised. The mother was counseled to "amuse" the child during his penitential experience in the tub in order to prepare him, by the cheerful endurance of this ordeal, to cope with future tribulations.[94] In a rare book of poetry for children by the English authors, Charles and Mary Lamb, one finds an early reference to cleanliness as a factor in child life:

> All-endearing cleanliness,
> Virtue next to godliness,
> Easiest, cheapest, needful'st duty,
> To the body health and beauty,
> Who that's human would refuse it,
> When a little water does it?[95]

Early Americans inherited a distinct aversion to water as an impure beverage which was generally believed to have a malevolent effect on the drinker, and this repugnance doubtless lessened the desire to use water for any other purpose.[96] It is a matter of record that Colonial children entertained the traditional misgivings about persistent scourings and scrubbings at the hands of their elders. The old *School of Good Manners,* which followed every avenue of child life, summarily dismissed the whole subject in one sentence: "Come not to the table without having your Hands and Face washed, and your Head combed."[97] Despite the strict discipline of the time, several sources reveal children of sufficient spirit to resist any efforts of their elders to make them "clean and decent." Under the trying circumstances attending an ordinary scrubbing perhaps the attitude of "Dirty Jack" towards personal cleanliness was understood, if not excused, by his contemporaries:

> His friends were much hurt,
> To see so much dirt,
> And often and well did they scour;
> But all was in vain,
> He was dirty again
> Before they had done it an hour.

When to wash he was sent,
He reluctantly went,
With water to splash himself o'er,
But he left the black streaks
All over his cheeks,
And made them look worse than before.[99]

The care of the teeth was another phase of Colonial child health that was pitifully neglected. The child was simply told, "If you will keep your teeth from rot, pluc, or aking, wash the mouth continually with Juyce of Lemons, and afterwards rub your teeth with a Sage Leaf and wash your teeth after meat with faire water."[99] There were of course no dentists in Colonial America, and no real knowledge of dental care. After the Revolution, when dental surgery began to receive some attention, authorities advised children to preserve their teeth by washing them night and morning with a brush, and by rinsing the mouth after each meal with clean water.[100] Others directed them to use salt and water daily, but only as a mouth wash; for they declared that "all brushing and scraping" of the teeth was dangerous and did "great mischief."[101] Some children chewed charcoal, or used chalk and camphor or some other powder on their brush as a dentifrice; others cleaned their teeth by rubbing them with a primitive brush made usually of a dogwood twig chewed into a fibrous swab.[102]

One Philadelphia authority, Dr. Dewees, regretted the fact that most parents attached no importance to the care of the child's "milk" teeth. Under the delusion that these first teeth would soon be lost and therefore did not merit attention, adults frequently neglected the mouths of the young. Dewees was among the few professionals who advised the removal by a skillful dentist of the child's loose or decayed teeth or stumps of teeth if they ached, "in order to prevent the formation of gum-boils." For these, he pointed out, would injure the second teeth.[103]

From this examination of the meager records of child care some estimate may be made of the dangers that beset childhood in the Colonial and early national periods. The diseases incidental to a newly opened country, the general ignorance of hygiene, the lack of competent medical skill, uncleanliness, and improper dress and diet combined to rob the country annually of a high percentage of its children. After the Revolution, medical authorities on both sides of the Atlantic sought for decades to discover why society was thus "ruthlessly weeded," and to take preventive measures.

Although no remarkable achievements may be noted for this period, the first three decades of the nineteenth century, in marked contrast to the Colonial era, reveal a slow but steady improvement in the attitude of the American adult towards the problem of child welfare. This advance in both the theory and practise of child care was conditioned partly by the progress made in scientific knowledge, and partly by the higher living standards which left mothers more time to devote to the care of their families. With the increased interest in child welfare stimulated by the economic and scientific advancement of the age, improved methods for the management of the young were given wide publicity, even if they were not universally accepted and put into practice by 1835.

[1] Richard H. Shryock, *The Development of Modern Medicine*, pp. 78-85.

[2] Oliver P. Chitwood, *A History of Colonial America*, pp. 578-81.

[3] Shryock, *op. cit.*, pp. 86, 87.

[4] Edward Eggleston, *The Transit of Civilization from England to America in the Seventeenth Century*, pp. 48-50.

[5] *Ibid.*, p. 51.

[6] *Ibid.*, pp. 52, 53; see also Henry C. Lea, ed., *A Century of American Medicine*, pp. 6-16.

[7] *Ibid.*, p. 61.

[8] *Ibid.*, pp. 64-68.

[9] *Ibid.*, pp. 69-73.

[10] William P. Dewees, M. D., *A Treatise on the Physical and Medical Treatment of Children*, p. 145.

[11] *Original Poems for Infant Minds*, p. 40.

[12] William Darton, *Chapter of Accidents and Remarkable Events: Containing Caution and Instruction for Children*, pages unnumbered.

[13] *Ibid.*

[14] *The Post Boy*, pages unnumbered.

[15] *Little Prattle Over a Book of Prints*, pages unnumbered.

[16] Nathan Bayley, *English and Latine Exercises for School Boys*, p. 152.

[17] *A Little Pretty Pocket-Book*, first Worcester edition, by Isaiah Thomas, pp. 7-9.

[18] Benjamin Coleman, *A Devout Contemplation on the Meaning of Divine Providence in the Early Death of Pious and Lovely Children*, p. 5.

[19] Noah Webster, *Elements of Useful Knowledge*, p. 184.

[20] George Fisher (pseud.), *The American Instructor*, Preface.

[21] *Ibid.*, p. 344.

[22] *Ibid.*

[23] *Ibid.*, p. 345.

[24] William Mavor (Fordyce), *The Catechism of Health*, p. 58.

[25] Mrs. A. G. Whittelsey, ed., "The Right Education of Youth," *The Mother's Magazine*, VIII (1840), 271.

[26] Fisher, *op. cit.*, pp. 369, 370.

[27] *Ibid.*, pp. 347, 348.

[28] *Ibid.*, p. 348.

[29] *Ibid.*, pp. 348, 349.

[30] *Ibid.*, pp. 362, 363.

[31] Walter Harris, *A Treatise on the Acute Diseases of Infants*, pp. 153-55.

[32] R. C. Faust, *Catechism of Health for Use of Schools*, p. 20.

[33] Christian Augustus Struve, M. D., *A Familiar View of the Domestic Education of Children during the Early Period of Their Lives*, pp. 33, 34.

[34]Dr. G. Ackerley, *On the Management of Children in Sickness and in Health,* second edition, p. 64.

[35]Lydia H. Sigourney, *Letters to Mothers,* p. 73.

[36]Mavor, *op. cit.,* Preface.

[37]John Hersey, *Advice to Christian Parents,* p. 86.

[38]Theodore Dwight, *The Father's Book,* p. 43. See also *Letters to a Young Student in the First Stage of a Liberal Education,* p. 41.

[39]*Original Poems for Infant Minds,* p. 74.

[40]The very mistakes condemned in the hygienic literature probably indicate how children actually did live. This was undoubtedly true not only of diet, but of all other phases of regimen.

[41]Ackerley, *op. cit.,* p. 58.

[42]*Ibid.,* pp. 59, 60.

[43]*Ibid.,* p. 60.

[44]James Nelson, *An Essay on the Government of Children,* p. 133.

[45]*Ibid.,* p. 124.

[46]Theodore Dwight, *op. cit.,* p. 128.

[47]*The Cries of New York, Printed and sold by Samuel Wood at the Juvenile Bookstore,* p. 41. This work also gives a quaint account of the sanitary measures in force at this time by explaining to children the office of the "Bell-Man":

> "This man on his cart,
> As he drives along,
> His bell doth swing
> Ding, dong, ding, dong.

When the warm season commences, as one means for the preservation of health, the citizens are not allowed to throw into the streets the offal of any animal, husks of corn, pea-pods, or any kind of garbage, dead rats, cats, or shells, but the servants have them ready in baskets or pails, and when they hear this man's bell turn out, and empty them into his cart. Such part as is fit for hogs or cows to eat he preserves and discharges the rest off the end of the dock into the river."

[48]Nelson, *op. cit.,* p. 133.

[49]*Ibid.,* p. 128.

[50]Dewees, *op. cit., pp.* 205-7.

[51]Nelson, *op. cit.,* pp. 127-9.

[52]As quoted in Hersey, *op. cit.,* p. 88.

[53]Nelson, *op. cit.,* p. 86.

[54]As quoted by John Ruhrah, *Pediatrics of the Past,* p. 430.

[55]William Buchan, *Domestic Medicine,* p. 15.

[56]Dewees, *op. cit.,* p. 175.

[57]Dwight, *op. cit.,* p. 43.

[58]Hersey, *op. cit.,* p. 85.

[59]Ackerley, *op. cit.,* p. 67.

[60]Eliza Ware Farrar, *The Young Lady's Friend,* p. 193.

[61]Christian A. Struve, *op. cit.,* p. 431.

[62]John Hersey, *op. cit.,* p. 84.

[63]William A. Alcott, ed., *The Moral Reformer and Teacher on the Human Constitution,* p. 50.

[64]*Ibid., pp.* 85, 86.

[65]*Ibid.,* p. 52.

[66]*Ibid.,* p. 82.

[67]Nelson, *op. cit.,* p. 138.

[68]*Ibid.,* pp. 140, 141.

[69]Alcott, *op. cit.,* p. 24.

[70]*Ibid.,* p. 25.

[71]Nelson, *op. cit.,* p. 139.

[72]William Faux, *Memorable Days in America*. In Reuben G. Thwaites, ed., *Early Western Travels, 1748-1846,* 30 vols. and Index (1904-1906), XI (1905), 226.

[73]Ackerley, *op. cit.,* p. 71.

[74]Mrs. A. G. Whittelsey, ed., "On Sleep," *The Mother's Magazine,* VIII (1840-43) 187.

[75]Nelson, *op. cit.,* pp. 109, 110.

[76]Lydia H. Sigourney, *op. cit.,* p. 78. In their poetry for children, Charles and Mary Lamb picture the pride experienced by a little boy on the day he cast away his "long coats" and put on the "manly breeches":

> Sashes, frocks, to those that need 'em—
> Phillip's limbs have got their freedom—
> He can run or he can ride,
> And do twenty things beside,
> Which his petticoats forbad;
> Is he not a happy lad?
> Now he's under other banners,
> He must leave his former manners;
> Bid adieu to female games,
> And forget their very names.
> Puss in corner, hide and seek,
> Sports for girls and punies weak!

(Charles and Mary Lamb, *Poetry for Children, entirely original,* p. 34.)

[77]Eliza Ware Farrar, *The Young Lady's Friend,* pp. 97, 98. See also Mavor, *Catechism of Health,* pp. 21, 22.

[78]G. Ackerley, *op. cit.,* pp. 68, 69.

[79]Mavor, *op. cit.,* pp. 22, 23.

[80]Ackerley, *op. cit.,* pp. 68, 69.

[81]C. A. Struve, *op. cit.,* p. 303.

[82]*Ibid.,* pp. 304, 305.

[83]Ackerley, *op. cit.,* p. 61.

[84]D. Gilbert, *The Mother's Magazine,* VIII, 270.

[85]John Robertson, *Observations on the Mortality and Physical Management of Children,* p. 188.

[86]Ackerley, *op. cit.,* p. 69.

[87]Quoted by Elizabeth A. Wilson, "Hygienic Care and Management of the Child in the American Family Prior to 1860" (M. S. thesis, Duke University, 1940), p. 135.

[88]Samuel K. Jennings, *The Married Lady's Companion; or The Poor Man's Friend,* pp. 145-416.

[89]Alcott, *op. cit.,* p. 48.

[90]As quoted in Wilson, *op. cit.,* p. 142; Singleton, *Letters from the South and West,* p. 93.

[91]Farrar, *op. cit.,* p. 163.

[92]*A Little Pretty Pocket-Book,* p. 42.

[93]Wilson, *op. cit.,* pp. 92, 93.

[94]*Ibid.,* p. 94.

[95]Lamb, *op. cit.,* p. 31.

[96]Earle, *Customs and Fashions in the Old New England,* pp. 302-5.

[97]Moodey, *School of Good Manners.*

[98]*Original Poems for Infant Minds,* p. 38.

[99]Earle, *op. cit.,* p. 302.

[100]Mavor, *op. cit.,* p. 53.

[101]Buchan, *op. cit.,* p. 305.

[102]Earle, *op. cit.,* p. 302.

[103]Dewees, *op. cit.,* p. 191.

SNARES

OF THE

OLD DELUDER

"Let thy Recreation be Lawful, Brief, and Seldom." This terse injunction found in the *School of Good Manners* epitomized the attitude of adults towards play in Colonial days, but not that of children. Boys and girls, despite this edict, followed at least furtively the natural bent of childhood, sublimely heedless of the prevailing conviction that a desire for play was a "snare of the Old Deluder" or another evidence of their "corrupt nature." According to the record, little Americans, among them Sammy Mather and the children of Judge Sewell, from within the very stronghold of Puritanism itself, displayed, to the dismay of their parents, "an inordinate love of play." These children contrived to amuse themselves with a variety of games, indifferent to the scornful stand of their elders for such foolish and sinful waste of time.

This condemnation of the universal love of play was partly conditioned by the poverty, the incessant labors, the dangers and privations incidental to Colonial life, as well as by a religion that glorified thrift and industry. Until well after the Revolution most adults had little time and less inclination to indulge in pastimes. The grim struggle for existence on the borders of an unexplored wilderness furnished sufficient occupation for the minds and bodies of these more responsible members of American society. A disapproving attitude—exalted to a virtue by necessity—kept a tenacious hold on the American mind, for as late as 1814, a little book named *The Seasons* bore this warning to young and old:

Unless care and labor are taken to keep down the evil propensities of little children to anger, idleness, *and too much play*, they will grow up in evil habits; and instead of being useful members of society they will be pests and burdens; will drag out an unprofitable existence here, and must expect in the coming world, that their lot will be among the miserable.[1]

An enthusiasm for play was classed by some adults as a temporary weakness or a passing defect of the childish character which, like many disagreeable habits, would eventually be outgrown or lost with the milk teeth. In the ensuing interval, until the seriousness of life was fully appreciated, the follies of youth and their yearnings for pleasures must be tolerated or suppressed as occasion demanded. Other adults bitterly deplored an enthusiasm for play as a childish inclination to evil—the sad result of original sin. Quite aptly, then, did Dr. Watts in his collection of *Divine Songs* express the popular sentiment on this head. Witness the sense of shame and grief he put into the child's complaint of his love of sports:

> How senseless is my heart and wild,
> How vain are all my thoughts!
> Pity the weakness of a child,
> And pardon all my faults.[2]

Another little book, *A Present to Children,* printed in New London in 1783, underscored the popular theory that play was a waste of time and that the love of it was an unfailing sign of a perverted nature. In somber tones little readers were warned:

Improve your time. When you play do it because God gives you leave. Learn to get good and do good in your plays. Don't learn foolish songs by heart, nor read them. Some songs are made for your play; not too solemn, that so you may say them in your sports without being profane and have no occasion to learn worse.[3]

As a whole, the moral songs in this work were dedicated to the apparently impossible task of directing the child's natural inclination to play into more profitable channels. Indicative of the conflict between the two worlds—that of adulthood with its moral repression for the playful minor members of society, and that of childhood with its passive resistence to unnatural restraint and gloom—the *Present* gives illuminating glimpses of the limited emotional life of the Colonial child. The lines "On Good Company" convey the impression that, even at this early stage of our national social development, halos were not the universal adornment of American youth, notwithstanding the stern, unyielding pietism with which their lives were surrounded:

> How many Children do I see
> With Noise and Folly fill the Street?
> They're lewd, call wicked Name and lye,
> Quarrel and rail at all they met.

With those who fear my God I'll walk,
And their dear Conversation court,
Often we'll mingle serious Talk,
Nor lose Salvation in our Sport.[4]

Quite clearly also does "A Song for Little Miss" in this same volume define, on the one hand, the adult standards of industry and sobriety for the godly American girl and, on the other, reveal the little maid's interior anguish for her supposedly blamable love of toys. After a pathetic confession of the pleasure she derived from her "painted toys," and the rapture with which she "carest her jointed babies and hugged them to her breast," or reveled in the "glittering shelves" and tiny "tables, plates, and chairs of her Baby-Room," she resolves:

> Fain would I guard this prattling Voice,
> These haughty Airs suppress;
> No more shall Baubles be my Choice
> Nor Plays nor Idleness.
>
> In Work my tender Hands, shall strive,
> And Wisdom watch my Tongue;
> My Lips shall learn, and in my Life,
> I'll copy out the Song.[5]

The "Plays" for boys, as depicted in this same work, were made the occasions for introspection, and were accompanied by suitable homilies exposing the vain and fleeting pleasures of this transitory existence. After learning how eagerly the boy rushed from school to his "marbles, whirling top, or bounding ball," the little reader could meditate on these lines:

> The changing Marbles to me show,
> How mutable all things below,
> My fate and their's may be the same,
> Dasht in an instant from the Game.
>
> Now on the Ice I shape the Slide,
> And smoothly o'er the Surface glide,
> I learn amidst the slipp'ry Play
> Most dangerous is the easiest Way.[6]

Happily for the young, the disparaging attitude of most adults for what was considered an excess of play had changed in some degree by the turn of the century. Not only did more secure economic conditions provide richer opportunities for the majority of Americans to relax a little; but the romanticism of the age had raised the child, as a distinct personality, to a position of some importance in the family. At the same time the strict principles of Puritanism had been somewhat mitigated. With this change in adult thinking came a partial shift in the popular attitude toward the child, expressed in this case by a desire to afford him amusement and recreation, at least to a limited degree. Instead of viewing the ordinary juvenile propensity for play as "a snare of the Old Deluder, Satan," many adults now saw the value of "rational and useful sports." Children's books reflected the change, and as a result there appeared such surprising sentiments as those expressed in *The Child's Spelling Book* of 1802:

> Youth to pastime is inclin'd
> Ever fix'd on play:
> Sport unbends the studious mind
> And makes the heart more gay.[7]

The idea of making "the heart more gay," or the indulgence of a mere personal gratification, was not yet widely considered the legitimate end of children's play. The goal was to refresh the bodily powers for a more successful discharge of duty. It was now a recognized fact, supported by the writing of medical authorities, that the constitution of the child's mind was such that it could not bear to be intensively employed on a given subject for a long time without interruption. It was also believed that in the attempt to keep it thus employed, far less was accomplished than might be gained with occasional relaxation; for the observation was made that under prolonged strain the energies of the young mind, instead of being improved, were definitely diminished. Hence, on the basis of an adult desire to obtain from the little men and women the greatest usefulness, amusements gradually became a recognized part of child life. Even under the new code, children were still told that they had no right to forget their accountability to God by refusing to acknowledge Him either in the selection of their amusements, or "in yielding themselves to them."[8]

A Catholic juvenile book of the times, in quite the same strain, declared that since recreation was necessary to relax the spirits, particularly of children, play then was not contrary to morals, but rather an act of virtue when it was done well. It was necessary above all things that the motive for playing be good; that the purpose be to recreate the mind, and to make the child more capable of labor which it could not be able to perform if it were always employed. Hence labor was again defined as the end of juvenile sport and recreation.[9]

In order to grow up "good and virtuous," small Christians were given three conditions to observe in their pastimes. The first was to observe moderation; for it was pointed out that excess in play rendered it no longer recreation, but rather employment which dissipated the spirits, enfeebled the powers of the body, and frequently ruined health by the "distempers" it caused. The second condition was not to have an "irregular affection" for amusements—the common fault of childhood. Plainly, this affection made children fall into excess, kept them from applying themselves seriously to labor, and, when at study, continually diverted their minds to sports. The third condition was to avoid all games of chance which, on the testimony of St. Augustine in his *Confessions,* were considered a fruitful source of juvenile delinquency, because youth played these games out of covetousness, which was a criminal motive. Young readers were told of the temporal punishments that followed gamblers—the loss of time and money, and the ruin of families.[10]

Despite the cautious acceptance of juvenile recreation as a necessity—simply as a means of enabling children to perform best the grim business of life—most adults of 1835 were still far from understanding the modern approach to this important subject. Today busy parents consider building block houses, cutting and pasting pictures, blowing soap bubbles, scribbling with crayons, or "dressing up," as a variety of interests to keep little ones absorbed and "good" and out of the way. On the other hand, play means something else to the modern educator; to him it incorporates such aims as the development and control of muscles, the exercise of the imagination, and the growth of creative expression. In the early nineteenth century, as the literature of the age proves, these points of view were for the most part nonexistent.[11]

In reference to children's amusements of early days, Theodore Dwight sounded a typical note when he advocated that playthings, sports, and games should always be connected with some useful end. Surprisingly enough, he longed for the time when "good men would devote due attention" to the improvement of toys and games for children, in which field there was much room for the exercise of ingenuity, talent, and learning. In fact, he advised fathers to use their own judgment in selecting and inventing toys, until such time as the toyshops and bookstores were better supplied with objects appropriate to the needs of children in rational sports.[12]

Since toys for "useful amusements" were scarce, this author advised that boys be permitted to witness the operation of various trades, because he noticed that they invariably enjoyed standing beside carpenters, masons, or stonecutters to watch the unfolding mysteries of their work. With equal fervor he dwelt at length on the pleasant moments boys might spend wandering about the "solitary but busy" lofts of mills, or watching the operations of domestic looms in retired homes. On fine mornings, he remarked, boys loved to observe the movements of fishermen with their nets and to rejoice with them in their catch; or they eagerly followed the plowman through the fresh furrows, and "heard his wisdom on crops and seasons."[13]

As girls were usually better furnished with useful work and amusement than were boys, this author believed it would have been a "happy thing" for many lads if they had been supplied with some substitute for needlework and knitting, since these "useful amusements" made the evenings pass in peaceful pleasure without interruptions to conversation or reading. It was advocated that the boys' daily schedule be as systematically divided as that of the girls between domestic cares and useful activities.[14] The record does not show what the youthful male reactions were to such recommendations, but it does contain the words a small boy scornfully addressed to his sister, who was trying to spin his top. From his reply interesting inferences may be drawn of boyish aversions to the play patterns of the genteel female:

> A top my dear girl is ill chosen for you.
> Go take up your doll, to your baby house go,
> And there your attention much better bestow!
> Leave the Pegtop behind and behave like a miss,
> And I'll give you this picture, these nuts, and a kiss.
> And should I sit on a stool with a needle and thread,
> And dress up Miss Dolly and put her to bed?
> Or do you not think 'twould be pleasant to see,
> Master Neddy turned fribble, and pouring out tea?[15]

Some idea of what constituted the "useful pleasures" of little girls has been left by another writer of the period whose work advised mothers to teach their daughters to knit, to weave bobbins, watchguards, and chains, and to become adept in all kinds of sewing, so that, according to tradition, the devil might not find in their homes employment for idle hands.[16] In almost every family the girls had a "stint" of sewing to do daily; some cross-stitched the alphabet large and small, the figures up to ten, and their name and age in bright-colored wools or silks on canvas; others embroidered slippers or made crocheted bags of twine for carrying their luncheons and other school properties.[17]

Such tasks were not always congenial to the little maids, nor were they always classified by them as "play"; a fact that can be gathered from the very frank inscription deliberately stitched into a sampler by Patty Polk of Maryland, in 1800. Patty left a permanent record of the rebellion that seethed in her young heart when she daringly cross-stitched the words, "Patty Polk did this and she hated every stitch she did in it. She loves to read much more." Then to atone for her unladylike outburst, this studious child bowed to convention and patriotically embroidered on a white tomb the initials G. W. in honor of the Father of her Country, and surrounded the whole with garlands of forget-me-nots.[18]

Indeed, among the more enlightened parents of the last century there were some who recognized in play a natural outlet for the abundant energies of childhood, and who sought to direct this power into proper channels. These adults, in advance of their age, understood that what was commonly considered an innate love of mischief was nothing more than the bubbling activity of youth seeking outlet and expression. The busy hands and brains of children, then as now, were restless for employment—ever seeking something to do—and if they were not furnished with what was useful and innocent, they invariably got into mischief.

To harness this energy, as well as to point the moral of charity, adults fostered, even in the very little, a desire to help others, on the theory that the young were supposed to be happy when they thought themselves useful. Children were encouraged to assist their elders, although such exertions at times probably caused as much trouble as profit. It is recorded that little ones were sent with their baskets on their arms and in the name of peaceful pleasure to pick peas for dinner, to weed the garden, or to feed the chickens, although constant supervision was necessary to prevent such disasters as their pulling up flowers as well as weeds. In the house, too, various small tasks were found to "amuse children innocently." To avoid habits of listlessness or of useless play, little girls dusted chairs and wiped spoons, while their brothers carried firewood and water or ran errands. After these useful pursuits had been accomplished, the attention and skill of the girls might be turned to such "ornamental work" as the making of boxes and baskets as gifts for their friends.[19]

In her *Juvenile Anecdotes*, Pricilla Wakefield gives an intimate description of the "useful amusement" in which a number of little girls engaged:

I was pleased at seeing a little group of girls sitting around a large table, busily employed at needlework; by the cheerfulness of their countenances and the assiduity in their occupations, I guessed they were performing some voluntary task, and enquired whether they were making their dolls new suits . . . or whether the baby house was to be furnished anew. . . . They smiled at my enquiry and the eldest replied that they were making clothes for the poor . . .

and that they made up different things according to their choice. Sometimes they made a complete dress for an infant; one selecting the cap for her share, another a little shirt, a third a printed cotton gown, and a fourth a flannel waistcoat; when the whole suit was finished, it was granted as a peculiar reward to any of them . . . to find some poor helpless babe, who stood in need of such a gift.[20]

In this same book the author described a garden contrived to offer boys various kinds of amusements. In one part was a lawn on which they might play at bowls, trap-ball, or such active sports. Among some tall trees was fixed a rope swing which was supposed to contribute equally to their health and happiness; while in an obscure corner, sheltered by thick shrubs, stood a small building furnished as a carpenter's shop where the boys might prove their skill and ingenuity by making useful objects. Boardwalks were laid for the accommodation of hoops and skipping ropes; and a small piece of ground was allotted to the children to cultivate as they pleased. There they sowed seeds and planted shrubs, cultivated their miniature garden with small spades, hoes, and rakes, and in due season had "a showing of flowers and vegetables."[21]

Although Colonial adults usually did not raise serious objections to the "form" of the games played by their children (such, for instance, as the abhorrence with which New Englanders regarded playing cards and dice), early Americans did begrudge youth the "time" spent in amusements, except that which was necessary to prevent "bodily weakness and infirmity." This distinction must be kept in mind if one is to understand the prevailing sentiment that held it proper to utilize the child's inclination to perpetual motion by his "studies and stints in due season," with no definite allowance for playtime. Early in the nineteenth century the editor of a little book, *Remarks on Children's Play,* frequently observed that the "little innocents" in a city were much to be pitied for the want of "safe and suitable room in the pure air to exercise and recreate themselves." He was far from wishing to encourage too much play, for he wrote:

> Tho' all work and no play makes Jack a dull boy,
> Yet all play and no work makes him a mere toy.[22]

The author of *Youthful Recreations* declared that he did not know who this Jack was, but since he did assent to the principle that youth was the time to obtain a "stock of health," and health was best promoted by moderate exercise, he warned little readers:

> For he who sits by the fire all day,
> And never goes abroad to play,

May keep himself from being cold,
But may not live till he is old.[23]

In order to guarantee the blessings of old age, the boys and girls of the land were advised to engage in some "rational recreation." This writer moreover admonished: "Children will remain more apt for instruction, if we do not break the spring of their capacity for it, by too eagerly overstraining; nay they may enjoy it perpetually, if we but have the art of mixing it with their bodily exercise." To play with the battledore and shuttlecock or with a trap and ball was good exercise; and he went on to say that not only the children of the wealthy, but even those of the poor who were compelled to pick cotton, card wool, or to spin and reel all day, should have at least one hour morning and evening for some youthful recreation. He also pointed out that the children of the poor, who could not afford to buy toys, could at least play at hopscotch.[24]

Although games and toys were accepted as part of the child's equipment for the business of life, this concession was made with some reservations. Witness the admonitions found as late as 1822:

They can employ themselves indoors with their tops to unbend the mind from their studies, when the storm, howling without, forbids their chasing the hoop, or tossing the ball; and in clear cold winter mornings, driving the whip-top has a good effect to exercise the arms and body, and of giving a free circulation to the blood. We would here remind our little readers, that although we recommend divers kinds of plays, as rational, innocent, etc., yet we would wish to be understood that we are far, very far, from being willing to encourage more of any kind, than simply and alone to unbend the mind, invigorate the body, that they may again return to their studies, or other useful employments with fresh energy and vigor.[25]

Among the books of quiet games for the entertainment of children were: *The Whim Wham: or Evening Amusement for all ages and sizes; Being an entire set of riddles, charades, questions, and transportations, by a friend of innocent mirth,* and also *The Puzzling Cap, a Choice Collection of riddles in familiar verse, with a curious cut to each.* The last-named work was not all nonsense; for here and there among the riddles it supplied the child with a moral lesson. For example, under the picture of a barrel of beer were the following lines obliquely preaching temperance:

My habitation's in a wood,
And I'm at any one's command;
I often do more harm than good,
If once I get the upper hand.[26]

A new game was published in Philadelphia in 1806, under the title: *Geographical, Statistical, and Political Amusement; by which may be obtained a general and particular knowledge of the United States. In a series of interesting games on a map designed for the purpose.* The purpose was to help the child remember the relative importance of states in their area and population, cities, rivers, and mountains, and to stimulate an interest in national geography. It was also meant to convey to those unacquainted with such mysteries the process of electing the highest officials, such as the President and Vice President. That the geographical information at this date was meager is shown by the section on the comparatively new state of Ohio, which read: "The time of the first settlement unknown, but presumed to be about the year 1790 . . . area in square miles exclusive of Lakes, 39,128. Exports unknown." In other items the information was more specific and exact. For instance, the child was told that the Navy had twenty vessels of 560 guns; and that the public debt of the United States was $74,247,991.[27]

Amusements which led to exercise in the open air were considered to have the advantage over all others, and certain writers during the feminist movement of the early nineteenth century advocated that no difference should be made in the outdoor sports of girls and boys. If health and cheerful spirits were as necessary for one as for the other, then such sports as gardening, skating, and snow-balling were as good for girls as for boys. To the objection that such play would make girls rude and noisy, these authors replied that such would not be the case if influences "within doors favored gentleness and politeness"; and that even if there were any dangers of this sort, it was easier to "acquire elegance" in after life than it was to regain lost health.[28]

While little ones were thus exposed to the quiet delights of "rational play," older boys and girls helped to relieve the shortage of manpower by such useful frolics as apple bees and cornhusks, or by spinning bevies and quilting parties. The youth who voluntarily united to assist a neighbor in any emergency that required dispatch were amply repaid at the conclusion of their tasks, not only by the stores of refreshments, but generally by that ever attractive diversion—a "ball."

Of all coöperative pastimes in this scheme of "exchanging works," the husking bee offered perhaps the most rollicking amusement. After the Indian corn had been gathered from the fields and deposited in heaps in the cornhouse, an evening was appointed for the husking. Those who were invited assembled early, took their seats in rows or circles at strategic points, and attacked the monstrous heaps before them. The ears were stripped with a dextrous hand and cast into a general pile, while the husks were thrown behind the operators. During this process, if a boy found an ear of red corn, he had the privilege of kissing the girl of his choice. This was a pleasant tradition which usually inspired most boys to come provided with one or more red ears in their pockets. While the husking was in progress, songs, jests, and laughter lightened the labor. Cider circulated freely to stimulate the workers to their best efforts and to prepare them for the "banquet and ball" which were regularly arranged to climax these occasions.[29]

Besides useful recreations of economic value to families, there were others that were supposed to offer an educational or aesthetic advantage to children. Only by an examination of this "rational play" that adults imposed on children at the beginning of the last century can the modern reader appreciate to what lengths the patience of youth must have been tried by the boring "amusements" in vogue. The prevailing ideas of adults on the merits of "educational play" were frequently sugar-coated in verse for youthful consumption. A typical example of this "improvement" propaganda is found in the lines entitled "Holidays":

> He found that employment created enjoyment,
> And past the time cheerful away;
> That study and reading, by far were exceeding
> His cakes, his toys, and his play.[30]

Among the classics in this field, the little volume, *Garden Amusements for Improving the Minds of Little Children,* illustrates the recreational diet of the times. Built around a slight story, this work deals with the habits of plants and vines, earthworms, butterflies, bees, ants, snails, and birds. The author remarks that the questions which even very little children put to those about them, by way of gathering knowledge of what they see and hear, fully prove that the "youthful mind is open at an early age to receive instruction." Parents were advised not to waste time, but to avail themselves of this desire in their children to teach them little by little everything they should know. The modern reader is reassured to find that during the recital of an obviously tiresome homily on plants, "little Ann" plainly became bored and hungry:

One plant hath an oily nature, another is watery; one flower is of a red colour, another is green or yellow; and some of both. One fruit is sweet, another is bitter; one shrub is prickly, another is smooth; one root is wholesome, another is poisonous; one tree is lofty, another is low. And thus is proved to us both the wisdom and goodness of God, the Almighty Author; so that we may truly say, "O Lord! how manifold are thy works, in thy wisdom thou hast made them all; the earth is full of thy riches!

Little Ann seemed tired of what I was saying, and, by her looks toward the grape vine, gave me to understand what she wished. I love to please children, and to be beforehand, if possible with them, in gratifying their innocent desires. I soon gathered for them a bunch each. . . . But while they were thus happy in the enjoyment, I thought it proper to mix instruction with it.

"You see, dear Ann, what a poor dry stick this is, on which those grapes grow; should you have thought, my dear, had you looked upon it in the winter season when no leaves or fruit appear, that it would ever be capable of affording such delicious fruit?" Ann said, "No, I should not." "Well, then my dear, let you and I learn never to judge of things by appearances alone. Many a man like this vine may look poor and unpromising, and yet capable of doing us very great acts of kindness."[31]

Pictures have always been a perennial delight for children, hence a number of picture books were published at the opening of the last century for the "amusement and instruction" of the young. Although the motive for producing these works was undoubtedly good, the results were decidedly bad, until several writers were driven to open rebellion against the practice of placing disproportionate pictures in the hands of boys and girls. Engravings of animals on large cards were in much demand at this time; but the aim of having objects in proportion was utterly disregarded by most illustrators. It frequently happened that when a child had been given at the same time a small image of an elephant and a large one of a mouse, he naturally came to the conclusion that both creatures were of the same size. Mary Jane Kilner was among the first to voice disapproval of the old form and content of juvenile books as sources of "amusement and entertainment" for the young: "Though the sentiments should always be suited to their simplicity, they ought to be expressed with propriety, since a taste for elegance may be insensibly acquired; and we should always endeavour to present them with proper models of imitation."[32]

When the fundamentals of design were thus outraged, Lydia M. Child was among those who sent up the plea for better illustrated juvenile books: "No matter how coarse or common they are, but let them be correct imitations of nature; if they be graceful as well as correct, so much the better."[33] The adult world slowly awakened to the realization that the sort of pictures children saw had an important effect in forming their tastes; that good tastes were of no less consequence than fine feelings, lofty principles, and good sense.

In the process of crystallizing aesthetic values for youth, the diminutive volume, *A Picture Book for Children*, may easily have acted as a catalytic agent. This book was precisely what it was stated to be on the title page, and carried beneath each picture a line or two of text containing a moral precept, platitude, or explanation. For instance, a cut of a mirror bore the obvious label: "We cannot see ourselves in this glass." On the other hand, what looked like a discouraged robin had the remarkable comment attached: "This turkey looks as if she had been in a shower of rain—perhaps she is not very well." A picture of a man and woman sitting back to back on a bench before a fireplace gave the counsel: "It is not genteel to sit back to back—always look at a person when you speak to him." Undoubtedly the book's most important contribution to the world was the injunction found under a picture of a mother and daughter: "Old folks should never forget they were once young."[34]

The title of another book, *Amusement for Good Children by G.S.C., or an Exhibition of Comic Pictures by Bob Sketch; Be Merry and Wise,* might be misleading to the modern reader. The author sought to remedy the moral ills of youth by poking fun and ridicule at the violators of social amenities. For instance, one of its poorly illustrated stories recounted a quarrel over the styles of the day by two "belles"—Miss Fanny Furbelow, an "old Maid" who had never changed her fashions since her youthful days, and Miss Dolly Dabcheek, a young "flirt" who changed to new styles at their yearly appearance. In a manner typical of the age, girlish readers were told that the dress of both belles was preposterous, although each regarded her own as perfect. From these premises, the child was to draw the supposedly sound conclusion that "Fashion, the whimsical child begot by Folly and Fancy, made many a ridiculous figure of those who pay too great attention to her various modes."[35]

A Peep into the Sports of Youth and the Occupations and Amusements of Age likewise gave some interesting sidelights on early juvenile recreation. This book endorsed cricket wholeheartedly as the "most pleasing" of the youthful sports, because in this diversion "healthful exercise and exciting amusements were most happily connected." Seesawing, on the other hand, was spurned as a useless pastime, and little horsemen were warned that they had "better be mindful of their tasks, than mounted on a dangerous plank where they would ride long before they got home."[36] In accordance with the spirit of an age that extolled industry, the book closed by dividing praise between the "industrious Dolly who rose just as day broke in the East and forthwith began her churning," and the no less "diligent Mary who at the first song of the lark pumped and heated water for her household tasks," as described in the verse:

> With some she scours the dressers smart,
> Or mops the kitchen bricks;
> And in the kettle sings apart,
> Above the crackling sticks.[37]

According to this book, "peep shows" were in that day an irresistible attraction of childhood. A description was given of a patriotic display calculated to inspire the hearts of young Americans: "Here is Master Curious and his sister spending their holiday money at the show box. They are now taking a view of the battles fought by the great and glorious Washington."[38] The international situation of the next decade was similarly reviewed for the child's pleasure; and the American pastime of "twisting the British lion's tail" was clearly indicated. For example, *Peter Pry's Puppet Show* gave in their order the following explanatory verses, under sketches of a bull dressed in men's clothing and smoking a pipe, a representation of a huge bear, and a miniature figure of Napoleon in a bird cage guarded by an English peasant.

> Here's Johnny Bull from England come,
> Who boasts of being a sailor,
> But Yankee tars will let him know
> He'll meet with many a failure.
>
> Here's Bruin next from Russia come,
> Don't let him you affright, Sir,
> Tho in his manner rather rough
> You'll find him here polite, Sir.
>
> Now here is somebody indeed!
> You'll know him I'll engage, Sir,
> If not, I'll tell you who it is—
> 'Tis Boney in a cage, Sir.[39]

As early as 1785, Isaiah Thomas published for dramatization in schools several plays for children. Among them was *Beauty and the Monster,* a comedy based on a fairy story by Stéphanie-Félicité de Genlis, the author of the *Theater of Education.* The closing lines of this work, addressed to the audience, gave the excuse for the play's existence: "Virtuous hearts, never complain of your fate: and may this example teach you to know that goodness and benevolence are the surest means of pleasing and the only claims to love."[40] In another play, *Hagar in the Desert,* the same author had the Angel Gabriel address the mother, Hagar, with reassuring advice which might reflect for us the current adult attitude toward the child: "Hagar, rejoice from henceforth in happiness unchangeable: God sent me to try you. He is satisfied and all your troubles are at an end. Train up your child in virtue: inspire him with the fear and love of God. This is the most acceptable sacrifice your gratitude can offer."[41]

The "spectacle of Cinderella, calculated to arrest the attention and to show virtue in her own image and vice as a deformity," was listed among the happiest tales that could possibly be selected for dramatization to instruct and amuse the generation of 1790. Such performances were advertised as highly deserving of liberal patronage, because they kept morals in view, and held virtue forth in such fascinating colors. The last scene of this favorite fairy tale was described in verse for the child:

> No longer his illness the Prince did endure;
> A smile from Cinderella completed his cure;
> The Queen to his nuptials did gladly consent,
> The sisters were pardoned and all were content.[42]

After the first decade of the new century the pleasure incidental to the production of a child's play was set aside for the more useful "training in speaking of single pieces, or the acting of single scenes." John Hamilton Moore expressed the sentiments of an age which reveled in the art of "elocution." The long title of his work gave the aim and object of those who substituted in the child's recreational life for the delightfully dramatized fairy stories of preceding years[43] what now seem tedious "selections from celebrated authors." Commenting on this action, the author said: "Though the acting of plays at school has been universally supposed a very useful practice, it has of late years been much laid aside." The advantages arising from the production of juvenile plays were no longer judged equal to the inconveniences necessitated and to the "long interruptions to the common school duties occasioned by the preparation of a play." It was also observed that the prevailing sentiment of most plays did not sufficiently recommend them to the guardians of youth.[44]

Thus the sober business of life continually intruded on the child's pursuit of happiness; but it seems that the "best-laid plans" of those who sought to prevent the youth's amusements from engrossing his time and thoughts came to naught before the avalanche of nonsense rhymes that began to inundate juvenile reading early in the century. This nonsense began with verses for the infant; the youngest reader could find in *Old Dame Margery's Hush-a-Bye,* under the picture of a mother cuddling her baby, the following rhyme:

> Great A, little a, Bouncing B;
> The cat's in the cupboard, and he can't see.[45]

Although the realists did their best to exclude such books as *Dame Trot and Her Comical Cat* from the shelves of children's libraries, the prodigious feats of the cat, Grimalkin, must have enchanted many little boys and girls. A cat that could not only prepare a feast for her mistress or play cards with the dog, Spot, and teach him to dance, but could also dress herself so that those who saw her "look'd, admir'd, and curtsied low," certainly merited a place among the children's friends. They could read of Grimalkin's costume:

> A hat and feather then she took,
> And stuck it on aside;
> And o'er a gown of crimson silk,
> A handsome tippet tied.[46]

Another book of nonsense rhymes of equal appeal to the young was *The Comic Adventures of Old Mother Hubbard and Her Dog,* in which fifteen hand-colored "elegant copperplate engravings" offered a special attraction. Since this has been one of the most popular jingle books of childhood, some variations of it have survived to our time. One particularly interesting scene of the old version described Mother Hubbard's dog in the verse:

> She went to the market to buy a sheep's head,
> When she came back he was sick in his bed.
> She ran away quick to call Dr. Hulse,
> When she came back he was feeling his pulse.[47]

In this group also belonged the rhymed version of the old familiar story of *Jack and the Bean Stalk,* which at that time was called *The History of Mother Twaddle and the Marvelous Achievements of Her Son Jack.* Jack's timely warning by the damsel "with a cap all of lace" that the giant would kill and eat him that night undoubtedly sent shivers of delight up juvenile spines:

> Soon as Jack saw him fall, he crept from the bed,
> Then snatched a large knife and chopped off his head.
> Thus he killed this great man, as he loudly did snore,
> And never again was a giant seen more.[48]

Stories of adventure, particularly the English tales reprinted in this country, such as those of Robin Hood and his merry men, furnished stimulating entertainment for American boys who loved

> To read how Robin Hood and Little John,
> Brave Scarlet, stately, valiant, bold, and free,
> Each of them did bravely, boldly play the man,
> While they did all reign beneath the Greenwood tree.

Bishops, Friers [sic], and Monks, likewise many more,
Parted with their gold to increase their store,
But ne'er would be guilty of robbing the poor.[49]

Perhaps it was the popularity of this tale that inspired "a Citizen of Philadelphia" to write "an original story of adventure," the scene of which was laid in the castle of Vauban in Burgundy. The tale related the experiences of Henry and Louis Boileau at the hands of the murderous Count de Vauban, after they had been lost exploring the wonders of his mysterious old castle. Prison, chains, dagger-wounds, and long fevers were but the prelude to the boys' escape when the castle burned; while their heroism during captivity led both lads to riches and a romantic marriage. The last sentence of this story indicates the appeal such fiction might have held for the peace-loving youth of Philadelphia: "No foe to domestic tranquility ever passed their threshhold, no intestine uneasiness inhabited their retirement, but as far as possible for humanity they enjoyed permanent and unalloyed happiness."[50]

The festivities of a people are assumed to reflect their national or sectional character, hence the various states of the country, except those of New England where Christmas was rejected as a feast, followed, as a part of the English heritage, a definite cycle of holidays. This yearly round of religious feasts and national holidays highlighted the recreational life of American boys and girls in an era that offered little excitement. Not only were the holidays themselves unusually welcome pauses— free from the small irksome duties of other days—but for the junior members of the household the weeks of eager anticipation heightened the enjoyment of their sumptuous dinners and gay family reunions.

The child's participation in the celebration of Christmas was curtailed for many decades in New England by the moral discipline and religious tenets of Puritanism, which were incompatible in many respects with the traditional feasts of the mother country. Among the early Colonial penal enactments of Plymouth was one that defined the stand of that section on the question of amusements: "No one shall keep Christmas, or any saint-day, read common-prayer, make mince pies, dance, play cards, or play on any instrument of music, except the drum, trumpet, and Jew's harp."[51]

Cotton Mather denounced Christmas festivities in strong terms: "Tis an evident affront unto the grace of God for men to make the birth of our holy Saviour an encouragement and an occasion for very unholy enormities. Can you in your consciences think that our holy Saviour is honored by mirth, by long eating, by hard drinking, by lewd gaming, and by rude revelling?"[52] Despite this attitude, some communities such as Narragansett, which was settled by wealthy Anglicans, observed two weeks of Christmas visiting and feasting on the part of the planters and their slaves alike.[53]

The frequent and rigid observance of days of "fasting and abstinence and the mortification of the flesh," which New Englanders set apart for themselves, further manifested the resistance to Anglican feast days. In prosperity or adversity, in peace or war, a general fast was their favorite mode of expressing thanks or contrition. Whether the occasion was joyful or sorrowful, a day of fasting, humiliation, and prayer was authorized, on which day all servile labor, and "recreation inconsistent with the solemnity of the said day and all creature comforts were absolutely forbidden by law."[54] But this solemn prohibition did not prevent many children from regarding "Fast Day" merely as a time when they were permitted to eat at random unlimited quantities of molasses gingerbread instead of sitting down to their regular meals.[55]

Thanksgiving, which was definitely a New England feast, was observed with fitting ceremonies and sports as the climax of the year's activities. This holiday may have originated as a substitute for Christmas, for it took place late in the autumn after the harvest had been gathered. Generally the first or second Thursday of December was appointed by the Governor for this purpose, and a copy of his proclamation was read by every clergyman on the preceding Sunday. On Thanksgiving day the people, dressed in their finest, assembled in the churches to listen to appropriate sermons, and to join in prayers and hymns. These devotions occupied about two hours of the morning; and the rest of the day was given to feasting, games, football for boys, and a variety of amusements for adults.[56]

Children found the Thanksgiving dinner the most attractive feature of the day because most tables were supplied with an abundance of fish and fowl, meat and game, as well as with a host of dainty desserts led by the traditional pumpkin pie. Apprentices from the city, who were allowed to visit their homes but once or twice a year, were sure to be present to share these delights. This feast was therefore a jubilee that drew together the members of the same family who had long been separated. As a "ball" invariably closed the day's celebration, eager excitement must have prevailed among the village lads and lasses.[57]

Thanksgiving was not celebrated with the same strictness in the towns south of New England, nor was it enjoyed with the same zest. Although the churches held appropriate services, these exercises were not followed by any extraordinary feasting and rejoicing. This attitude was probably conditioned by the general introduction of other holidays, especially Christmas, which was kept by Christians of other denominations; but it was celebrated with particular solemnity by the people of New York.[58]

Many of the Dutch customs and distinct observances of the early settlers were still prevalent as late as 1835 in the city and state of New York. The readiness with which the English copied the festivities of a Dutch Christmas, New Year's, and Paas led to the observation that the "jolly Saint Nicholas on a dark night was unable to distinguish his own legitimate urchins from those of pure English blood. And as a result, he good-naturedly distributed his gifts to all with no distinctions except those that arose from superior conduct." Notwithstanding the fact that the population of the middle and southern states included representatives from almost every nation on the globe, there was little dissimilarity in their holiday amusements.[59]

New Year's Day, the first feast of the yearly cycle, was observed not only as one of the Christmas holidays, but also "as a landmark in the journey of life, an inn or stopping place for refreshments, at which the wayworn traveller pauses with delight, and then passes forward with renovated hope and vigor."[60] On that day the heads of most households liberally dispensed spiced beverages and cakes to all visitors, and petty disputes and jealousies were temporarily forgotten in the exchange of "Happy New Year" greetings.

A contemporary account of New Year's celebrations gives a glimpse of the children's participation in the joys of that day, near Philadelphia: "Some gambolled and tumbled on the frozen Delaware; others played at hurley with crooked sticks, with which they sometimes hit the ball, and sometimes each other's shins." A few of the boys who were fortunate enough to own a pair of skates enjoyed that sport in which they were "emulated by some half dozen little urchins with smooth bones fastened to their feet, skating away with a gravity and perseverance worthy of better implements." The author declared these lads made the "frost-bit ears of winter glad with the sounds of mirth and revelry . . . and that the icy mirror of the noble Delaware reflected as light hearts as ever beat together in the new world."[61]

Easter or the Paas, by which term the merry schoolboys of the middle states understood nothing more or less than Easter Monday, the "day of cracking eggs," was next in the cycle of the great feasts. In this section the ancient practice of dyeing eggs was widely practised. Paas eggs dyed in a variety of bright colors were displayed for sale on Easter Monday by grocers and hucksters. For centuries the egg had expressed the idea of the resurrection of Christ; for the chick emerging from its shell symbolized Our Lord ascending from the grave to a new life.

Descendants of the Dutch developed, in connection with the Paas celebration, a new game that was believed to be peculiar to the United States. Both parties in preparation equipped themselves with the "munitions of war," which were in this case a dozen or more eggs carefully selected and scientifically tested by tapping the "butts" and "points" (the large and small ends) against the front teeth to make sure that the shells were hard and strong. The challenger then enclosed an egg in one hand with only the "point" or "butt" visible as the choice might be. As the egg generally protruded some distance below the circling thumb and fingers, the lower end was supported by the palm of his other hand. Holding the egg in this manner, the boy challenged his opponent to hit it with the point or butt of another egg; the egg that cracked after one or more trials became *ipso facto* the prize of the victor. In this manner, hundreds of eggs usually exchanged hands within a short time; and since the crack which they had received did not lessen their intrinsic value, the victors made some profit by the sale of their winnings.[62]

Human beings, even in childhood, are prone to take advantage of their fellow creatures, hence it is not surprising to learn that artificial eggs, curiously made of wood, marble, or other hard substances, were often used with such cleverness as to deceive the eye of an unsuspecting youth. The deluded one would find himself suddenly stripped of his capital without being able to account for his losses. Records testify that when such tricks were detected, retribution overtook the young villain with lightning speed.[63]

The fourth of July seems to have been a far more welcome holiday for boys and girls in the early 1800's than it is in modern times. Cannons were fired off at morning and noon, and bells rang joyously; while in some places there were firecrackers or torpedoes to endanger the life and limbs of the young. After watching a military parade march through the main street and seeing the display of colors, children decked in their Sunday clothes attended the church services in which a blessing was asked on the nation. Some statesman of more or less importance delivered an oration in which much was usually said about "this universal Yankee nation." It is recorded that young people at noon devoured amazing quantities of fried chicken and cake at the public dinners; and in the evening from some vantage point they watched the rockets that were sent skyward from their own or a neighboring town. After completing this program, children went wearily to bed with the comfortable feeling that they had been good patriots.[64]

Undoubtedly it was Christmas, the closing holiday of the year, which eclipsed all other festivals by the gayety and splendor of its celebration in all sections except New England. A stranger in the city of New York described in phrases that have a delightfully familiar tone, the "pleasing and effective spectacle" of the streets on Christmas Eve:

Whole rows of confectionary stores and toy shops, fancifully, and often splendidly decorated with festoons of bright silk drapery, interspersed with flowers and evergreens, are brilliantly illuminated with gas-lights. . . . During the evening until midnight, these places are crowded with visitors of both sexes and all ages; some selecting toys and fruit for holiday presents; others merely lounging from shop to shop to enjoy the varied scene. But the most interesting and most delightful of all, is the happy and animated countenances of the the children on this occasion. Their joy cannot be restrained, but bursts out in boisterous mirth, or beams from their countenances in sunny smiles, which are still more expressive.[65]

The Christmas season in the rural districts, where homeborn pleasures were obviously the only ones at hand, still afforded children the highest degree of satisfaction and joy. The boys and girls of a family carefully selected a gigantic yule log long before the day came on which they were to drag it home. With appropriate ceremony on Christmas Eve they rolled this log upon the hearth, and placed before its crackling flames supplies of nuts, cakes, and cider. Children, according to the tradition of the particular family, hung their stockings to be filled by Santa Clause either on the mantelpiece or at the foot of their beds.[66] A contemporary story illustrates the practice:

On Christmas Eve, little Charles hung his stocking carefully by the chimney corner, and after saying his prayers, got into bed and soon fell asleep. Charles dreamed that he was in bed peeping at his stocking over the bed-clothes, when he saw a very pleasant-looking gentleman come down the chimney on a nice little pony. His hair was made of crackers, and as he came nearer to the lamp that stood on the hearth, pop went off one of the crackers, then another, and then another. But Saint Nicholas was not a bit frightened; he only rubbed his ears, patted the pony to keep him quiet, and laughed till he showed the concave of his great mouth full of sugar plums.[67]

Most of the active motion games played by early American children were of old English origin. These were accompanied by rhymed formulas such as "London bridge is falling down, etc.," which had been transmitted from generation to generation. In this process of handing down the rhymes and rules of juvenile play, the printed word had practically no part. Since the tradition was almost wholly oral, the rhymes of American children differed slightly from the form of the same game played in

Great Britain. A few games were also borrowed from Ireland, France, and Germany, but these formed only a small portion of the stock in trade of American youth.

Boys' games, impelled by some mysterious force, succeeded one another with little variation at fixed times every year; a phenomenon which can hardly be explained except as a matter of instinct in some measure conditioned by the climate and by the traditions of the mother country. As a matter of fact, in all the states from Maine to Georgia, the first play "time" of the year was marble-time. Thus in New England, when the snow had hardly melted, boys scooped out the necessary holes and "knuckled at taw" on the oozing ground, while at that very time the lads of Georgia were absorbed in the same game.[68]

Subsequent to the period for marbles, the appropriate series of sports in New York was explained by the adage: "Top-time's gone, Kite-time's come, and April Fool's Day will soon be here." In Georgia the succession was kites, tops, and hoops. In that region, too, the season for popguns was determined by the time when chinaberries were ripe; for then the pith of the elder reed was ripe enough to be pushed out, and the empty stalk could be used for the barrel of the weapon. Baseball was the special holiday game for the New England Fast Day on the first of April, just as football was their regular amusement for Thanksgiving afternoon.[69]

To determine who was to be "It" or who had the onerous duty of commencing a game, an amazing variety of counting-out rhymes was used by children in the different parts of the country. A child told off the words of a rhyme by tapping every player; and the one on whom the last word fell was "out." Often each player in a small group put his finger on the brim of an inverted hat, and the words were told off on the fingers. This rite in either form was repeated until only one child was left; he was then obliged to lead the game.[70] Most of these rhymes made no sense, but were mere gibberish of unmeaning sounds with rhythm the most important quality. The following examples illustrate this jargon and give the locality in which it was most popular:

> 1 2 3 4
> Mary at the kitchen door
> 5 6 7 8
> Mary at the garden gate.
> (Massachusetts)
>
> Eny, meny, mony, mine,
> Hasky, pasky, daily, ine,
> Agy, dagy, walk.
> (Connecticut)

Apples and oranges, two for a penny,
Takes a scholar to count as many;
OUT, out goes he.

Three potatoes in a pot
Take one out and leave it hot.

Red, white, and blue,
All out but you.
(Philadelphia)

Monkey, monkey, bottle of beer,
How many monkeys are there here?
1 2 3 You are he.

Intry mintry cutry corn,
Apple seed and apple thorn,
Wire brier limber lock,
Five geese in a flock:
Set and sing by the spring,
O U T, out.
(Massachusetts to Georgia)[71]

The origins of this childish lore belong for the most part to medieval
England—to the days before religious distinctions existed—hence there
were no striking contrasts in the ordinary amusements of American children, either in the North or South, or in the descendants of Puritan,
Quaker, or Anglican. The old active games were usually accepted by
Americans as part of the tradition of their ancestors. Certain timeworn
sports of youth were maintained even in Puritan localities, with the
result that some of the grace, music, and gayety of merry England survived to brighten the formality and gloom of the child's existence.[72]

The volume of works on children's games and sports produced in the
middle section, and particularly in the Philadelphia area, suggests that
active play was either more in keeping with the tastes of this region or
that the publishers of this locality were more concerned with supplying
children's recreational needs. At any rate, more than three times as many
works on juvenile sports were published in the middle states as in New
England, where amusement of a quiet nature, such as stories, was supplied by the publishers. As already indicated, the active sports so attractive to the young were perpetuated there chiefly by an oral tradition.

Youthful Sports, published in Philadelphia in 1802, contained not only
practical descriptions of active sport, but also gave warning of the dangers lurking in them for young players. An idea of the fearful and
awful caution behind recreational advice can be gathered from the rules
for such apparently harmless frolics as "Blind-man's Buff." The direc-

tions began with the plea: "Stop him! he is running against the wall! Blindman's Buff is a rather dangerous play unless it be in some open place, or very large room. It seems to be very amusing! How they laugh! But if the blinded boy should fall down and break his nose, what then!"[73] In "Peg Top," the author tells of a child who nearly lost a toe "by a violent blow from one of these tops"; so he concluded: "Surely then, Peg Top is hardly safe." He also observed that in trundling hoops, little boys were so taken up with their play that they were often heedless where they drove.[74] Directions for the use of the bow and arrow gave extravagant warning:

> Bend well your bow, your skill to try,
> Then shoot the target in the eye!
> 'Tis better thus to be employed,
> Than have the birds for nought destroyed.
>
> Children are fond of variety; and this play will do
> If care be taken not to shoot each other, or to
> Kill birds wantonly. It will not answer at all in
> The crowded streets of New York.[75]

The aim of many writers evidently was to instill a regard for caution in the heart of youth; for in such works as *A Mother's Remarks on a Set of Cuts for Children,* a variety of "harmless sports" were described and recommended. Among those for boys, looking through a microscope held high place—a diversion which reflected the growing popularity of science as well as the attempts then being made to harmonize religion and science in current thought. Budding scientists were told that many animals were so small as to be invisible to the human eye, but, with the assistance of a magnifying glass, observers could see the goodness and wisdom of God in the most minute insects.[76]

Some reform writers at the beginning of the century objected to girls' playing with dolls because they thought such toys led to a love of dress and finery. The majority of children's books, however, listed the dressing of a doll by an "industrious little girl" as the "most innocent amusement for tender youth, and the most agreeable to their future employ." Making dolls' gowns and hats not only stimulated the child's imagination and afforded her a useful experience in "neat sewing," but it was thought that the rocking and crooning to a doll—as a creature from the world of "make-believe"—developed strong affections in the little owners.[77]

Pets were supposed to have a good effect on youth for this same reason; and the feeding and care of such animals as dogs, cats, lambs, or rabbits was encouraged because it aroused kindness and stimulated a love of

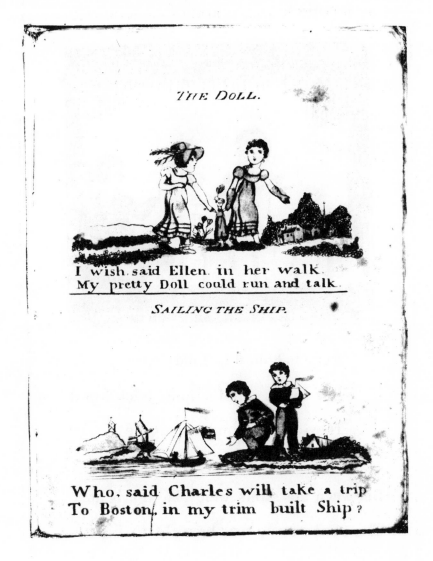

From JUVENILE PASTIMES IN VERSE, 1830

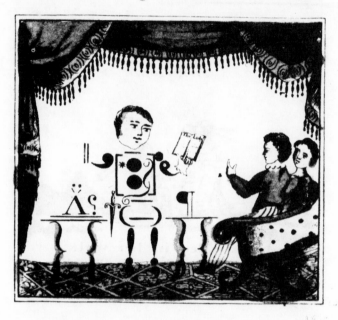

"Ev'ry lady in this land

"Has twenty nails upon each hand

"Five & twenty on hands & feet

"And this is true without deceit."

But when the stops were plac'd aright,

The real sense was brought to light.

From PUNCTUATION PERSONIFIED; OR POINTING
MADE EASY, 1831

usefulness in children. There were frequent references to this pastime in the books of children's amusements; for instance, *The Seasons* has this passage:

The feeding of chickens is a very pleasing business for little children. What a pretty sight they make when they are fed, or when their mother hovers over them. And the little chicks if they are hungry or have lost their mother have a language to tell their distress, which makes tender little children feel for them.[78]

The care of pets was also employed to foster humanitarian virtues in children. One finds in the juvenile literature early in the century evidence of the same humane trends which later appeared in the national social reforms of the 1800's. In a little book entitled *Limed Twigs,* for example, the child was told to deny himself the pleasure of keeping rabbits, pigeons, and other wild creatures penned up in cages, since it was their nature to frisk about and fly at will in search of food.[79] The story of *The Tame Goldfinch* was a favorite among the publishers of children's moralistic tales for several decades. The woeful account of Louisa Manner starving her goldfinch through neglect ended with this lesson to careless youth:

Mr. Manners regarded her with a severe look and reprimanded her on account of her negligence, observing that if he had twisted off the bird's neck when he bought it, the cruelty would have been small indeed, when compared to that of suffering it to perish with famine.

Louisa stood over the bird, clasping her hands with unutterable grief. . . . Mrs. Manners was deeply affected by her daughter's unfeigned sorrow, and pleaded so powerfully as to obtain her forgiveness; but whenever she was guilty of any giddiness or inattention, the bird (which was stuffed for that purpose) was immediately produced, and everyone exclaimed, "She had forgot the barbarous death of the Tame Goldfinch."[80]

Cruelty to animals was further denounced in *Æsop's Fables,* especially in the story of the mischievous boys who threw stones at the frogs in a pond, and were reproached in turn by one of the victims: "Children, you should consider, that though this may be sport to you it is death to us." The "Application" of this fable declared that the cruel practice many children had of throwing stones at harmless birds and other creatures, of torturing flies, setting dogs on cats to worry them, or in any way afflicting an animal for sport showed that their education had not been of the proper sort. They were unfeeling children with depraved morals; and such callousness, if continued, would end in brutality and tyranny.[81]

Children of this country played various kinds of ball games including football, cricket, stool-ball, fives, baseball, tip-cat, and trap-ball.[82] This sport was advocated for schoolboys as an "excellent exercise to unbend the mind and to restore to the body that elasticity and spring which the close application to their studies had a tendency to blunt."[83] In this age of caution, football, although popular with boys, was given only a half-hearted approval by adults. "This play is not so desirable as some others of the kind; for in the hurry to kick the ball, boys sometimes hurt each other sadly."[84] An old description of "Fives" is typical of the verses for other forms of ball games:

> With what force the little ball
> Rebounds, when struck against the wall;
> See how intent each gamester stands!
> Mark well his eyes, his feet, his hands!
>
> *Rule of life*
> Know this (which is enough to know)
> Virtue is happiness here below.[85]

Even in Colonial days horseback riding was not only a pleasure enjoyed by most children, but a necessity as well, because other means of travel were few and inconvenient. Hence a number of children's manuals were published in the eighteenth century dealing with the "art of riding and reducing the horse to proper obedience, as well as necessary directions for a journey." Young riders were warned to heed the golden rule of this art: "Mad men and mad horses never will agree together."[86] Although horseback riding was still considered in 1835 a healthful exercise for both sexes, as well as a favorite "rational sport," it was steadily losing ground to the pleasures of "the more luxurious modes of travel on steamboats and railroad cars."[87] But boys still had their ponies and learned to ride them early, as can be inferred from such verses as the following:

> I gracefully sit in saddle with ease,
> To manage my poney with art;
> My toes I hold in, and I keep tight my knees;
> I have my whole lesson by heart.
>
> I low hold my bridle, and steady and still,
> Nor wriggle nor sidle about;
> I lean myself forward, when going up hill
> And downhill lean backward no doubt.[88]

"Skipping the rope" has now been taken over by the girls as their own, but in the early days this game was considered a "pretty play for active boys."[89] By the 'thirties a concession was made in favor of the equally active little maids: "Little boys and girls can amuse themselves in this play with much propriety. In cities especially where play ground is scarce, this exercise is very commendable."[90] For the sake of economy little boys were advised "never to skip with their shoes off" as that practice wore out stockings very fast—"a waste that all good children should endeavor to avoid."[91]

The method of playing the well-known game "I Spy" varied somewhat from the procedure followed today. According to the old rules, six or eight boys stayed at "home," on the base, while an equal number hid themselves within a given district. At a signal, those on base went in search of the hiders; and when a seeker spied a lad in his hiding place, he called out: "I spy Tom Brown. Home for Tom Brown!" Then the boy spied rushed forth and caught, if he could, any one of the seekers and rode home on his back.[92]

On the index of outlawed games were those that were condemned as being either too rough or too cruel, hence not proper for children. Wrestling was described as a "violent and dangerous exercise" that might easily produce broken or dislocated bones. Fishing and bird-nesting, although alluring pastimes for many boys, were branded as "detested sports that owed their pleasure to another's pain."[93] "Badger the Bull" or "Bait the Bear" was thought so "foolish and dangerous a game that not one word could be said in its favor." An interesting description of this old favorite of the boys is given in *Youthful Sports:*

A boy kneels down on the ground and has another to stand over him to guard him from the blows of the rest. . . . . Some boys stand around with their handkerchiefs twisted up, and tied in a knot at one end, to strike the harder; while he that is to bear the blows sits in the middle, with his arms over his head, to defend it from their attacks, until his keeper may catch an assailant, who lies down in his turn. Boys should be taught not to look upon any sport as a pleasure which has been attended with some bad consequences;—at best it tends to wear out the handkerchiefs, and to make children careless about their clothes, which are not made without much labour, nor procured without much expense.[94]

In a typical book of juvenile pastimes forty-five games were described, of which all but three were for boys; while eight others—swinging, bathing, jumping rope, hunting the slipper, riding on hands, threading the needle, tossing balls, and shuttlecock—were recommended either for boys or girls as "profitable and suitable to occupy the reasonable time allowed as a respite from the needle or study." In the accounts of the three diversions reserved exclusively for girls—dressing dolls, blowing soap bubbles, and cup and ball—the description of the last game not only indicates the contemporary attitude towards the female sex, but definitely sets the proper bounds for girls' amusements. The game cup and ball is characterized as a "trifling diversion as there seems not much to be gained by it on the score of exercise; it is fit only for girls to amuse themselves with, and for them only in rainy weather, or on a very hot day. It requires a steady hand and a nice eye for the player to be expert in catching the ball in the point of the ivory handle."[95] Older girls were told to amuse themselves by reading, and by the study of natural science—especially by "arranging flowers, by walking abroad in solitude, or by useful and cheerful conversations with their friends."[96]

Dancing was always a favorite amusement for older children; young people in towns and villages assembled at every opportunity to "trip merrily to the sound of music." Many of these dances, by their very names, reflected the historical trend of the times. For example, in a *Choice Collection of New and Approved Country Dances of 1796*, there were directions given young Americans for performing *The Democratic Rage, The President, De La Bastille,* and *Génet's Recal.*[97] Even in New England, dancing masters taught little boys and girls their steps as a part of a liberal education; for this complicated art was everywhere regarded as a pleasant accomplishment as well as a solemn business in good society. Hence it is recorded that when a Philadelphia girl, who was taking part in a country dance, spoke for a minute to a friend and consequently forgot her turn, the master of ceremonies rushed to her saying: "Give over, Miss. Take care what you are about. Do you think you came here for your pleasure?"[98]

The vanity and dissipation which at times accompanied dancing brought it into disrepute; and the controversy on its merits as a juvenile pastime raged bitterly in children's books. As a mere exercise, dancing raised no objections; but on moral grounds it was charged with bringing the sexes together in circumstances "unfavorable to the cultivation of female delicacy." It was blamed for monopolizing the thoughts of youth with preparations days before the event occurred, and with stealing hours ordinarily given to sleep and rest. As dancing was believed by some to foster vanity and "to work up the mind to a feverish excitement," it was also condemned on the score that it was followed by "a state of body and mind which for a time at least forbade any useful exertion."[99] Denunciation of this pleasure was futile, nevertheless, in an age which offered so little other excitement and so few opportunities for social gatherings.[100]

Children's balls and parties were common occurrence by the 'thirties, and though reformers were grieved to see "innocent creatures thus early trained to vanity and affectation," their protests were likewise futile. Lydia M. Child particularly deplored those balls "where children in imitation of their elders in the fashionable world, ate confectionery, stayed up late, dressed in finery, talked nonsense, and affected what they did not feel."[101]

While it is true that early American children played a variety of games, they did not have an equal assortment of toys. During most of this period such orthodox playthings as boys and girls did enjoy were imported from Europe and especially from England. Dolls of various kinds were first on the list of these juvenile importations, ranging from small jointed wooden figures to the more elaborate creations with a kid body and china head—dressed for the most part like adults of the period.[102] Since these puppets required homes, there were also intriguing "baby houses" fully equipped with tiny figures, furniture, and cooking utensils. All kinds of military apparatus had its age-old appeal in these days; toy bows and arrows were used in spite of the warnings found in little books; and pop-guns with pellets of clay, or slings made to send missiles a distance, were always popular with boys, if not with their families. Small warriors, armed with little wooden swords, stepped to martial music furnished by elder pipes, cow-horn trumpets, or by regular drums. Troops of dashing tin or wooden soldiers, painted and dressed in gay uniforms, were reviewed by many little American boys as the climax of their hopes and dreams.[103]

The English "penny toys," sold in this country during the nineteenth century by the Yankee peddlers, included carved wooden horses mounted on wheels that could be pulled about by the child, or bright-colored jumping jacks on a stick, whose arms and legs jerked frantically when a string was pulled, as well as toy acrobats who could whirl around a wooden bar and "never pause for breath." Among the mechanical toys of painted wood were small merry-go-rounds that revolved to wheezy tunes as a handle was turned, birdcages that squeaked when the top was pressed, and boats, "occupied by ladies and gentlemen," which swung blithely from a crossbeam.[104]

There are only a few allusions to specific toys in the children's books of this period, but among the references is a good description of "The Wax Doll," a work which shows that these toys were an established institution with little girls as early as 1804:

> Mamma now brought her home a Doll of wax,
> Its hair in ringlets white and soft as flax;

Its eyes could open, and its eyes could shut,
And on it with much taste its clothes were put.

* * * * *

She plac'd it in the sun,—misfortune dire:
The wax ran down as if before the fire!
Each beauteous feature quickly disappeared,
And melting left a blank all soil'd and smeared.[105]

Most American girls were mercifully spared the loss of their dolls in the above manner, for either the poverty of their parents or their remoteness from toyshops prevented the purchase of such treasures. Always, in the serious business of play, children have naturally copied the objects which surrounded them, and have imitated the activities of adults. Thus these little ones who were denied the artistic toys of the shops cleverly supplied their play needs by objects of their own manufacture. There are records of little country girls whose imagination and busy fingers contrived cows of fir-cones, and tiny chairs, sofas, and cradles of prickly burdock balls, as well as cups and saucers of acorns. These little maids could fashion dolls of small sticks—without arms and legs or features, to be sure—but gorgeously costumed in hollyhock skirts and petunia bonnets! No less ingenious were they in exploiting the recreational facilities of a neighboring hill; for there is evidence to show that in the fantastic world of make-believe the stony ledges of the hillside might readily become the winding stairs up castle towers with breakfast rooms and boudoirs on the landings. There the little girls could set tables with bits of broken glass and china for imaginary guests; or the young mothers might leave their weather-beaten rag families asleep beneath mullein-blankets or plantain-coverlets while they amused themselves on the lofty turrets at the summit.[106]

Skillful little boys made kites and reed fifes, pegged together carts from bits of wood, or whittled ingenious toys for themselves and others. Very small lads galloped miles on broomstick horses; while others, a little older, expertly managed hobby-horses fashioned from a long-necked squash that had been bridled and placed on four sticks. There are also records of numerous sham battles fought by determined youth armed with wooden swords and reed popguns; others of a more tranquil nature fastened smooth bones to their shoes for skates, or coursed down hills on homemade sleds.[107]

Children learned early that their talents were not given them solely for pleasure, but rather for the sober business of life. It was almost a universal assumption that one's faculties were to be diligently employed either at work or at some "rational sport," and not merely squandered in idleness and frivolous pursuits.[108] To early American children, play was indeed a part of the business of life, but always a minor part. Boys and girls at this period were quite adept at mixing work and play, and one may recognize in many phases of our modern morale—either in athletics or in warfare—traces of that vibrant energy and grim drive for victory which animated the youth of former days in such competitive frolics as corn huskings and spinning bevies.

The majority of young Americans whose parents could not afford expensive imported toys lost nothing in constructing playthings for themselves. Thus left to their own devices in childhood, they proved especially resourceful in later life. The crude creations of youth were undoubtedly supplied by the childish imagination with the qualities demanded by their age and talents. Since fineness of form is indeed of small importance to the young, and the instinct for destruction is always strong within them, those absurd playthings which the early children fashioned for themselves best answered their quickly changing whims. In deference to the play instinct, which abhors relics of its recent past, either the girl's flower-dressed doll or the boy's squash horse conveniently fell to pieces and disappeared as soon as it had satisfied some fleeting need. Such were the capacities of youthful imaginations and the impetus given to creative genius by work and play that early American boys and girls, in the serene orbit of their simple childhood experiences, could dream dreams of greatness and lay the groundwork for the miracles of art and science wrought by succeeding generations.

[1]*The Seasons*, p. 21. Italics are mine. The mutual appraisal of the worlds of adulthood and childhood is further revealed by the inscription on the frontispiece of a small book entitled *A Peep Into The Sports of Youth*: "The cradle age is that of helplessness. In a few years after, when we get the use of every faculty, we think that old folks are fools, while they, by experience, know that we are so." See *A Peep Into The Sports of Youth, And The Occupations And Amusements of Age*, Frontispiece.

[2]Isaac Watts, *Divine Songs For The Use of Children*, p. 22.

[3]*A Present to Children*, Part of the Dedication.

[4]*Ibid.*, p. 10.

[5]*Ibid.*, pp. 13, 14.

[6]*Ibid.*, p. 15.

[7]*A Child's Spelling Book*, p. 51.

[8]*The Daughter's Own Book*, pp. 123-25.

[9]W. E. Andrews, *The Catholic School Book*, p. 187.

[10]*Ibid.*, p. 188.

[11]Edgar W. Knight, *Twenty Centuries of Education*, pp. 494-96.

[12]Theodore Dwight, Jr., *The Father's Book*, p. 97.

[13]*Ibid.*, pp. 106, 107.

[14]*Ibid.*, p. 108.

[15]Mary Jane Kilner, *The Memoirs of a Peg Top*, pp. 88, 89.

[16]Sigourney, *op. cit.*, pp. 246, 247.

[17]Caroline Hewins, *A Mid-Century Girl and Her Books*, p. 19.

[18]As quoted in Ethel S. Bolton and Eva J. Coe, *American Samplers*, p. 96.

[19]Lydia Maria Child, *The Mother's Book*, pp. 61, 62.

[20]Pricilla Wakefield, *Juvenile Anecdotes founded on facts. Collected for the Amusement of Children*, p. 81.

[21]*Ibid.*, pp. 114-16.

[22]*Remarks on Children's Play*, p. 2.

[23]*Youthful Recreations*, pages unnumbered.

[24]*Ibid.*

[25]*Children's Amusements*, p. 15. See also Mrs. Teachwell (pseud.), *Rational Sports in Dialogues passing among Children of a Family*.

[26]*The Whim Wham;* see also *The Puzzling Cap*, pp. 10, 11.

[27]*Geographical, Statistical, and Political Amusement; by which may be obtained a general and particular knowledge of the United States. In a series of interesting games on a map designed for the purpose*, pp. 10, 11.

[28]Child, *op. cit.*, pp. 58, 59.

[29]Horatio Smith, *Festivals, Games and Amusements, Ancient and Modern*, pp. 328, 329.

[30]*Original Poems for Infant Minds, By Several Young Persons*, I (1816), 91.

[31]*Garden Amusements for Improving the Minds of Little Children*, p. 8.

[32]Mary Jane Kilner, *The Adventures of Pincushion*, Preface, v.

[33]Child, *op. cit.*, pp. 54, 55.

[34]*A Picture Book for Little Children*, pages unnumbered.

[35]*Amusements for Good Children by G. S. C.*, pp. 17, 18.

[36]*A Peep into the Sports of Youth and the Occupations and Amusements of Age*, pp. 11-15.

[37]*Ibid.*, p. 30.

[38]*Ibid.*, p. 29.

[39]*Peter Pry's Puppet Show. Part Second. There's a Time for Work and a Time for Play*, pages unnumbered.

[40]Stéphanie-Félicité de Genlis, *The Beauty and the Monster, A Comedy from the French*. Extracted from the *Theatre of Education*, p. 36.

[41]Madame Leprince de Beaumont, *The Beauty and the Monster*, p. 31.

[42]Charles Perrault, *Cinderella; or the Little Glass Slipper, Illustrated with elegant engravings*, p. 16; see also *Cinderella, or the Little Glass Slipper, A Grand Allegorical Pantomimic Spectacle as performed at the Philadelphia Theatre*, pp. 1-12.

[43]John Hamilton Moore, *The Young Gentleman and Lady's Monitor, and English Teacher's Assistant; being a collection of select pieces from our best modern writers calculated to facilitate the reading, writing, and the speaking of the English language with elegance and propriety*, title page.

[44]*Ibid.*, p. 8.

[45]*Old Dame Margery's Hush-a-Bye*, pages unnumbered.

[46]*Dame Trot and Her Comical Cat*, pages unnumbered.

[47]*Comic Adventures of Old Mother Hubbard and Her Dog*, pages unnumbered.

[48]*The History of Mother Twaddle, and the Marvelous Atchievements of her son Jack, by H. A. C.*, pages unnumbered.

[49]*The Life and Death of Robin Hood, complete in twenty-four songs*, p. 1.

[50]*Adventures in a Castle, An Original Story, Written by a Citizen of Philadelphia*, p. 72.

[51]Smith, *op. cit.*, p. 321.

[52]As quoted by Abram Brown, "The Ups and Downs of Christmas in New England," in *New England Magazine*. New Series, vol. 29 (1904), 483.

[53]*Ibid.*, p. 484.

[54]Smith, *op. cit.*, p. 322.

[55]Lucy Larcom, *A New England Girlhood*, p. 98.

[56]Horatio Smith, *op. cit.*, pp. 322, 323.

[57]*Ibid.*, p. 324.

[58]*Ibid.*

[59]*Ibid.*, p. 331. Although William Penn, in a quarrel with the governor of New York, hinted that the custom of observing holidays "savoured not only of popery, but paganism," this idea was set aside by most of his colonists, particularly by the Germans, with the result that the observance of Christmas, for example, suffered little if any sea change.

[60]*Ibid.*, p. 332.

[61]*Ibid.*

[62]*Ibid.*, p. 336.

[63]*Ibid.*, p. 337.

[64]Larcom, *op. cit.*, p. 98.

[65]Smith, *op. cit.*, pp. 339, 340.

[66]*Ibid.*, p. 341.

[67]*The Christmas Dream of Little Charles*, pp. 3-6.

[68]Newell, *op. cit.*, pp. 175, 176.

[69]*Ibid.*, p. 176.

[70]*Ibid.*, pp. 194, 195.

[71]*Ibid.*, pp. 199-202; See also *Mother Goose's Melody, or Sonnets for the Cradle*, pp. 21-25; *Peter Prim's Profitable Present to Little Misses and Masters of the United States*, pp. 14-16. The Connecticut rhyme, "Eny meny, etc.," according to Alexander J. Ellis, is an imitation of a curious old Gipsy system of counting from one to ten:— "unemi, dunemi, troemi, ronemi, donemi, etc."' The Philadelphia version went:

> Eny, meny, mony, mite,
> Butter, lather, bony strike,
> Hair cut, froth neck,
> Halico, balico,
> We, wo, wack. (See Newell, *op. cit.*, p. 199.)

[72]William Wells Newell, *Games and Songs of American Children*, pp. 1-3.

[73]*Youthful Sports*, p. 40.

[74]*Ibid.*, pp. 43, 44. See also *Tommy Lovechild, Pretty Poems in Easy Language for the Amusement of Little Boys and Girls*, p. 3.

[75]*Juvenile Pastimes in Verse*, p. 13.

[76]*A Mother's Remarks on a Set of Cuts for Children*, Part 1, p. 83.

[77]Child, *op. cit.*, p. 57; see also *A Mother's Remarks*, p. 85; *Useful Sports*, p. 31; Esther Singleton, *Dolls*, Introduction, v.

[78]*The Seasons*, p. 14; see also Peter Kalm, "Colonial Pets" in Albert B. Hart, *Colonial Children, Source Readers in American History No. 1*, p. 82.

[79]Ann and Jane Taylor, *Limed Twigs to Catch Young Birds*, p. 116.

[80]*The Tame Goldfinch or the Unfortunate Neglect*, p. 35.

[81]*Aesop's Fables*, p. 5.

[82]*Juvenile Pastimes in Verse*, p. 4; See also *Remarks on Children's Play*, pp. 30-33.

[83]*Children's Amusements*, p. 9.

[84]*Juvenile Pastimes in Verse*, p. 11.

[85]*A Little Pretty Pocket-Book*, p. 46.

[86]Philip Astley, *The Modern Riding-Master*, p. 21.

[87]Dwight, *op. cit.*, p. 105.

[88]Adelaide O'Keefe, *Original Poems*, p. 4.

[89]*A Little Pretty Pocket-Book*, p. 56.

[90]*Juvenile Pastimes in Verse*, p. 16.

[91]*A Little Pretty Pocket-Book*, pp. 56, 57.

[92]*Remarks on Children's Play*, p. 34.

[93]*Ibid.*, pp. 42, 43.

[94]*Youthful Sports*, p. 53.

[95]*Remarks on Children's Play*, p. 40.

[96]*The Daughter's Own Book, or Practical Hints*, p. 132.

[97]*A Collection of New and Approved Country Dances*, pp. 1-16.

[98]As quoted in Alice M. Earle, *Child Life in Colonial Days*, pp. 110, 111; see also Noah Webster, *Elements of Useful Knowledge*, third edition, p. 206.

[99]*The Daughter's Own Book, or Practical Hints*, pp. 128, 129.

[100]Child, *op. cit.*, p. 60; See also Earle, *op. cit.*, p. 110.

[101]Child, *op. cit.*, p. 60.

[102]Earle, *op. cit.*, p. 361. Dolls were also sent to this country from France and England as models of the latest fashions prevailing in those countries either for ordinary or for ceremonial dress. After fulfilling this mission, the fashion dolls were consigned to little girls for real play. See Earle, *op. cit.*, p. 365.

[103]C. Geoffrey Holme, *Children's Toys of Yesterday*, p. 7. See also Elizabeth Godfrey, *English Children in the Olden Time*, p. 72.

[104]Holme, *op. cit.*, pp. 112-19.

[105]*Original Poems for Infant Minds*, p. 53.

[106]Lucy Larcom, *A New England Girlhood*, pp. 29, 30. See also Child, *op. cit.*, p. 55; Grober, *op. cit.*, pp. 1-4.

[107]Horatio Smith, *op. cit.*, p. 333.

[108]Archer, *Rousseau on Education*, p. 89.

SUMMARY

This study, by an examination of the various aspects of child life as revealed in juvenile literature, has indicated the changing status of the American child during the Colonial and early national periods. The curve of that status begins with the gradual emergence of the child from a submerged position in an adult world and ends with his occupying a place of honor as a cherished social entity, charged only with the responsibilities of an immature human being. The recognition of the child as a distinct personality constitutes the first revolution of juvenile life in our national history. This revolution, disquieting as it was to some writers of the early nineteenth century, was to put the prelude to the phenomenal developments which have transformed childhood in the last fifty years.

Religion for the Colonial child was not confined to the life of the spirit; one does not read very far into the juvenile literature of the period before he discovers the sovereignty of religion in every phase of child life. Not only were his education, manners, and morals motivated by theological concepts, but even his recreation and hygienic care were conditioned by the same principles.

Although children of every faith were expected to "walk in the ways of the godly and to wage war with the devil," they had no special religious status, but shared that of their elders. The foundations of their transitory existence rested on the lesson so early and so often heard— "Our days begin with trouble here, our life is but a span." Since this other-worldly attitude was consciously fostered, what now seems to have been a morbid pietism overshadowed the young and tended to confine their activities to the awful duty of an early spiritual conversion as the preparation for an untimely death. The Colonial boy and girl repeatedly heard such warnings as, "You Children are daily liable to the stroke of Death; in the midst of seeming health you may drop down and die." Since, in this pioneer society, such utterances were indeed far from fiction, the child was left to ponder the frightful implications of his impending doom.

The decline of Puritanism, the growth of skepticism, and the influence of deistic philosophy, as well as the emotional reactions of the American Revolution, combined to change the religious status of the child. The spiritual standards of the young American shifted from their early theological foundations to a mild moral basis. This new status, which stressed the temporal expediency of good conduct, was soon characterized by a steadily increasing disregard for variations in points of Protestant dogma. By blurring their former sharp theological distinctions and by fostering a new spirit of toleration according to the "live and let live" concept, Protestant sects were able ultimately to merge and cross various denominational traditions.

Deism also tended to eliminate the element of fear from the spiritual life of many early American children by changing the basis of ethics from a sense of sin to a desire for happiness, and by repudiating the idea of evil as a part of the natural order. Instead of emphasizing the importance of dogmatic instruction in the religious training of the young, a new spirit of indifference to doctrinal variations fostered the belief that "one religion is as good as another." By contemplating the order and grandeur of nature, youth was led to the conviction that life is essentially good and that the universe is governed by a beneficent God who might be approached by many avenues of worship.

By 1835, theological concepts were being gradually displaced in religious training by rules for good conduct or by moral stories calculated to develop the natural virtues into habits of honesty, industry, and sobriety—all of which were judged essential to the good of American society. A comfortable code of ethics and certain fixed standards for temporal prosperity were supplanting those stern theological tenets which had demanded personal sanctity according to a specific creed and had laid firmly the religious foundation of early American childhood. The Colonial child's well-defined conceptions of the duties owed to God, to his fellow men, and to himself—those black and white dogmatic patterns by which he had "lived and breathed and had his being"—were fading into vague uncertain hues. The little books indicate that much of the direction and vitality that had previously conditioned the child's religious experience was lost in the misty shadows that confused the spiritual life of later decades.

Manners and customs in every colony were based on the authority of God as manifested in the Bible, and on the national traditions as discovered in the American cultural heritage. Parents and "superiors" exercised their acknowledged authority and ruled children with a relentless hand. The burning zeal of Colonial adults for a more perfect way of life inspired them to eradicate from childhood all that was judged frivolous and vain by the stringent standards of the times. As a result of this rigid exercise of power, the narrow circle of childhood was hedged in by the barriers of minute regulations. The young were bound by a formidable code of manners and drilled in the "art of decent behaviour."

A change of disciplinary standards was apparent by the close of the American Revolution. Some adults realized that coercion itself was not discipline; and although they might subdue children by the fear of the rod, such exercise of authority contributed little to the formation of a noble character. Adults' attitudes henceforth turned from their original severity to an appeal to reason as the guiding force in youthful conduct. When a new freedom supplanted the petty tyranny of Colonial days, children were gradually permitted opportunities to make decisions for themselves, and also to accept the results of their own judgments. Those adults who deplored the "unhappy restraint" of Colonial days thus abandoned the use of formal precepts and the rod for the force of moral suasion. The practice of concealing rules of conduct in didactic tales helped to shape the mind and heart of the young. Although the adult world was still convinced that a "little good Breeding may do the Children some Good," violence was repudiated as a factor in producing that "decent behaviour" or the poise and dignity so highly cherished in the last century. Most Americans of the growing democracy believed that since true politeness was the result of education and habit and not inherent in the nature of the child, good manners could accordingly be produced in a hovel as well as in the home of the rich.

The emphasis of the Colonial educational system was also directed by far-reaching social forces from religious to secular interests. Although most of the schools were still church-controlled and accordingly cherished the classical traditions, by 1776 some offered vocational training and all were gradually introducing useful subjects into the curriculum. This secularization of education, once begun, proceeded steadily to its logical conclusion, even though it was for years viewed with suspicious distrust by many Colonial scholars. Since the chief aim of education was to fit children adequately for their probable vocation in life, such responsible agents as the church, the school, and the home assisted year by year in the steady injection of secular interests into juvenile training.

On the other hand, certain positive forces operative by the first quarter of the nineteenth century not only aided the "rise of the common man," but incidentally stimulated an interest in a democratic system of instruction. Accelerated means of transportation and communication, the growth of cities and towns, the development of the factory system, the aggressive spirit of the frontier, and an incipient proletarian consciousness continually centered public attention on the necessity of a free elementary school system.

The hygienic care of the Colonial child was given meager consideration, for parents and educators were handicapped by a lack of scientific knowledge. Since the belief persisted that demons exerted an influence over bodily health, ministers at times gave medical as well as spiritual aid. In direct contrast to the present generation, so solicitous in matters of child care, parents of the Colonial era committed the fate of their children in health, as in death, to the will of Providence. The rates for child morbidity and mortality were extremely high, hence the natural reaction of godly people was to resign themselves to the inevitable as best they could, and to give the cross under which they bowed a spiritual significance. In the poor health and early deaths of their "pious children," they therefore consoled themselves with the reflection that salvation depended "not on the length of time," but on an effectual coöperation with divine grace. Hence many were able to say: "Blessed are the Dead in Christ, that are soon passed from Sin and Sorrow here, to the Eternal Fulness of Holiness and Comfort in the Presence of God forever."

The progress made in the nineteenth century by the medical profession in anatomical and pathological studies, as well as the advance in sanitary reform and the rise in standards of living, resulted in a marked improvement in the lot of the young. Adult education in child care also relieved little ones of many of the sufferings incidental to frontier life, and reforms in sanitation eliminated much disease and many health hazards from American homes. Although superstition and "kitchen physick" still held forth, regular physicians, overcoming their prejudice against pediatrics, were consulted with greater frequency and confidence by adults. As a result of improved standards of living, many mothers had more leisure to devote "to the wants and infirmities of their children." By all these factors medical authorities were heartened to face the stupendous problems of child welfare; preventive measures were taken to control the diseases incidental to a newly settled country, and to dispel the general ignorance of hygiene, as well as to correct the improper diet and dress which had previously threatened youthful lives. The advance in child welfare by 1835 was, however, but a minor victory, for there were many Americans who still clung to the ancient traditions of "kitchen physick" and others who hesitated to place much confidence in natural and material aids.

An examination of the function of play in the organization of early American life reveals the most remarkable change in adult attitudes. From the Colonial warning to the young to let their recreation be "lawful, brief, and seldom," this adult philosophy shifted by the third decade of the nineteenth century to the approbation of a mild program of "rational play" in the interests of juvenile health and efficiency. Whether

BIBLIOGRAPHY

GUIDES

Barry, Florence V., *A Century of Children's Books*, New York, 1923.
Darton, F. J. H., *Children's Books in England: Five Centuries of Social Life*, London, 1933.
Field, E. M., *The Child and His Book*, London, 1892.
Field, Walter Taylor, *Fingerposts to Children's Reading*, Chicago, 1918.
Gardner, Emelyn E., and Ramsey, Eloise, *A Handbook of Children's Literature*, New York, 1927.
Griffin, G. G., *Writings on American History*, Washington, 1906-30.
Halsey, Rosalie V., *Forgotten Books of the American Nursery*, Boston, 1911.
James, Philip, *Children's Book of Yesterday*, ed. C. Geoffrey Holme, New York, 1933.
Jordan, Alice M., "Early Children's Books" *Bulletin of the Boston Public Library*, XV, Boston, April 1940.
Moore, Annie E., *Literature Old and New for Children*, New York, 1934.
———, *New Roads to Childhood*, New York, 1923.
———, *The Three Owls; a Book about Children's Books*, New York, 1924.
Rosenbach, A. S. W., *Early American Children's Books*, Portland, Maine, 1933.
Smith, E. S., *A History of Children's Literature, A Syllabus with Selected Bibliographies*, New York, 1937.
Tuer, A. W., *Stories from Old Fashioned Children's Books*, New York, 1900.
———, *Pages and Pictures from Forgotten Children's Books*, New York, 1899.
Weekes, Blanche E., *Literature and the Child*, New York, 1935.
Welsh, Charles, "Early History of Children's Books in New England," *New England Magazine*, XX. Boston, 1899, 146-60.
Wilson, H. W., *Children's Catalogue*, 3d rev., New York, 1937.

SECONDARY WRITINGS

GENERAL WORKS

Adams, James Truslow, *Provincial Society 1690-1763*, New York, 1938.
Andrews, Charles M., *Colonial Folk Ways, A Chronicle of American Life in the Reign of the Georges*, New Haven, 1919.
Andrews, Charles M., *Colonial Background of the American Revolution*, New Haven, 1924.
Bamberger, Florence, E., *Effects of the Physical Make-up of a Book upon Children's Selection*, Baltimore, 1922.
Bossard, James H., *Social Change and Social Problems*, New York, 1938.
———, *Marriage and the Child*, Philadelphia, 1940.
Chitwood, Oliver P., *A History of Colonial America*, New York, 1931.
Greene, E. B., *Foundations of American Nationality*, New York, 1935.
Hart, Albert B. (ed.) *Source Readers in American History*, vols. 1-4 New York, 1925.

the controlling motive of the new attitude was to refresh and invigorate the child's bodily powers and thus make him more competent in the performance of his tasks, or whether it was simply to afford youth periods of unalloyed joy—"to make the heart more gay"—play was ordinarily kept at the minimum requisite for the peace of families. Although amusements varied with the age, sex, and the natural bent of the individual child, moderation, on moral grounds, was considered of the highest importance in any recreation. Not all adults had accepted in its entirety Rousseau's exhortation, "Love childhood; look kindly on its play, its pleasures, its lovable instincts. . . . "

The major conclusion from this investigation is that the era of the American Revolution marked the beginning not only of the political freedom of the American people, but also of the emancipation of the American child. Some adults in the early national period still failed to penetrate the child's mind and to recognize his needs as fully as later generations were to do, but the status of the child advanced with the growth of the country toward democratic goals. It is now clearly evident to the student of society that childhood thus forged ahead and shared the progress of the "more perfect government," until by 1835 the foundation of that freedom and self-expression which characterizes both today had been established.

"Life, liberty, and the pursuit of happiness" had special connotations for children in the minds of many thoughtful Americans by the beginning of the nineteenth century. This formula of the Founding Fathers was interpreted by social reformers to mean the freedom of children to live as immature human beings with special needs and definite rights that had to be respected by grown-ups. It also meant the freedom of little ones to pursue happiness according to the ideals of childhood, and not, as previously, in conformity with adult behavior patterns. Impelled by the humanitarianism of the age, most adults agreed that children had the right to develop spiritually, socially, and mentally by a gradual process. Parents and guardians no longer expected their small charges to leap at one bound from infancy into maturity in order to play the role of "little men and women" without the stabilizing interlude of carefree childhood.

McMaster, John Bach, *History of the People of the United States from the Revolution to the Civil War*, 8 vols., New York, 1891-1910.

Nettles, Curtis P., *The Roots of American Civilization*, New York, 1939.

Nicholas, and Nicholas, *The Growth of American Democracy*, New York, 1939.

Sanders, Jennings B., *Early American History*, New York, 1938.

RELIGION

Bates, Ernest S., *American Faith, Its Religious, Political, and Economic Foundations*, New York, 1940.

Burtt, Edwin A., *Types of Religious Philosophy*, New York, 1939.

Curtis, J. G., "Saving the Infant Class," *Scribner's Magazine*, New York Nov. 1929, 564-70.

Fleming, Sanford, *Children and Puritanism*, New Haven, 1933.

Green, E. B., "The Anglican Outlook on the American Colonies in the Early Eighteenth Century," *American Historical Review*, XX, October, 1914, 64-85.

Hall, Thomas C., *The Religious Background of American Culture*. Boston, 1930.

Haroutunian, Joseph, *Piety Versus Moralism, The Passing of New England Theology*, New York 1932.

Homan, Walter J. *Children and Quakerism*, Berkeley, Calif., 1939.

Hough, Lynn H., *The Christian Criticism of Life*, New York, 1941.

McConnell, S. D., *History of the American Episcopal Church*, Milwaukee, 1916.

Manross, William W., *A History of the American Episcopal Church*, New York, 1936.

Maynard, Theodore, *The History of American Catholicism*, New York, 1941.

Morais, Herbert M., *Deism in Eighteenth Century America*, New York, 1934.

Sweet, William Warren, *The History of Religions in America*, New York, 1930.

MANNERS AND MORALS

Bolton, Ethel S. and Coe, Eva J., *American Samplers*, Boston, 1921.

Brooke, Iris, *English Children's Costume Since 1775*, London, 1930.

Calhoun, Arthur W., *A Social History of the American Family from Colonial Times to the Present*, 3 vols., Cleveland, 1917.

Earle, Alice M., *Child Life in Colonial Days*, New York, 1924.

———, *Costume of Colonial Times*, New York, 1894.

———, *Customs and Fashions in Old New England*, London, 1893.

———, *Home Life in Colonial Days*, New York, 1910.

Furness, Clifton J., *The Genteel Female*, New York, 1931.

Godfrey, Elizabeth, *English Children in the Olden Time*, New York, 1907.

Goodsell, Willystine, *A History of the Family as a Social and Educational Institution*, New York, 1924.

Hewins, Caroline M., *A Mid-Century Girl and Her Books*, New York, 1926.

Horace, Elisha S., *Men and Manners in America One Hundred Years Ago*, New York, 1876.

Larcom, Lucy, *A New England Girlhood,* Cambridge, 1889.
Reed, Ruth, *The Modern Family,* New York, 1929.
Rhodes, Lillian, *The Story of Philadelphia,* New York, 1900.
Schouler, James, *Americans of 1776,* New York, 1906.
Stoddard, Lothrop, *The Story of Youth,* New York, 1928.
Sweetzer, Kate Dickinson, "The American Girl," *D.A.R. Magazine,* No. 9 LIII, Philadelphia, September, 1919.
Ware, John F., *Home Life: What it is, and What it Needs,* Boston, 1866.

EDUCATION

Archer, R. L., *Rousseau on Education,* London, 1928.
Brambaugh, Martin G., *The Life and Works of Christopher Dock,* Philadelphia, 1908.
Brewer, Clifton H., *A History of the Religious Education in the Episcopal Church to 1835,* New Haven, 1924.
Burns, James A., *The Growth and Development of the Catholic School System in the United States,* New York, 1912.
Butterweck, Joseph, and Seegers, J. Conrad, *An Orientation Course in Education,* New York, 1933.
Comenius, John, *Orbis Pictus,* London, 1777.
Curti, Merle, *The Social Ideas of American Educators,* New York, 1935.
Dexter, Edwin G., *A History of Education in the United States,* New York, 1904.
Eby, Frederick, and Arrowood, Charles F., *The Development of Modern Education in Theory, Organization, and Practice,* New York, 1941.
Eversall, Harry Kelso, *Education and the Democratic Tradition,* Marietta, 1938.
Ford, Paul L., *The New England Primer,* New York, 1897.
Graves, Frank P., *Great Educators of Three Centuries,* New York, 1912.
Guernsey, Lucy Ellen, *School-days in 1800; or, Education As It Was a Century Since,* Philadelphia, 1875.
Johnson, Clifton, *Old Time Schools and School-Books,* New York, 1904.
Knight, Edgar W., *Twenty Centuries of Education,* Boston, 1940.
Monroe, Paul, *Founding of the American Public School System,* New York, 1940.
Noble, Stuart G., *A History of American Education,* New York, 1938.
Tuer, Andrew, *The History of the Hornbook,* 2 vols., New York, 1898.
Woody, Thomas, *Educational Views of Benjamin Franklin,* New York, 1931.
——, *A History of Women's Education in the United States,* 2 vols. New York, 1929.

HEALTH

Eggleston, Edward, "Some Curious Colonial Remedies," *American Historical Review,* V. December, 1899, 199,-206.
Lea, Henry C., (ed.), *A Century of American Medicine,* Philadelphia, 1876.
Ruhrah, John, *Pediatrics of the Past,* New York, 1925.

Shryock, R. H., *The Development of Modern Medicine,* Philadelphia, 1936.
Wilson, Elizabeth Andrews, "Hygienic Care and Management of the Child in the American Family Prior to 1860." Unpublished M. S. thesis, Duke University, 1940.

RECREATION

Grober, Karl, *Children's Toys of Bygone Days,* New York, 1928.
Holme, C. Godfrey, ed., *Children's Toys of Yesterday,* New York, 1932.
Newell, William Wells, ed., *Games and Songs of American Children,* New York, 1883.
Singleton, Esther, *Dolls,* New York, 1927.

CONTEMPORARY JUVENILE LITERATURE

RELIGION

Barbauld, Anna Letitia, *Hymns in Prose for the Use of Children,* New York, 1814.
Burder, George, *Early Piety, or Memoirs of Children Eminently Serious, Interspersed with familiar Dialogues, Prayers, Graces, and Hymns,* Baltimore, 1821.
Coleman, Benjamin, *A Devout Contemplation on the Meaning of Divine Providence, in the Early Death of Pious and Lovely Children. Preached upon the Sudden and Lamented Death of Mrs. Elizabeth Wainwright, Who Departed this life, April 8, 1714. Having just completed the Fourteenth Year of Her Age,* Boston, 1714.
Curious Hieroglyphic Bible, Worcester, Mass., 1788.
Davies, Samuel, *Little Children Invited to Jesus Christ, A Sermon Preached in Hanover County, Virgina, May 8, 1758,* Boston, 1761.
Doddridge, Phillip, *The Principles of the Christian Religion: Divided into Lessons and adapted to the Capacities of Children,* Worcester, Mass., 1805.
Fuller, Samuel, *Some Principles and Precepts of the Christian Religion by One of the people called Quakers,* Philadelphia, 1753.
Gallaudet, Thomas H., *The Child's Book of the Soul,* Hartford, 1831.
Gregory, John, *A Father's Legacy to His Daughters,* Norwich, 1785.
Hendley, George, *A Memorial for Children, being an authentic account of the Conversion, Experience, and Happy Deaths of Eighteen Children. Designed as a Continuation of Janeway's Token,* New Haven, 1806.
Heywood, Henry, *Two Catechisms by Way of Question and Answer: designed for the Instruction of the Children of the Christian Brethren who are commonly known and distinguished by the name of Baptists,* Charles-Town, 1749.
Hill, Hannah, *A Legacy for Children, being some of the Last Expressions and Dying Sayings, of Hannah Hill, Junr. of the City of Philadelphia, in the Province of Pennsylvania, in America, Aged Eleven and near Three Months,* Philadelphia, 1717.
Janeway, James, *A Token for Children. Being an Exact Account of the Conversion, Holy and Exemplary Lives and Joyful Deaths of Several Young*

Children, Philadelphia, reprinted and sold by B. Franklin and D. Hall, 1747. To the original English edition Cotton Mather added the *Token for the Children of New England.*

Keach, Benjamin, *War with the Devil; or the Young Man's Conflict with the Powers of Darkness,* New York, 1707.

Lane, Jeremiah, *A Few Drops of Choice Honey, extracted from Old Comb of a very ancient Hive,* Exeter, 1794.

Lewis, John, *The Catechism Explained by Way of Question and Answer, and Confirmed by Scripture Proofs, 35th edition,* London, 1787.

Mackarsie, John, *The Children's Catechism: or an Help to the more easy Understanding of the Doctrine taught in our Confession of Faith, and catechisms larger and shorter,* Philadelphia, 1780.

Mason, William, *The Closet Companion, or an Help to Serious Persons,* Hartford, 1815.

———, *The Pious Parent's Gift, or a plain and familiar sermon wherein the Principles of the Christian Religion are proposed and clearly represented to the minds of Children,* Hartford, 1815.

Mather, Cotton, *Magnalia Christi Americana,* vol. 11, Hartford, 1820.

Mavor, William, *The Mother's Catechism, or First Principles of Knowledge and Instruction,* Leicester, Eng., 1815.

Moodey, Samuel, *Judas the Traitor Hung up in Chains. To give Warning to Professors that they Beware of Worldlymindedness, and Hypocrisy; Preached at York in New England,* Boston, 1714.

Oakman, John, *Moral Songs for the Instruction and Amusement of Children, Intended as a Companion to Dr. Watts' Divine Songs,* London, 1802.

Penn, William, *Fruits of a Father's Love. Being the Advice of William Penn to His Children Relating to Their Civil and Religious Conduct,* Philadelphia, 1727.

Phillips, Samuel, *The Orthodox Christian: or, a Child Well-Instructed in the Principles of the Christian Religion,* Boston, 1738.

Pilkington, Mary, *Biography for Boys; or, Characteristics calculated to impress the youthful mind with an admiration of Virtuous Principles, and a detestation of Vicious Ones,* Philadelphia, 1809.

———, *Biography for Girls; or, Moral and Instructive Examples for the Female Sex,* Philadelphia, 1809.

Porteus, Bielby (Bishop of London), *A Summary of the Principal Evidence for the Truth and Divine Origin of the Christian Revelation, Designed for the Use of Young Persons,* Worcester, Mass., 1808.

Potter, John, *The Words of the Wise,* Philadelphia, 1768.

Prince, Thomas, *Morning Health No Security against the Sudden Arrest of Death before Night. A Sermon,* Boston, 1727.

Sampson, Ezra, *Beauties of the Bible, being a selection from the Old and New Testaments with various remarks and brief dissertations, designed for the use of Christians in general, and particularly for the use of schools, and for the Improvement of youth,* New York, 1802.

Secker, William, *A Wedding Ring fit for the Finger, Or, the Salve of Divinity on the Sore of Humanity . . . laid open in a Sermon in Edmonton by William Secker, Preacher of the Gospel,* Boston, 1705

Smith, Frederick, *A Letter to the Children and Youth of the Society of Friends,* Philadelphia, 1906.

Taylor, Ann and Jane, *Hymns for Infant Minds, We use great plainness of speech,* Newburgh, 1820.

——, *A Selection of Hymns for Infant Minds,* Boston, 1820.

Taylor, John, *Verbum Sempiternum, The Third Edition with Amendments,* Boston, 1755.

Vincent, Thomas, *An Explicatory Catechism; or, an Explanation of the Assemblies Shorter Catechism,* Boston, 1729.

Watts, Isaac, *Divine Songs, Attempted in an Easy Language for the Use of Children,* Boston, 1774.

Westminister Assembly of Divines, *A Shorter Catechism,* Boston, 1762.

Witherspoon, John, *A Sermon on the Religious Education of Children, Preached in the Old Presbyterian Church in New York to a very numerous audience,* Elizabeth-Town, 1789.

SUNDAY SCHOOL LITERATURE

American Suday School Union, *First Lessons on the Great Principles of Religion, Designed to be used in Infant Sabbath Schools and Private Homes,* Philadelphia, 1833.

——, *The Glass of Whiskey,* Philadelphia, 1825.

——, *Memoirs of an Infant Scholar,* Philadelphia, 1838.

——, *The Six-Penny Glass of Wine,* Philadelphia, 1833.

——, *The Youth's Friend, No. 33,* Philadelphia, 1826.

——, *Youth's Penny Gazette, vol. III,* Philadelphia, 1833.

American Tract Society, *The History of Ann Lively and Her Bible,* New York, c. 1830.

——, *A New Picture Book,* New York, c. 1830.

New Jersey Sunday School Journal, vol. 1, Princeton, 1827.

Sunday and Adult School Union, *Milk for Babes or a Catechism in Verse for the Use of Sunday Schools,* Philadelphia, 1824.

Anonymous, *The Children's Bible, or an History of the Holy Scriptures,* Reprinted in Philadelphia, 1763.

——, *A Father's Advice to His Child; or, the Maiden's Best Adorning,* Exeter, 1792.

——, *The Happy Child, or A Remarkable and Surprising Relation of a Little Girl,* Boston, 1774.

——, *A Present to Children, consisting of several New and Divine Hymns and Moral Songs,* New London, 1783.

——, *The Prodigal Daughter,* Boston, 1771.

——, *The Rule of the New Creature, To Be Practiced Every Day, in all the Particulars of It Which are Ten,* Boston, 1682.

——, *Take Your Choice; or, the Difference betwen Virtue and Vice shown in Opposite Characters,* Philadelphia, 1804.

——, *Wisdom in Minature or the Young Gentleman and Lady's Magazine. Being a Collection of Sentences Divine and Moral. Embellished with Cuts,* Philadelphia, 1805.

MANNERS AND MORALS

Cameron, Lucy Lyttleton, *The Polite Little Children*, Andover, 1820.

Chambaud, Louis, *Fables Choisis*, Philadelphia, 1796.

Chesterfield, Philip D.S., *Principles of Politeness and of Knowing the World*, Norwich, 1785.

Cooper, Charles, *Blossoms of Morality Intended for the Amusement and Instruction of Young Ladies and Gentlemen*, Philadelphia, 1810.

Darton, William, *The First, Second, Third Chapter of Accidents, and Remarkable Events: Containing Caution and Instruction for Children*, Philadelphia, 1807.

Earl, Alice M. (ed.), *Diary of Anna Green Winslow, A Boston Girl of 1771*, Boston, 1894.

Edgeworth, Maria, *Idleness and Industry*, Philadelphia, 1804.

———, *The Parents' Assistant; or, Stories for Children, 3 vols*. London, 1796.

Farrar, Eliza Ware, *The Young Lady's Friend*, Boston, 1837.

Follen, Eliza Lee, *Little Songs for Little Boys and Girls*, Reprinted in Boston, 1833.

Francis, C. S., *The True Mother Goose*, Boston, 1842.

Franklin, Benjamin, *The Way to Wealth; or Poor Richard Improved, Industry Leads to Wealth*, New York, 1814.

Goodrich, Samuel G., *Peter Parley's Tale about the State and City of New York, illustrated by a map and many engravings. For the use of schools*, New York, 1832.

L'Estrange, Robert, *A History of the Life of Aesop; to which is added a choice Selection of Fables with Instructive Morals for the the Benefit of Youth*, Philadelphia, 1798.

Moodey, Eleazer, *The School of Good Manners, fifth edition*, New London, 1754.

Murray, Hannah and Mary, *The American Toilet*, New York, c. 1825.

O'Keefe, Adelaide and Taylor, Ann and Jane, *Rhymes for the Nursery*, London, 1805.

———, *Original Poems for Infant Minds*, Philadelphia, 1816.

Oliver, Daniel, *The Foreign Visitant: containing interesting observations and remarks made by an Inhabitant of Terra Incognita, on the character and manners of the inhabitants of this earth, particularly in relation to the Lord's Day*, Boston, 1814.

Phillips, Richard, *A View of the Character, Manners, and Customs of the Inhabitants of the United States*, Philadelphia, 1810.

Anonymous, *Be Merry and Wise; or the Cream of Jests and the Marrow of Maxims, for the Conduct of Life*, Isaiah Thomas, Worcester, Massachusetts, 1786.

———, *The Brother's Gift; or, the Naughty Girl Reformed*, Worcester, Massachusetts, 1795.

———, *The Cries of New York*, New York, 1814.

———, *False Stories Corrected*, New York, 1814.

———, *A Father to His Daughter, The Daughter's own Book, or Practical Hints*, Philadelphia, 1815.

————, *History of Goody twoshoes,* Isaiah Thomas, Worcester, Massachusetts, 1787.

————, *History of Jack Idle and Dicky Diligent,* Philadelphia, 1806.

————, *History of Little Dick,* Philadelphia, 1807.

————, *History of Little Fanny, exemplified in a Series of figures,* Philadelphia, 1825.

————, *Jack Halyard and Ishmael Bardus,* Wendell, Massachusetts, 1828.

————, *Jack Dandy's Delight: or the History of Birds and Beasts; in Verse and Prose,* Worcester, Massachusetts, 1788.

————, *Juvenile Biographer; containing the Lives of Little Masters and Misses; including a Variety of Good and Bad Characters,* Worcester, Massachusetts, 1787.

————, *Lilliputian Masquerade, Occasioned by the Conclusion of Peace between those potent Nations, the Lilliputians and the Tommythumbians,* Worcester, Massachusetts, 1795.

————, *Little Prattle over a Book of Prints, With Easy Tales for Children,* Philadelphia, 1808.

————, *Little Pretty Pocket-Book, First Worcester Edition by Isaiah Thomas,* Worcester, Massachusetts, 1787.

————, *Mother Goose's Melody: or Sonnets for the Cradle Reprinted by Isaiah Thomas,* Worcester, Massachusetts, 1794.

————, *Nurse Truelove's New-Year Gift: or, The Book of Books for Children. Adorned with Cuts,* Worcester, Massachusetts, 1788.

————, *Picture of New York,* New York, 1825.

————, *Post Boy,* Philadelphia, c. 1807.

————, *Present to Children,* New York, c. 1830.

————, *Pretty New-Year's Gift; or, Entertaining Histories for the Amusement and Instruction of Young Ladies and Gentlemen in Winter Evenings,* Worcester, Massachusetts, 1786.

————, *School of Good Manners, Containing an Explanation of many terms used in moral philosophy and divinity,* New London, 1796.

————, *The Seasons,* New York, 1814.

————, *Silver Penny; or, the New Lottery Book for Children, by J. Horner, Esq., Fellow of the Royal Society of A.B.C.,* Philadelphia, 1806.

————, *Sugar Plum; or Sweet Amusement for Leisure Hours: Being an Entertaining and Instructive Collection of Stories embellished with Curious Cuts,* Worcester, Massachusetts, 1787.

————, *True Stories Related. By a Friend of Little Children,* New York, 1814.

————, *Useful and Necessary Companion in Two Parts,* Boston, 1708.

————, *Variety of Stories for Children,* New York, 1828.

————, *Vice in Its Proper Shape; or, The Wonderful and Melancholy Transformation of Several Naughty Masters and Misses into those Contemptible Animals which they most resembled in Disposition.* Worcester, Massachusetts, 1789.

Wisdom of Crop the Conjuror, Isaiah Thomas, Worcester, Mass., 1786.

Wisdom in Miniature; or the Young Gentleman and Lady's Pleasing Instructor, Being a Collection of Sentences, Divine, Moral, and Historical, Worcester, Mass., 1795.

————, *Young Lady's Parental Monitor,* Hartford, 1792.

EDUCATION

Andrews, W. E., *The Catholic School Book, containing easy and familiar lessons for the instruction of youth of both sexes, in the English Language and the paths of true religion and virtue*, Philadelphia, 1824.

Bailey, Nathan, *English and Latine Exercises for School Boys, Comprising, all the Rules of Syntax*, Boston, 1720.

Benezet, Anthony, *The Pennsylvania Spelling-Book; or, Youth's Friendly Instructor and Monitor*, Philadelphia, 1779.

Bingham, Caleb, *The American Preceptor; Being a Selection of Lessons for Reading and Speaking*, Boston, 1821.

——, *Juvenile Letters, Being a Correspondence between Children from eight to fifteen years of age*, Boston, 1803.

Burton, Richard, *Some Excellent Verses for the Education of Youth*, Boston, 1708.

Cooper, W. D., *The History of North America*, Albany, 1795.

Corry, John, *Biographical Memoirs of the Illustrious General George Washington*, New Haven, 1810.

Culman, Leonard, *Sententiae Pueriles Anglo-Latinae. Collected out of sundry Authors long since . . . for the first Entrers [sic] into Latin*, Boston, 1702.

Davidson, Robert, *Georgaphy Epitomized; or, a Tour Round the World; attempted in verse for the sake of the memory; and principally designed for the use of schools*. By an American, Philadelphia, 1784.

Dilworth, Thomas, *A New Guide to the English Tongue*, Philadelphia, c. 1770.

Dwight, Nathaniel, *A Short but Comprehensive System of Geography of the World: by way of question and answer*, Hartford, 1800.

Dwight, Timothy, *A Valedictory Address to the Young Gentlemen who commenced Bachelors of Arts, at Yale-College, July 25th, 1776*, New Haven, 1776.

Ely, John, *The Child's Instructor, consisting of easy lessons for children; on subjects familiar to them, in language adapted to their capacities*, Philadelphia, 1793.

Fenning, Daniel, *The American Youth's Instructor; or, a New and Easy Guide to Practical Arithmetic*, Dover N. H., 1795.

Fisher, George, *The American Instructor: or the Young Man's Best Companion, Containing Spelling, Reading, Writing, and Arithmetic. Ninth Edition revised and corrected by B. Franklin and D. Hall*, Philadelphia, 1748.

Fox, George, *Instructions for Right-Spelling and Plan Directions for Writing True English*, Philadelphia, 1702.

Franklin, Benjamin, *Proposals Relating to the Education of Youth in Pensilvania [sic]*, Philadelphia, 1749.

Frenau, Philip and Hugh Brackenridge, *A Poem on the Rising Glory of America; being an Exercise Delivered at the Public Commencement at Naussau-Hall, September 25, 1771*, Philadelphia, 1772.

Greenwood, James, *The Philadelphia Vocabulary; English and Latin*, Philadelphia, 1787.

Hall, John, *On the Education of Children While under the Care of Parents or Guardians*, New York, 1835.

Hodder, James, *Hodder's Arithmetic: or that Necessary Art Made Most Easy*, Boston, 1719.

Johnson, Benjamin, *The New Philadelphia Spelling Book: or a Pleasant Path to Literature*, Philadelphia, 1809.

Lamb, Charles and Mary, *Poetry for Chidren, entirely original*, Boston, 1812.

Martinet, Johannes F., *The Catechism of Nature for the Use of Children*. Translated from the Dutch by John Hall, Philadelphia, 1794.

Mavor, William, *Catechism of Animated Nature*, New York, 1821.

Milns, William, *The Well-Bred Scholar*, New York, 1797.

Moore, John Hamilton, *The Young Gentleman and Lady's Monitor, and English Teacher's Assistant*, New York, 1809.

O'Keefe, Adelaide, *Original Poems; calculated to improve the minds of youth and to allure it to Virtue*, Philadelphia, 1810.

Osborne, Henry, *An English Grammar adapted to the capacities of children*, Charleston, c. 1785.

Peters, Richard, *A Sermon on Education*, Philadelphia, 1751.

Philadelphia Society for the Establishment of Charity Schools, *Manual of the System of teaching Reading, Writing, Arithmetic, and Needle-Work in the Elementary Schools of the British and Foreign Society*, Philadelphia, 1817.

Sigourney, Lydia Huntley, *Tales and Essays for Children*, Hartford, 1835.

Simmons, John, *The Juvenile Class Book*. Compiled for the use of schools, No. 4, Philadelphia, 1832.

Taylor, Ann and Jane, *Limed Twigs to Catch Young Birds; or Easy Reading in Large Letters for Schools and Families*, Philadelphia, 1849.

Webster, Noah, *The American Spelling Book*, Fifth edition, Boston, 1793.

Webster, Noah, *A Dictionary of the English Language; Compiled for the use of the Common Schools in the United States*, Boston, 1807.

Webster, Noah, *Elements of Useful Knowledge*, New London, 1807.

———, *The Prompter; A Commentary on Common Sayings and Subjects which are full of common sense, the best, sense in the world*, Boston, 1798.

Weed, Enos, *The American Orthographer, in three books by a Physician and Surgeon in Difficult Cases*, Danbury, 1797.

Whittenhall, Edward, *A Short Introduction to Grammar for the Use of College and Academy in Philadelphia*, Philadelphia, 1762.

Williard, Samuel, *The Franklin Primer, Containing a new and careful selection of moral lessons*, Boston, 1802.

Anonymous, *The A B C with the Church of England Catechism*, Philadelphia, 1785.

———, *The American Letter-Writer: Containing a Variety of Letters on the most common Occasions in Life*, Philadelphia, 1793.

———, *Beauties of the New England Primer*, New York, 1814.

———, *The Book of the Sea for the Instruction of Little Sailors*, New York, c., 1835.

———, *Boy's Manual: Comprising a Summary of the Studies, Accomplishments, and Principles of Conduct Best Suited for Promoting Respectibility and Success in Life*, New York, 1837.

———, *Child's Spelling Book: Calculated to render Reading Completely Easy to Little Children; to impress upon their Minds the Importance of Religion, and the Advantages of Good Manners*, Hartford, 1802.

——, *Compendious History of the World from the Creation to the Dissolution of the Roman Republic*, 2 vols., Philadelphia, 1774.

——, *Das Neue Deutsche A B C—und Buchstabir—Büchlein für die Schulen aller Religionen in Nord-Amerika*, Baltimore, 1795.

——, *Easy Lessons for Children*, Philadelphia, 1794.

——, *Elements of Georgaphy Made Easy*, Philadelphia, 1825.

——, *The Fortune Teller*, Philadelphia, 1793.

——, *General Description of the Thirteen United States*, Reading, 1788.

——, *History of America, abridged for the use of Children of all Denominations*, Philadelphia, 1795.

——, *History of Animals*, Wendell, Massachusetts, 1828.

——, *The Infant's Grammar*, Baltimore, c. 1825.

——, *Instructive Alphabet*, New York, 1814.

——, *Lessons for Children from Two to Four Years Old, Part One*, Philadelphia, 1788.

——, *Lessons for Children of Four Years Old, Part Two*, Philadelphia, 1788.

——, *Letters to a Young Student in the First Stages of a Liberal Education*, Philadelphia, 1832.

——, *The Life of General George Washington*, Philadelphia, 1794.

——, *Little Sketch Book*, New York, c. 1835.

——, *Miscellanies, Moral and Instructive in Prose and Verse Collected from Various Authors for the Use of Schools and Improvement of Young Persons of Both Sexes*, Philadelphia, 1787.

——, *Natural History of Four-Footed Beasts* New York, 1795.

——, *The New England Primer*, Boston, 1749.

——, *New England Primer*, Hartford, 1800.

——, *The Pilgrims, or the First Settlers of New England*, Philadelphia, 1825.

——, *Progressive Primer Adapted to Infant School Instruction*, Concord, 1835.

——, *Punctuation Personified: or Pointing Made Easy*. By Mr. Stops, Steubenville, Ohio, 1831.

——, *The Remarkable Story of Augi: or a Picture of True Happiness*. First American Edition. Translated and reprinted by Isaiah Thomas, Jun., Worcester, Mass., 1796.

——, *Royal Primer Improved: Being an Easy and Pleasant Guide to the Art of Reading*, Philadelphia, 1783.

——, *Sententiae Pueriles: or, Sentences for Children, fitted to the fundamental rules of Latin Syntax*, Philadelphia, 1761.

——, *Seven Wonders of the World; and Other Magnificent Buildings*, New York, 1814.

——, *Tom Thumb's Picture Alphabet in Rhyme*, New York, c. 1835.

——, *Washington Primer: or First Book for Children*, Philadelphia, 1836.

——, *Wisdom in Miniature: or the Young Gentleman and Lady's Magazine*, Philadelphia, 1805.

——, *Wonderful History of an Enchanted Castle Kept by Giant Gumbo*, Albany, 1813.

——, *Youth's Cabinet of Nature*, New York, 1814.

HEALTH

Ackerley, G., *On the Management of Children in Sickness and in Health,* Second Edition, New York, 1836.

Alcott, William A., (de.), *The Moral Reformer and Teacher on the Human Constitution,* vol. 1, Boston, 1835.

Anonymous, *The Daisy; or, Cautionary Stories in Verse. Adapted to the Ideas of Children from four to eight years old,* Philadelphia, 1808.

Buchan, William, *Domestic Medicine: or, A Treatise on the Prevention and Cure of Disease by Regimen and Simple Remedies,* London, 1786.

Chavasse, Pye Henry, *Advice to Mothers on the Management of their Offspring during the periods of infancy, childhood, and youth,* New York, 1844.

Dewees, William, *A Treatise on the Physical and Medical Treatment of Children, Ninth Edition,* Philadelphia, 1847.

Faust, B. C., *Catechism of Health for the Use of Schools and for Domestic Instruction,* Boston, 1795.

Mavor, William, (Fordyce), *The Catechism of Health; containing simple and easy rules and directions for the management of children, and observations on the conduct of health in general; for the use of schools and families,* New York, 1815.

Struve, Christian Augustus, *A Familiar View of the Christian Education of Children during the Early Period of Their Lives, Translated from the German,* London, 1800

RECREATION

Aesop's Fables, New York, 1814.

Astley, Philip, *Modern Riding-Master: A Key to the Knowledge of the Horse and Horsemanship,* Philadelphia, 1776.

Dorset, Catherine Ann, *Peacock at Home: or Grand Assemblage of Birds,* Philadelphia, 1814.

de Genlis, Stéphanie-Félicité, *Beauty and the Monster, A Comedy from the French, Extracted from the Theatre of Education,* Worcester, Mass., 1785.

Kilner, Mary Jane, *Adventures of a Pincushion,* Worcester, Mass., 1788.

———, *Memoirs of a Peg Top,* Worcester, Mass., 1788.

Perrault, Charles, *Cinderella or the Little Glass Slipper, Illustrated with elegant engravings,* Philadelphia, 1822.

Roscoe, William, *The Butterfly's Ball and the Grasshopper's Feast,* London, 1807.

Sandham, Elizabeth, *Adventures of Poor Puss,* Philadelphia, 1809.

Smith, Horatio, *Festivals, Games, and Amusements, Ancient and Modern,* New York, 1831.

Teachwell, Mrs., (pseud.), *Rational Sports in Dialogues passing among Children of a Family,* London, 1783.

Wakefield, Pricilla, *Juvenile anecdotes founded on facts. Collected for the Amusement of Children,* Philadelphia, 1809.

Anonymous, *Adventures in a Castle, An Original Story Written by a Citizen of Philadelphia,* Harrisburg, 1806.

———, *Amusement for Good Children by G. S. C., Or an Exhibition of Comic Pictures by Bob Sketch. Be Merry and Wise,* Baltimore, 1806.

——, *Children's Amusements*, New York, 1822.

——, *Christmas Dream of Little Charles*, New York, 1835.

——, *Cinderella, or the Little Glass Slipper, A Grand Allegorical Pantomimic Spectacle as performed at the Philadelphia Theatre*, New York, 1807.

——, *Comic Adventures of Old Mother Hubbard and her Dog*, Philadelphia, 1817.

——, *Dame Trot and Her Comical Cat*, Philadelphia, 1814.

——, *Dances, A Collection of New and Improved Country*, Northampton, 1796.

——, *Garden Amusements for Improving the Minds of Little Children*, New York, 1814.

——, *Geographical, Statistical, and Political Amusement; by which may be obtained a general and particular knowledge of the United States. In a series of interesting games on a map designed for the purpose*, Philadelphia, 1805.

——, *History of Mother Twaddle, and the Achievements of her son Jack, by H.A.C.*, Philadelphia, 1814.

——, *Juvenile Pastimes in Verse*, New York, 1830.

——, *Life and Death of Robin Hood, complete in twenty-four songs*, Philadelphia, 1803.

——, *Mother's Remark on a Set of Cuts for Children, Part I*, Philadelphia, 1803.

——, *Old Dame Margery's Hush-a-Bye*, Philadelphia, 1814.

——, *Peep into the Sports of Youth, and the Occupations and Amusements of Age*, Philadelphia, 1809.

——, *Peter Prim's Profitable Present to Little Misses and Masters of the United States*, Philadelphia, c. 1821.

——, *Peter Pry's Puppet Show, Part Second*, Philadelphia, 1821.

——, *Picture Book for Little Children*, Philadelphia, c, 1812.

——, *Present to Children. Consisting of Several New and Divine Hymns and Moral Songs*, New London, c. 1783.

——, *Puzzling Cap, A Choice Collection of Riddles in familiar verse with a curious cut to each*, Philadelphia, 1805.

——, *Remarks on Children's Play*, New York, 1814.

——, *The Seasons*, New York, 1814.

——, *Tame Goldfinch or the Unfortunate Neglect*, Philadelphia, 1808.

——, *Tommy Lovechild, Pretty Poems in Easy Language for the Amusement of Little Boys and Girls*, Litchfield, 1808.

——, *Whim Wham: or Evening Amusements for all ages and sizes, being an entire set of riddles, charades, questions, and transportations, by a friend of innocent mirth*, Philadelphia, 1811.

——, *Youthful Recreations*, Philadelphia, 1810.

——, *Youthful Sports*, Philadelphia, 1802.

BOOKS ABOUT CHILDREN:

PARENTS' GUIDES, MANUALS, ETC.

Abbott, Gorham, D. *The Family at Home, or Familiar Illustrations of Various Domestic Duties*, Boston, 1834.

Abbott, John S., *The Child at Home; or, the Principles of Filial Duty Familiarly Illustrated, American Tract Society*, New York, 1833.

Babington, T., *A Practical View of Chirstian Education in Its Earliest Stages*, Boston, 1818.

Bonhote, Mrs., *The Parental Monitor*, Boston, c. 1800.

Burgh, James, *Rules for the Conduct of Life*, American reprint of London publication of 1767, Philadelphia, 1846.

Child, Lydia Maria, *The Mother's Book*, Baltimore, 1831.

Crocker, John, *Advice to His Children in Friends Library, XIV*, Plymouth, Eng., c. 1727.

Dwight, Theodore, *The Father's Book; or Suggestions for the Government and Instruction of Young Children on Principles Appropriate to a Christian Country*, Springfield, Mass., 1835.

Grant, Mrs., *Sketches on Intellectual Education and Hints in Domestic Economy Addressed to Mothers*, London, 1812.

Griffith, Mrs. Richard, *Letters Addressed to Young Married Women*, Philadelphia, 1796.

Harris, Walter, *A Treatise of the Acute Diseases of Infants* Translated from the Latin by John Martyn, London, 1742.

Hersey, John, *Advice to Chiristian Parents*, Baltimore, 1839.

Hoare, Louisa, *Hints for the Improvement of Early Education and Nursery Discipline*, Salem, 1826.

Jennings, Samuel K., *The Married Lady's Companion; or, The Poor Man's Friend*, Richmond, n. d.

Mather, Cotton, *Family Well-Ordered*, Boston, 1699.

Myres, James, (ed.), *The United States Catholic Almanac; or Laity's Directory*, Baltimore, 1836.

Nelson, James, *An Essay on the Government of Children Under Three General Heads: viz. Health, Manners, and Education*, London, sold by M. Cooper, New York, 1753.

Robertson, John, *Observations on the Mortality and Physical Management of Children*, London, 1827.

Rush, Benjamin, *Essays, Literary, Moral, and Philosophical*, Philadelphia, 1806.

Sewall, Samuel, *Diary 1674-1729*. Coll. of Mass. Hist. Soc. vols. V-VII. Boston, 1878. vol. I of series.

Sigourney, Lydia Huntley, *Letters to Mothers*, New York, 1829.

Smedley, Jacob, (ed.), *Hints for the Training of Youth; A Scrap Book for Mothers*, Philadelphia, 1875.

Tuttle, George, *A Parent's Offering; or, My Mother's Story of Her Home and Childhood, about 1800*, New Haven, 1844.

Whittelsay, Mrs. A. G. (ed.), *The Mother's Magazine vol. VIII*, New York, May 1840.

Anonymous, *Cares About the Nurserie*, Boston, 1702.

———, (J. G.), *A Small Help Offered to Heads of Families for Instructing Children and Servants*, Morris-Town, 1814.

———, (A Mother), *Thoughts on Domestic Education*, Boston, 1829.

INDEX

DE(